THIRD EDITION

RADIOLOGY 101

The Basics and Fundamentals of Imaging

Editor

William E. Erkonen, M.D.
Associate Professor Emeritus
Department of Radiology
Carver College of Medicine
University of Iowa Hospitals and Clinics
Iowa City, Iowa

Associate Editor

Wilbur L. Smith, M.D.
Professor and Chairman
Department of Radiology
Wayne State University Detroit Medical Center
Detroit, Michigan

Wolters Kluwer | Lippincott Williams & Wilkins
Health
Philadelphia · Baltimore · New York · London
Buenos Aires · Hong Kong · Sydney · Tokyo

Acquisitions Editor: Brian Brown
Product Manager: Ryan Shaw
Vendor Manager: Bridgett Dougherty
Senior Manufacturing Manager: Benjamin Rivera
Senior Marketing Manager: Angela Panetta
Design Coordinator: Teresa Mallon
Production Service: Aptara Corp.

© 2010 by LIPPINCOTT WILLIAMS & WILKINS, a WOLTERS KLUWER business
530 Walnut Street
Philadelphia, PA 19106 USA
LWW.com

Printed in China

Library of Congress Cataloging-in-Publication Data

Radiology 101 : the basics and fundamentals of imaging / editor, William
E. Erkonen ; associate editor, Wilbur L. Smith. — 3rd ed.
     p. ; cm.
  Includes bibliographical references and index.
  ISBN 978-1-60547-225-6 (alk. paper)
1. Radiography, Medical. 2. Diagnosis, Radioscopic. 3. Diagnostic
imaging. I. Erkonen, William E. II. Smith, Wilbur L. III. Title:
Radiology one hundred one. IV. Title: Radiology one hundred and one.
  [DNLM: 1. Diagnostic Imaging. 2. Radiology. WN 180 R1295 2009]
  RC78.R242 2009
  616.07'54—dc22

                                            2009021224

                                 10 9 8 7 6 5 4 3

To the students and practitioners in all the medical sciences who seek basic information about radiology.

CONTRIBUTING AUTHORS

Carol C. Boles, M.D.
Professor, Department of Radiology, Wake Forest University
Baptist Medical Center, Winston–Salem, North Carolina

David L. Bushnell, Jr., M.D.
Chief of Diagnostic Imaging, Veterans Administration
Hospital, Iowa City, Iowa; Associate Professor, Carver
College of Medicine, University of Iowa Hospitals and
Clinics, Iowa City, Iowa

William E. Erkonen, M.D.
Associate Professor Emeritus, Department of Radiology,
Carver College of Medicine, University of Iowa Hospitals
and Clinics, Iowa City, Iowa

Laurie L. Fajardo, M.D., M.B.A., F.A.C.R.
Professor and Head, Department of Radiology, Carver
College of Medicine, University of Iowa Hospitals and
Clinics, Iowa City, Iowa

Thomas A. Farrell, M.D., F.R.C.R., M.B.A.
Assistant Professor, Pritzker School of Medicine, University
of Chicago, Chicago, Illinois; Section Head, Interventional
Radiology, Department of Radiology, Evanston Hospital,
Evanston, Illinois

Edmund A. Franken, Jr., M.D.
Professor, Department of Radiology, Carver College of
Medicine, University of Iowa Hospitals and Clinics, Iowa
City, Iowa

Vincent A. Magnotta, Ph.D.
Associate Professor, Department of Radiology, Carver
College of Medicine, University of Iowa Hospitals and
Clinics, Iowa City, Iowa

Jeong Mi Park, M.D.
Professor and Director, Division of Breast Imaging and
Intervention, Director of Breast Imaging Fellowship,
Department of Radiology, Carver College of Medicine,
University of Iowa Hospitals and Clinics, Iowa City, Iowa

Yutaka Sato, M.D.
Professor, Director of Radiology Pediatrics, Department of
Radiology, Carver College of Medicine, University of Iowa
Hospitals and Clinics, Iowa City, Iowa

Wilbur L. Smith, Jr., M.D.
Professor and Chairman, Department of Radiology, Wayne
State University/Detroit Medical Center, Detroit Receiving
Hospital (3L8), Detroit, Michigan

Brad H. Thompson, M.D.
Associate Professor, Department of Radiology, Carver
College of Medicine, University of Iowa Hospitals and
Clinics, Iowa City, Iowa

The specialty of radiology has been around for over 100 years and has played a critical role in patient diagnosis and care. During the last 30 years the role of radiology in patient diagnosis and care has soared on the wings of extraordinary technologic advances. As you read this work, remember that diseases haven't changed a lot, but the way we look at them has due to these new and improved technologies.

All too often, educators incorrectly assume that the students know something about the subject that they are about to study. Therefore, the third edition of *Radiology 101* assumes that the reader's knowledge of radiology is at the most basic level.

The primary purpose of this book is to give the reader a "feel" for radiologic anatomy and the radiologic manifestations of some common disease processes. After reading this book, you will be better prepared for consultation with the radiologist, and this usually leads to an appropriate diagnostic workup. As one develops an understanding of what radiology has to offer, improved patient diagnosis and care are likely to follow. In addition, the reader will be able to approach an image without feeling intimidated. You might say, "it will prepare you for the wards and boards." The book is not intended to transform the reader into a radiologist look-alike. Rather, it is designed to be a primer or general field guide to the basics of radiology.

Anatomy is the language of radiology. A solid foundation in good old-fashioned normal radiologic anatomy is essential to understand the various manifestations of diseases on radiologic images. Thus, this book places heavy emphasis on images, stressing normal anatomy and commonly encountered radiologic pathology. We present clearly labeled images of normal anatomy from a variety of angles not only on radiographs but also on other commonly used imaging modalities such as computed tomography, magnetic resonance imaging, and ultrasonography.

Section I presents basic understandable discussions of how major imaging modalities function. Understanding how radiologic images are produced by the various imaging modalities is extremely helpful in understanding what their images portray. The strengths and weaknesses of the various modalities are described in clinical tips within the text (e.g., "What are the basic differences between T-1 and T-2 images and what are the clinical indications for each?").

Section II systematically examines the imaging of anatomic regions and major organ systems and contains extensive presentations of normal anatomy, normal anatomic variants, and commonly encountered pathology. Each chapter begins with an outline to make topics easier to locate, and the chapter concludes with a summary list of key points to remember. In general, the writing tends to be informal and dispenses common-sense tips and pointers freely (e.g., how to systematically examine or approach a chest radiograph and how to correctly position an image on the viewbox). We have attempted to make each chapter user-friendly by adding practical tips on how to radiologically approach common clinical problems such as abdominal trauma. This work should be an excellent resource for the beginner in all medical-allied fields.

We call the reader's attention to Chapter 4 that combines pediatric chest and abdomen, as they are the most frequently ordered pediatric images. All other pediatric images and text will be located in their appropriate chapter.

New to this third edition are many updates in each chapter to keep pace with this rapidly changing specialty. These changes will be found especially in the chapters involving nuclear imaging (PET/CT), computed tomography (multislice), magnetic resonance (DWI, t-MRI, MRS), sonography (FAST), abdominal imaging (CT urography), mammography (digital mammograms), and the many indications for interventional radiology.

ACKNOWLEDGMENTS

A deep debt of gratitude is owed to those people in the departments of the contributing authors who helped in one way or another to produce this book. We are also indebted to Radiology Technologist Scot Heery for some of the excellent images and to Librarian Nicole Jenkins, who was so helpful with references. Also, thanks are due to Jim Olson and his laboratory for many of the fine images.

A very special thanks to George El-Khoury, MD, Ronald Bergman, PhD, and Kathy Martensen, RTR, for their initial encouragement, suggestions, and general advice to get this book underway.

The skillful illustrations of Shirley Taylor, Carol Boles, MD, and the late Frank J. Sindelar are greatly appreciated. Brian Clarke provided the original drawings for Figures 9.1, 9.2, 9.18, 9.21, and 9.23. Their illustrations helped clarify difficult concepts.

■ CONTENTS

SECTION I ■ BASIC PRINCIPLES

SECTION II ■ DIAGNOSTIC RADIOLOGY

SECTION I ■ BASIC PRINCIPLES

CHAPTER 1 ■ RADIOGRAPHY, COMPUTED TOMOGRAPHY, MAGNETIC RESONANCE IMAGING, AND ULTRASONOGRAPHY: PRINCIPLES AND INDICATIONS

WILLIAM E. ERKONEN AND VINCENT A. MAGNOTTA

Very few of us take the time to study, let alone enjoy, the physics of the technology that we use in our everyday lives. Almost everybody drives an automobile, for instance, but only a few of us have working knowledge about what goes on under our car hoods. The medical technology that produces imaging studies is often met with a similar reception: we all want to drive the car, so to speak, but we don't necessarily want to understand the principles underlying the computed tomograms or magnetic resonance images that we study. Yet, a basic understanding of imaging modalities is extremely important, because you will most likely be reviewing images with a radiologist during radiologic consultations throughout your professional life. The results of these consultations will at times profoundly affect your making a clinical decision. Add to this the fact that the interpretation of imaging studies is to a considerable degree dependent on understanding how the images are produced. Here is where our analogy breaks down: One doesn't necessarily have to be a mechanic to be a skilled driver, but reaching a basic understanding of how imaging studies are produced is a necessary first step to viewing the studies themselves. This chapter is designed to demonstrate the elementary physics of radiologic diagnostic imaging.

RADIOGRAPHY

Radiographs are the most common imaging consultations requested by clinicians. So let's set off on the right foot by referring to radiologic images as *radiographs*, *images*, or *films*, but not *x-rays*. After all, x-rays are electromagnetic waves produced in an x-ray tube. It is acceptable for a layperson to refer to a radiograph as an x-ray, but the knowledgeable clinician

and health care worker should avoid the term. Your usage of appropriate terminology demonstrates *savoir-faire* (the ability to say and do the right thing) to your colleagues and patients.

Whenever possible, radiographs are accomplished in the radiology department. The number of views obtained during a standard or routine study depends on the anatomic site being imaged. The common radiographic views obtained are referred to as posteroanterior (PA), anteroposterior (AP), oblique, and lateral views.

The chest will be used to illustrate these basic radiographic terms, but this terminology applies to almost all anatomic sites. PA indicates that the central x-ray beam travels from posterior to anterior or back to front as it traverses the chest or any other anatomic site (Fig. 1.1). Lateral indicates that the x-ray beam travels through the patient from side to side (Fig. 1.2). When the patient is unable to cooperate for these routine views, a single AP upright or supine view is obtained. AP means that the x-ray beam passes through the chest or other anatomic site from anterior to posterior or front to back (Fig. 1.3). PA and AP radiographs have similar appearances. When the patient cannot tolerate a transfer to the radiology facility, a portable study is obtained, which means that a portable x-ray machine is brought to the patient wherever he or she is located. AP is the standard portable technique with the patient sitting or supine (Fig. 1.4).

Radiographs have traditionally been described in terms of shades of black, white, and gray. What causes a structure to appear black, white, or gray on a radiograph? Actually, it is the density of the object being imaged that determines how much of the x-ray beam will be absorbed or attenuated (Fig. 1.5). In other words, as the density of an object increases, fewer x-rays pass through it. It is the variable density of structures that

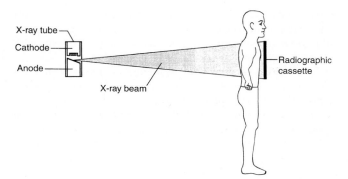

FIGURE 1.1 A posteroanterior chest radiograph. The patient's chest is pressed against the cassette with hands on the hips. The x-ray beam emanating from the x-ray tube passes through the patient's chest in a posterior-to-anterior or back-to-front direction. The x-rays that pass completely through the patient eventually strike the radiographic film and screens inside the radiographic cassette.

results in the four basic radiographic classifications: air (black), fat (black), water (gray), and metal or bone (white; Table 1.1). For example, the lungs primarily consist of low-density air, which absorbs very little of the x-ray beam. Thus, air allows a large amount of the x-ray beam to strike or expose the radiographic film. As a result, air in the lungs will appear black on a radiograph. Similarly, fat has a low density, but its density is slightly greater than that of air. Fat will appear black on a radiograph but slightly less black than do air. High-density objects such as bones, teeth, calcium deposits in tumors, metallic foreign bodies, right and left lead film markers, and intravascularly injected contrast media absorb all or nearly all of the x-ray beam. As a result, the radiographic film receives little or no x-ray exposure, and these dense structures appear white. Muscles, organs (heart, liver, spleen), and other soft tissues appear as shades of gray, and the shades of gray range somewhere between white and black depending on the structure's density. These shades of gray are referred to as *water density*.

Radiographic screens are positioned on both sides of the radiographic film inside the light-tight cassette or film holder (Fig. 1.6A). The chemical structure of the screens causes them to emit light flashes or to fluoresce when struck by x-rays

(Fig. 1.6B). Actually, it is the fluoresced light from the screens on both sides of the film that accounts for the major exposure of the radiographic film. The direct incident x-rays striking the radiographic film account for a small proportion of the film exposure. The use of screens decreases the amount of radiation required to produce a radiograph, and this in turn decreases the patient's exposure to radiation. *It is important to remember that both radiographic and photographic films respond in a similar manner to light and x-rays.*

Computed Radiography (Digital Radiography)

In conventional radiography, the radiographic image is recorded on film that goes through chemical processing for development. Computed radiography (CR) or digital radiography (DR) is the process of producing a digital radiographic image. Instead of film, a special phosphor plate is exposed to the x-ray beam. The image information is obtained by scanning the phosphor plate with a laser beam that causes light to be released from the phosphor plate. The intensity of the emitted light depends on the local radiation exposure. This emitted light is intensified by a photomultiplier tube and is subsequently converted into an electron stream. The electron stream is digitized, and the digital data are converted into an image by computer. The resulting image can be viewed on a monitor or transferred to radiographic film. The beauty of this system is that the digital image can be transferred via networks to multiple sites in or out of the hospital, and the digital images are easily stored in a computer or on a server. For example, a digital chest radiograph obtained in an intensive care unit can be transmitted to the radiology department for consultation and interpretation in a matter of minutes. Then the radiologist can send this image via a network back to the intensive care unit or to the referring physician's office. Of course, this digital information would be stored in a computer (server) for future recall. As this technology improves, it has become more and more important to the routine practice of medicine.

Contrast Media

Radiographic contrast media usually refer to the use of intravascular pharmaceuticals to differentiate between normal

FIGURE 1.2 A lateral chest radiograph. The x-ray beam passes through the patient's chest from side to side. The x-rays that pass completely through the patient eventually strike the radiographic film and screens. Note that the patient's arms are positioned as not to project over the chest.

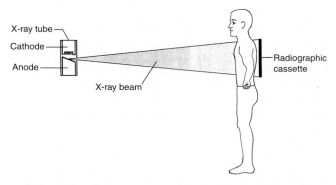

FIGURE 1.3 An anteroposterior chest radiograph. The x-ray beam passes through the patient's chest in an anterior-to-posterior or front-to-back direction. Note that the patient's hands are on the hips.

FIGURE 1.4 An anteroposterior portable chest radiograph with the patient either sitting (**A**) or supine (**B**). The x-ray beam passes through the patient's chest in an anterior-to-posterior direction. The x-ray machine has wheels and that allows it to be used wherever needed throughout the hospital.

and abnormal tissues, to define vascular anatomy, and to improve visualization of some organs. These high-density pharmaceuticals in conventional radiology depend upon chemically bound molecules of iodine that cause varying degrees of x-ray absorption. Soft tissues such as muscles, blood vessels, organs, and some diseased tissues often appear similar on a radiograph. Usually, when contrast agents are injected intravascularly to tell the difference between normal and abnormal tissues there is a difference in the uptake of the contrast media in the various tissues. Thus, the more the uptake of contrast media in a tissue, the whiter it appears, and this is called *enhancement.*

It is this enhancement or contrast that enables the viewer to detect subtle differences between normal and abnormal soft tissues and between an organ and the surrounding tissues. Also, it beautifully demonstrates arteries and veins.

The use of iodinated high osmolar contrast agents for radiographic studies through the years has led to complications due to this high osmolar load especially in infants and in individuals with compromised renal function. With high osmolar contrast agents, approximately 7% of the people developed reactions consisting of vomiting, pain at the injection site, respiratory symptoms, urticaria, and generalized burning sensation. However, a major advance occurred in the 1990s with the widespread adoption of low osmolar contrast agents (LOCAs) that substantially reduced the risk of osmolar reactions. LOCAs improved the comfort of administration and decreased the frequency of annoying and sometimes life-threatening reactions. LOCAs did not completely eliminate the incidence of serious contrast reaction and nephropathy. If

a patient has had a prior reaction, one should consult with one's radiologist to weigh the benefit versus the risk and possible alternative imaging considered especially in patients with diabetes, vascular disease, or renal dysfunction.

There are many uses for iodinated compounds in radiographic examinations such as in *angiography, myelography, arthrography,* and *computed tomography (CT). Angiography* is merely the injection of an iodinated contrast media directly into a vein or artery via a needle and/or catheter (see Chapter 11).

FIGURE 1.5 **A:** The level in the distal thigh through which the x-ray beam is passing in B. **B:** Cross section of the distal thigh at the level indicated in A. Notice that when the x-ray beam passes through air, the result is a black area on the radiograph. When the x-ray beam strikes bone, the result is a white area on the radiograph. If the x-ray beam passes through soft tissues, the result is a gray appearance on the film.

TABLE 1.1	

BASIC RADIOGRAPH FILM DENSITIES OR APPEARANCES

Object	Film density
Air	Black
Fat	Black
Bone	White
Metal	White
Calcium	White
Organs, muscles, soft tissues	Shades of gray

Arthrography is the injection of contrast media and/or air into a joint. Air may be used alone or in combination with these compounds to improve contrast. It has been used to image multiple joints such as rotator cuff injuries of the shoulder and to assess meniscus injuries in the knee. Since the advent of CT and magnetic resonance imaging (MRI), the arthrogram has become less important. *Myelography* is the placement of contrast media in the spinal subarachnoid space, usually via a lumbar puncture. This procedure is useful for diagnosing diseases in and around the spinal canal and cord. Because of the advent of the less invasive CT and MRI modalities, the use of myelogram studies has been decreasing.

In the past, orally ingested tablets containing iodinated compounds were used to visualize the gallbladder (oral cholecystogram). These orally administered compounds were removed from the blood by the hepatic cells, then excreted into the biliary tree and concentrated in the gallbladder. This study provided information about gallbladder function and the presence or absence of filling defects such as calculi and tumors. However, this method for imaging the gallbladder is rarely used since ultrasonography imaging became widely available. Ultrasonography is especially useful in acute situations.

The excretory urogram is another examination that is rarely used. This was the method of choice when searching for a wide variety of urinary tract pathologic conditions as well as anatomic and physiologic information. This study uses intravenously injected ionic high and low osmolar iodinated compounds that are excreted by the kidneys. However, this method for imaging the genitourinary system has for the most part been replaced by computer technology.

Another type of contrast media is used for the gastrointestinal (GI) tract. A heavy metal–based compound (usually barium) defines the mucosal pattern very well. To accomplish a GI contrast examination, the barium sulfate suspension is introduced into the GI tract by oral ingestion (upper GI series) or through an intestinal tube (small bowel series) or as an enema (barium enema). When air along with the barium is introduced into the GI tract, the result is called a double-contrast study. Barium studies are safer, better tolerated by patients, and relatively inexpensive compared with the more invasive GI endoscopic studies. Barium studies can be effective in diagnosing a wide variety of GI pathology, as they are quite sensitive and specific.

When the integrity of the GI tract is in question, there exists a potential for catastrophic extravasation of the barium into the mediastinum and peritoneum. In these situations, bar-

ium studies are contraindicated and a water-soluble iodinated compound should be used. As a general rule, images produced with water-soluble contrast agents are less informative than barium studies, because the water-soluble agents are less dense than barium and result in poorer contrast.

In MRI standard iodinated contrast agents are of no use. Instead, we use magnetically active compounds such as gadolinium or other metals with unpaired electrons (paramagnetic effects) to enhance imaging certain disease processes. Gadolinium does not produce a magnetic resonance (MR) signal but does cause changes in local magnetic fields by inducing T1 shortening in tissues where it has localized. It is useful for imaging tumors, infections, and acute cerebral vascular accidents. Although the principles of MRI and CT differ, the practical outcomes are similar. They both cause lesion enhancing or in other words a lesion is whiter than the surrounding tissues (Fig. 1.7).

Gadolinium generally has a low risk for reactions and/or nephropathy, but it can cause a severe connective tissue disorder, *nephrogenic sclerosing fibrosis (NSF)*. NSF occasionally occurs in patients who are on dialysis or have a creatinine clearance less than 30 mg/dL. This disease is a very serious

FIGURE 1.6 **A:** An open radiographic cassette containing one sheet of radiographic film and two intensifying screens. A radiographic screen is positioned on each side of the film, and the screens emit a light flash (fluoresce) when struck by an x-ray. Also, some x-rays directly strike the radiographic film. This combination of light flashes from the screens and x-rays directly striking the film causes the radiographic film to be exposed. This is similar to photographic film. **B:** Cross-sectional illustration of a radiographic cassette. Note the lead foil in the back of the cassette that is designed to stop any x-rays that have penetrated the full thickness of the cassette. The curved arrows represent light flashes that are created when x-rays strike the screens.

FIGURE 1.7   Sagittal, coronal, and axial anatomic planes.

- Median or midsagittal plane
- Coronal plane
- Axial or transverse (cross-sectional plane)

complication and is similar to scleroderma. The takeaway lesson on gadolinium is *to consult with your radiologist* on any patient with known renal failure or a history of NSF before requesting a contrast-enhanced MRI examination.

COMPUTED TOMOGRAPHY

Computed tomography involves sectional anatomy imaging or anatomy in the sagittal, coronal, and axial (cross-sectional, transverse) planes. These terms, which can be confusing, are clearly illustrated in Fig. 1.7. Sectional anatomy has always been important to physicians and other health care workers, but the newer imaging modalities of computed tomography (CT), magnetic resonance imaging (MRI), and ultrasonography (US) demand an in-depth understanding of anatomy displayed in this manner.

CT, sometimes referred to as computerized axial tomography (CAT) scan technology, was developed in the 1970s. The rock group The Beatles gave a big boost to CT development when it invested a significant amount of money in a business called Electric Musical Instruments Limited (EMI). It was EMI engineers who subsequently developed CT technology. Initially, EMI scanners were used exclusively for brain imaging, but this technology was rapidly extended to the abdomen, thorax, spine, and extremities.

CT imaging is best understood if the anatomic site to be examined is thought of as a loaf of sliced bread; an image of each slice of bread is created without imaging the other slices (Fig. 1.8). This is in contradistinction to a radiograph, which captures the whole loaf of bread as in a photograph.

The external appearance of a typical CT unit or machine is illustrated in Fig. 1.9. CT images are produced by a combination of x-rays, computers, and detectors. A computer-controlled couch transfers the patient in short increments through the opening in the scanner housing. In the standard CT unit, the x-ray tube located in the housing (gantry) rotates around the patient, and each anatomic slice to be imaged is

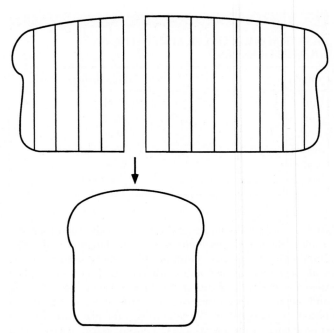

FIGURE 1.8   Illustration of how CT technology creates an image of a single slice of bread from a loaf of sliced bread without imaging the other slices.

exposed to a pencil-thin x-ray beam (Fig. 1.10). Each image or slice requires only a few seconds; therefore, breath holding is usually not an issue. The thickness of these axial images or slices can be varied from 1 to 10 mm depending on the indications for the study. For example, in the abdomen and lungs we commonly use a 10-mm slice thickness because the structures are large. A slice thickness of only a few millimeters is used to image small structures like those found in the middle and inner ear. An average CT study takes approximately 10 to 20 minutes depending on the circumstances.

As in a radiograph, the amount of the x-ray beam that passes through each slice or section of the patient will be inversely proportional to the density of the traversed tissues. The x-rays that pass completely through the patient eventually strike

- X-ray tube gantry
- Opening in gantry
- Patient couch

FIGURE 1.9   A standard CT scanner or machine. The patient couch or cradle is fed through the opening in the x-ray tube gantry or housing, and the anatomic part to be imaged is centered in this opening. The x-ray tube is located inside the gantry and moves around the patient to create an image.

FIGURE 1.10 **A:** Illustration of how the x-ray tube circles the patient's abdomen to produce an image (slice) as shown in B. **B:** Demonstration of how a CT scan creates a thin-slice axial image of the abdomen (*arrows*) without imaging the remainder of the abdomen.

detectors (not film), and the detectors subsequently convert these incident x-rays to an electron stream. This electron stream is digitized or converted to numbers referred to as CT units or Hounsfield units; then computer software converts these numbers to corresponding shades of black, white, and gray. A dense structure, such as bone, will absorb most of the x-ray beam and allow only a small amount of x-rays to strike the detectors. The result is a white density on the image. On the other hand, air will absorb little of the x-ray beam, allowing a large number of x-rays to strike the detectors. The result is a black density on the image. Soft tissue structures appear gray on the image.

This CT digital information can be displayed on a video monitor, stored on magnetic tape, transmitted across computer networks, or printed on radiographic film via a format camera.

Because CT technology uses x-rays, the image densities of the anatomic structures being examined are the same on both CT images and radiographs. In other words, air appears black on both a CT image and a radiograph and bone appears white on both modalities. One major difference between a radiograph and a CT image is that a radiograph displays the entire anatomic structure, whereas a CT image allows us to visualize slices of a structure. Another major difference is that in radiography the x-rays that pass through an object are recorded

TABLE 1.2

SOME COMMON INDICATIONS FOR CT IMAGING

Trauma
Intracranial hemorrhage (suspected or known)
Abdominal injury, especially to organs
Fracture detection and evaluation
Spine alignment
Detection of foreign bodies (especially in joints)
Diagnosis of primary and secondary neoplasms (liver, renal, brain, lung, and bone)
Tumor staging

on film, whereas in CT the x-rays are recorded by devices called detectors and converted to digital data.

CT imaging is accomplished with and/or without intravenously injected contrast media. The intravenous contrast media enhance or increase the density of blood vessels, vascular soft tissues, organs, and tumors as in a radiograph. This enhancement assists in distinguishing between normal tissue and a pathologic process. Contrast media are not needed when searching for intracerebral hemorrhage or a suspected fracture or for evaluating a fracture fragment within a joint. However, contrast is used when evaluating the liver, kidney, and brain for primary and secondary neoplasms. A few of the common indications for CT imaging are listed in Table 1.2. Whenever possible, oral GI contrast agents are administered prior to an abdominal CT to delineate the contrast-filled GI tract from other abdominal structures.

High-Resolution Computed Tomography

High-resolution computed tomography refers to CT studies that result in thin slices that are approximately 1.0 to 2.0 mm thick. This technology has become very useful in the diagnosis of parenchymal lung diseases.

Helical or Spiral Computed Tomography

Helical or spiral CT technology is similar to standard CT but with a few new twists. In helical or spiral CT, the patient continuously moves through the gantry while the x-ray tube continuously encircles the patient (Fig. 1.11). This combination of

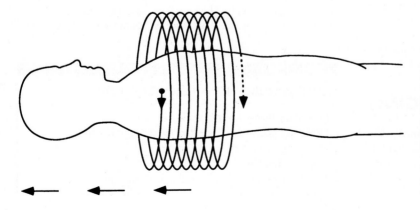

FIGURE 1.11 A helical or spiral CT scanner. The x-ray tube continuously circles the patient while the patient couch moves continuously through the opening in the x-ray tube gantry. The combination of continuous patient and x-ray tube movement results in a spiral configuration, hence the name "helical." In a standard CT or nonhelical scanner, the patient couch moves in short increments toward the gantry opening and stops intermittently to allow the x-ray tube to move around the patient. Thus, the x-ray tube moves around the patient only when the couch is stationary.

TABLE 1.3

ADVANTAGES AND DISADVANTAGES
OF MULTISLICE CT

Advantages
Static and cine or movie images
Noninvasive
Rapid filming results in decreased motion artifact
Good spatial resolution
Disadvantages
Expensive
Limited availability

TABLE 1.4

ADVANTAGES AND DISADVANTAGES OF MRI

Advantages
Static and cine or movie images
Multiple plane images
Good contrast
No known health hazards
Good for soft tissue injuries of the knee, ankle, and shoulder joints
Disadvantages
More expensive than CT
Long scan times may result in claustrophobia and motion artifacts
Limited availability

the patient and x-ray tube continuously moving results in a spiral configuration. This technology can produce 1 slice per second, and the slice can vary in thickness from 1 to 10 mm. The resolution and contrast of these images are better than on standard CT images, resulting in improved images in areas such as the thorax and abdomen.

Multislice/Dynamic Computer Tomography

The early conventional CT scanners had only a single row of detectors, thus only one tomographic slice or image was generated with each rotation of the x-ray tube around the patient. The current state of the art is multislice CT. This equipment has multiple contiguous rows of detectors that yield multiple tomographic slices with only one rotation of the x-ray tube around the patient. There can be as many as 128 detector rings in one CT unit, thus resulting in multiple image slices of a 15-cm segment of anatomy. Hence, large volumes can be scanned in short periods of time, and the slice thickness varies depending on the structure being imaged. For example, one rotation around the cervical spine encompassing the base of the skull to T3 would take 11 seconds. Subsequently, with software this data can immediately create a three-dimensional (3-D) reconstruction and even a cine. The resulting 3-D image can be rotated with the mouse either to the right or to the left. Also, structures such as the ribs may be edited out of the images.

This increased speed of volume coverage by the multislice CT is especially beneficial in CT angiography or dynamic CT. For example, in CT angiography or dynamic CT the multislice scanner can cover the entire abdominal aorta in 15 seconds. Following a bolus injection of contrast media, serial angiographic images of the aorta or any area of interest can be made to observe the movement of contrast media through the area of interest during the arterial and venous phases. Some advantages and disadvantages of the multidetector CT are listed in Table 1.3.

MAGNETIC RESONANCE IMAGING

Magnetic resonance imaging (MRI) or magnetic resonance (MR) is another method for displaying anatomy in the axial, sagittal, and coronal planes, and the slice thicknesses of the images vary between 1 and 10 mm. MRI is especially good for coronal and sagittal imaging, whereas axial imaging is the forte of CT. One

of the main strengths of MRI is its ability to detect small changes (contrast) within soft tissues, and MRI soft tissue contrast is better than that found on CT images and radiographs.

CT and MR imaging modalities are digital-based technologies that require computers to convert digital information to shades of black, white, and gray. The major difference in the two technologies is that in MRI the patient is exposed to external magnetic fields and radio frequency waves, whereas during a CT study the patient is exposed to x-rays. The magnetic fields used in MRI are believed to be harmless. The assessment of fetal exposure to MRI is a developing and evolving field, and the U.S. Food and Drug Administration has not established the safety of MRI for fetal imaging. While most studies have shown that MRI is safe for the fetus, several animal studies have suggested that there is the potential for teratogenic effects during early fetal development. The safety concerns to the fetus are primarily related to teratogenesis and acoustic damage. Therefore, MRI should be used cautiously, especially during the first trimester. However, maternal safety is the same as that for imaging a nonpregnant patient.

MR scanning can be a problem for people who are prone to develop claustrophobia, because they are surrounded by a tunnellike structure for approximately 30 to 45 minutes. Some of the advantages and disadvantages of MRI are summarized in Table 1.4. There are a few contraindications for an MRI study, and these are listed in Table 1.5.

The external appearance of an MRI scanner or machine is similar to that of a CT scanner with the exception that the opening in the MRI gantry is more tunnellike (Fig. 1.12). As in CT, the patient is comfortably positioned supine, prone, or decubitus on a couch. The couch moves only when examining the extremities or areas of interest longer than 40 cm. The

TABLE 1.5

CONTRAINDICATIONS FOR MRI STUDIES

Pregnancy unless an emergency
Cerebral aneurysms clipped by ferromagnetic clips
Cardiac pacemakers
Inner ear implants
Metallic foreign bodies in and around the eyes

patient hears and feels a jackhammer-like thumping while the study is in progress.

The underlying physics of MRI is complicated and strange-sounding terms proliferate. Let's keep it simple: *MRI is essentially the imaging of protons.* The most commonly imaged proton is hydrogen, as it is abundant in the human body and is easily manipulated by a magnetic field. However, other nuclei can also be imaged. Because the hydrogen proton has a positive charge and is constantly spinning at a fixed frequency, called the *spin frequency,* a small magnetic field with a north pole and a south pole surrounds the proton. Remember that a moving charged particle creates a surrounding magnetic field. Thus, these hydrogen protons act like magnets and align themselves within an external magnetic field much like nails in a magnetic field or the needle of a compass.

While in the MRI scanner, or magnet, short bursts of radio frequency waves are broadcast into the patient from radio transmitters. The broadcast radio wave frequency is the same as the spin frequency of the proton being imaged (hydrogen in this case). The hydrogen protons absorb the broadcast radio wave energy and become energized or *resonate,* hence the term magnetic resonance. Once the radio frequency wave broadcast is discontinued, the protons revert or decay back to their normal or steady state that existed prior to the radio wave broadcast. As the hydrogen protons decay back to their normal state or relax, they continue to resonate and broadcast radio waves that can be detected by a radio wave receiver set to the same frequency as the broadcast radio waves and the hydrogen proton spin frequency (Fig. 1.13). The intensity of the radio wave signal detected by the receiver coil indicates the numbers and locations of the resonating hydrogen protons. These analog (wave) data received by the receiver coil are subsequently converted to numbers (digitized), and the numbers are converted to shades of black, white, and gray by computers.

For example, there are many hydrogen atoms and protons present in fat, and the received radio wave signal will be intense or very bright. However, there is much less hydrogen in bone cortex, and the received radio wave signal is of low intensity or black. The overall result is a 3-D proton density plot or map of the anatomic slice being examined. Now comes the complicated part. The received radio wave signal intensity from the patient is determined not only by the number of hydrogen atoms but also by the T1 and T2 relaxation times. If the radio receivers listen early during the decay following the discontinuance of the radio wave broadcast, it is called a T1-weighted sequence. In a T1 image, the fat is white and the gray soft tissue detail is

FIGURE 1.12 Illustration of an MRI scanner. Notice that its external appearance is similar to that of a CT scanner. The main difference, of course, is that there is a magnetic field rather than an x-ray tube around the gantry opening.

excellent. If the radio receivers listen late during the decay, it is called a T2-weighted sequence wherein the water in soft tissues is now a lighter gray and fat appears gray. The simplest way to think of T1 and T2 is as two different technical ways to look at the same structure. This is analogous to the PA and lateral radiographs being two different ways to view a bone or the chest. We tend to use T1 imaging when seeking anatomic information. T2 imaging is helpful when searching for pathology, because most pathology tends to contain considerable amounts of water or hydrogen and T2 causes water to light up like a light bulb. In general, T1 images have good resolution and T2 images have better contrast than T1 images.

Although human anatomy is always the same no matter what the imaging modality, the appearances of anatomic structures are very different on MR and CT images. Sometimes it is difficult for the beginner to differentiate between a CT image and an MR image. The secret is to *look to the fat.* If the subcutaneous fat is black, it is a CT image as fat appears black on studies that use x-rays. If the subcutaneous fat is white (high-intensity signal), then it has to be an MRI. Next, *look to the bones.* Bones should have a gray medullary canal and a white cortex on radiographs and CT images. The medullary canal contains bone marrow, and the gray is due to the large amount of fat in bone marrow. On a T1 MR image nearly all of the bone appears homogeneously white, as the bone marrow is fat that emits a high-intensity signal and appears white. Also, on MRI the cortex of the bone will appear black (dark or low-intensity signal), whereas on CT images the cortex is white. Soft tissues and organs appear as shades of gray on both CT and MR. Air appears black on CT and has

FIGURE 1.13 The general principles of MRI physics. The frequencies of the radio wave transmitter, the radio wave receiver, and the spin frequency of hydrogen atom protons are the same.

TABLE 1.6

A COMPARISON OF STRUCTURE APPEARANCES ON IMAGES[a]

		MRI	
Object	CT and radiographs	T1	T2
Air	Black	Dark	Dark
Fat	Black	Very bright	Intermediate to dark
Muscles	Gray	Dark	Dark
Bone cortex	White	Dark	Dark
Bone marrow	Gray	Bright	Intermediate to dark
Gadolinium		Very bright	Bright

[a]On MR images, the words dark, low-intensity signal, and black are synonymous; bright, high-intensity signal, and white are synonymous; and intermediate-intensity signal and gray are synonymous.

a low-intensity signal (black or dark) on MR. Table 1.6 compares the appearances of various structures on MR and CT images.

Magnetic Resonance Angiography

Magnetic resonance angiography (MRA) is a special noninterventional study that can image vessels without using needles, catheters, or iodinated contrast media. As a general rule, flowing blood appears black on most MR images, but by using a special imaging technique (gradient-echo pulse sequence) the arterial and venous blood appears as a high-intensity signal, or bright (Fig. 1.14). This procedure takes approximately 10 minutes, and 3-D images of the vasculature can be reconstructed with the digital information. MRA has been effective for imaging arteries and veins in the head and neck, abdomen, chest, and extremities. Gadolinium is the contrast media utilized when imaging smaller vessels, as in the distal extremities. However, as a general rule, contrast media is not needed for imaging larger blood vessels.

Functional Magnetic Resonance Imaging

This procedure gives us a good way to assess brain and cardiac function as oxygenated and deoxygenated blood cause magnetic signal variations that can be detected by MRI scanning. This makes it possible to identify areas that are active or inactive such as in the brain. Functional magnetic resonance imaging (fMRI) is good for cognitive tests. fMRI is used in normal controls to study how the brain functions and has been used extensively for presurgical planning.

fMRI is a technique that sensitizes the acquired signal intensity to changes in regional blood flow that occur while performing a cognitive task. The primary method for collecting fMRI data is the blood oxygenation level dependence method. A change in the relative hemoglobin oxygenation generates the underlying signal that is acquired during a rapid dynamic acquisition using a T2-weighted echo-planar imaging sequence. The signal intensity time series acquired during the dynamic acquisition is correlated with a description of the task being performed.

With the limited coverage required to study the brain during fMRI studies, the couch remains in a static position and the patient remains immobile.

Functional Cardiac Magnetic Resonance Imaging

Several methods have been employed to assess cardiac function using MRI. Cine studies acquire the MRI signal and reconstruct images across several phases of the cardiac cycle. From these images, it is possible to measure left ventricle volume and ejection fraction. Tagging sequences place a series of lines or grid across the image using selective spatial presaturation pulses (spatial modulation of magnetization). This is performed prior to a cine-imaging sequence. The change in the grid positions can be used to extract information regarding myocardial contraction and strain. Other techniques such as delayed contrast enhancement can be used to distinguish infarct from viable myocardium. Normal myocardial tissue will appear dark on this sequence while areas of bright signal within the myocardium are regions of infarct/scar.

Diffusion Weighted Imaging Magnetic Resonance

Because free diffusion of protons is inhibited by cell membranes, diffusion weighted imaging magnetic resonance (DWIMR) is particularly sensitive to cellular injuries of multiple etiologies. In DWIMR the abnormal motion of water molecules in the brain is detected from the additional loss in the dephasing signal as the water molecules diffuse through the tissues. As a result, DWIMR is routinely used in the diagnosis of ischemic stroke and can reliably detect hypoxic ischemia within minutes of symptom onset (Fig. 1.15).

FIGURE 1.14 **A:** MRA axial image of the circle of Willis arteries (normal). **B:** MRA coronal image of the carotid arteries (normal).

Magnetic Resonance Spectroscopy

Magnetic resonance spectroscopy (MRS) is a method that evaluates the metabolite concentrations in the body. In this technique, the signal from protons contained within water is suppressed, and the protons in various metabolites such as N-acetyl aspartate (NAA), choline, creatine, and lactate are detected. The signal from these metabolites is approximately 1000 times smaller as compared with the signal from water. Therefore, voxels on order of 1 cc are used. This technique is often used to evaluate lesions to determine whether they are cancerous, since tumors have been shown to have an elevated concentration of choline with a reduction in NAA (Fig. 1.16). MRS has also been used to diagnose acute stroke by showing an increase in lactate. MRS is also useful for looking at disorders of metabolism and inflammatory diseases.

FIGURE 1.15 Three slices from a diffusion weighted MRI scan in a patient with an acute stroke. The bright area shows the region of infarct and ischemia.

FIGURE 1.16   A patient with a tumor. **A:** An anatomical T1-weighted image showing the tumor mass. The arrow shows the region where the MRS data were collected. **B:** Graph of metabolite concentrations. The graph shows increased choline and reduced NAA. These are typical findings for MRS studies in tumors.

ULTRASONOGRAPHY

Ultrasonography (US) is another useful diagnostic imaging tool that is noninvasive and does not use x-rays or radiation. US has significantly improved the diagnosis, treatment, and management of a number of diseases. Some common areas where US imaging is used are listed in Table 1.7. US has achieved excellent patient acceptance because it is safe, fast, painless, and relatively inexpensive when compared with the other imaging modalities. The advantages and disadvantages of US are listed in Table 1.8.

Ultrasound technology produces sectional anatomy images or slices in multiple planes much like CT and MRI. An US machine consists of an ultrasound wave source, a computer, and a transducer (Fig. 1.17). The US machine emits high-frequency sound waves, ranging from 1 to 10 MHz, whose frequencies are considerably above the human ear's audible range of 20 to 20,000 Hz. Short bursts of these high-frequency sound waves are alternately broadcast into the patient via the transducer,

and some of the reflected sound waves from the body tissues are intermittently received by the transducer (Fig. 1.18). The acoustic impedance (Z) of a structure determines the amount of sound energy transmitted and reflected at its boundary (Z = tissue density $\times$ sound velocity). When a sound wave encounters an acoustic interface or the boundary between two media of different acoustic impedance, the sound waves may be absorbed, deflected, or reflected (Fig. 1.19).

The analog sound waves that are reflected directly back to the transducer are subsequently digitized. Next, a computer converts this digital information to an image with shades of black, white, and gray. US, like MRI and CT, depends on computer technology to store digital information and subsequently converts it to an image.

Normal organs and tissues have their own characteristic echo pattern, whereas diseased organs and tissues have altered

TABLE 1.7

SOME COMMON IMAGING APPLICATIONS FOR DIAGNOSTIC US

Obstetrics
Pediatric brain
Testicle and prostate
Female pelvis
Chest for pleural fluid drainage
Abdomen (kidney, pancreas, liver, and gallbladder)
Vascular disease
Rotator cuff of the shoulder

TABLE 1.8

ADVANTAGES AND DISADVANTAGES OF US DIAGNOSTIC IMAGING

Advantages
  Multiple plane imaging including obliques
  Safe—no known biological harm at diagnostic sound
    frequency levels
  Painless (noninvasive)
  Less expensive than CT and MRI
  Equipment cost is less than that of CT and MRI
  Real time or cine is possible
  Very portable
Disadvantages
  Requires technical skill or is operator dependent
  Not good for bone and lung imaging

FIGURE 1.17 A US unit, an ultrasonographer, and the patient. The transducer is centered over the abdomen. The ultrasonographer moves the transducer with the right hand while making technical adjustments on the US unit with the left hand.

echo patterns. Solid organs usually have a homogeneous echo pattern, whereas fluid-filled organs and masses such as the urinary bladder, cysts, some tumors, gallbladder, pleural effusions, and ascites have relatively fewer internal echoes.

The terminology used to describe an US image plane is slightly different from that used to describe CT and MR image planes. In US an axial view may be referred to as a transverse scan, and a sagittal view may be called a longitudinal scan or view (Fig. 1.20). As previously noted, a significant part of medicine is just learning the lingo.

While an US study is in progress, the images are viewed on a monitor. The monitor is analogous to a movie screen or television, and this viewing mode is called real time. This allows onlookers to observe a beating heart or the anatomy and movements of an intrauterine fetus. Also, static images may be reproduced on film by a format camera.

A small portable unit is now available for use in emergency situations. The laptop-sized computer is placed on a nearby flat surface. The transducer is approximately the size of one's

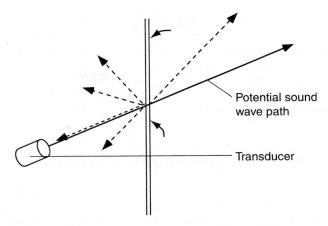

FIGURE 1.19 Illustration of what can happen to sound waves when they encounter an acoustic interface. An acoustic interface represents the intersection of two structures that possess different acoustic impedances or densities. When the sound waves are broadcast from the transducer (*solid black line*) and strike an acoustic interface (*curved arrows*), a number of things can happen to them such as the following: they can be reflected back to the transducer, be deflected away from the transducer, pass through the interface, or be absorbed at the interface.

hand and can be easily held over the area of interest to obtain urgently needed information such as when looking for abdominal fluid in trauma cases. This is called *FAST* or Focused Assessment with Sonography for Trauma.

TELERADIOLOGY

This term simply means the transmission of images from one site to another across telephone lines. This technology allows an image to be transferred to a radiologist's office or home for instant interpretation. Thus, a distant site without a radiologist present can transfer images to a radiologist at another site.

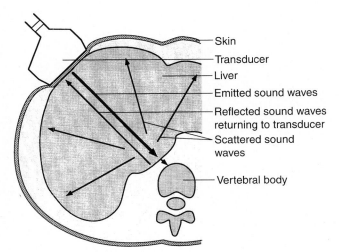

FIGURE 1.18 A transducer placed on the skin overlying the liver. The transducer broadcasts short bursts of high-frequency sound waves into the liver and deeper structures. Reflected sound waves are intermittently received by the transducer when it is not broadcasting sound waves. Note that some of the sound waves are deflected away from the transducer and are of no use for imaging.

FIGURE 1.20 Clarification of some of the terminology used to describe sectional anatomy planes on US images.

ALARA

ALARA is the acronym for "as low as reasonably achievable" and refers to radiation dose reduction for employees. It is an obligatory regulatory policy to protect employees wherein a radiation employee exposure should be less than 5 Roentgen Equivalent Man/year, but most departments commonly limit exposure to 10% of this amount.

PICTURE ARCHIVING SYSTEMS

The picture archive and computer system (PACS) is a comprehensive computer-based system designed to easily store and rapidly retrieve medical images. As one might expect, this is a challenging task as the size and number of images continue to grow rapidly. In recent years, the development of a standardized image format called Digital Imaging and Communications in Medicine (DICOM) has made the handling of medical images from a wide variety of modalities and manufacturers possible.

KEY POINTS

- There are four basic densities or appearances to observe on radiographs and CT images: *air*, which appears black; *fat*, which also appears black; *soft tissues and organs*, which appear gray; *and metal, calcium, and bone*, which appear white.
- Plain radiography images are produced by x-rays and radiographic film. CR or digital radiographs are produced by phosphor plates, x-rays, laser scanning, and computers. CT images are produced by x-rays, detectors, and computers. MR images are produced by magnetic fields, radio frequency waves, and computers. US images are produced by high-frequency sound waves, transducers, and computers.
- Sectional anatomy is the imaging of anatomy in multiple planes, including the axial plane (transverse or cross-sectional), the sagittal plane, and the coronal plane.
- A key to distinguishing an MRI image from a CT image is that the fat on an MRI appears white, whereas fat on a CT appears black. Look to the fat.
- T1 MR images tend to have excellent resolution and are, therefore, used to procure anatomic information. T2 MR images have better contrast than T1 images. T2 images cause water to light up; therefore, T2 imaging is frequently used when searching for pathology, as most pathology tends to contain a lot of water.
- The high resolution of CT makes it effective for imaging anatomy. MRI has high soft tissue contrast that makes it especially useful for soft tissue imaging.
- Commonly used contrast agents include barium sulfate, high and low osmolar iodinated compounds, ionic iodinated and nonionic (low osmolar) contrast media, air, and gadolinium. Images produced with water-soluble iodinated agents are generally less informative than barium studies, because they are less dense and result in poorer contrast.

Suggested Readings

Bushberg JT, Seibert JA, Leidholdt EM Jr, Boone JM. *Essential physics of medical imaging*. Philadelphia: Lippincott Williams & Wilkins, 2002.
Cherry SR, Sorenson JA, Phelps ME. *Physics in nuclear medicine*, 3rd ed. Philadelphia: WB Saunders, 1993.
Hashemi RH, Bradley WG. *MRI: the basics*. Baltimore: Williams & Wilkins, 1997.

SECTION II ■ DIAGNOSTIC RADIOLOGY

CHAPTER 2 ■ CHEST

WILLIAM E. ERKONEN AND BRAD H. THOMPSON

Chest pain, shortness of breath, and pneumonia are common presenting complaints for patients seeking medical care, especially through the emergency department. The workup or investigation of these symptoms usually necessitates an initial investigation with a chest radiograph. Therefore, it is not surprising that chest radiographs are by far the most commonly ordered examinations by family physicians and emergency room clinicians. Since all primary care physicians should be adept and comfortable reviewing chest films, it is our goal through this chapter to provide a primer on how to logically approach chest radiographs and to discuss those disease processes that are commonly encountered in daily practice.

TECHNIQUE

The chest radiographic examination is best accomplished within the radiology department, and a routine study consists of posteroanterior (PA) and lateral views. When the patient's condition precludes these routine views, a single portable anteroposterior (AP) view can be obtained. AP films can also be performed portably on those individuals unable to ambulate. It should be realized that portable films do not include lateral projections, which decrease sensitivity for detecting chest disease, and are also necessarily fraught with numerous technical limitations such as artificial cardiac magnification. For these reasons, every attempt should be made to request PA and lateral radiographs whenever possible. Illustrations for these radiographic techniques have been previously demonstrated in Chapter 1 (Figs. 1.1 to 1.4).

Chest radiographs are solely designed to provide optimal detailed information about the lungs and are not indicated for evaluation of suspected problems of ribs, shoulders, or the thoracic spine. In practice, one of the most common mistakes that occurs daily is the inappropriate request to evaluate for bony abnormalities such as rib fractures with chest films. These structures are poorly delineated on chest films and require formal dedicated radiographs in an effort to adequately evaluate these structures. Fortunately, the amount of radiation required for a routine two view radiological chest examination is small and not a threat to the patient. A routine plain film radiographic examination of the chest exposes the patient to 0.1 millisieverts (mSv) of radiation, which is similar to 10 days' exposure to environmental background radiation. In comparison, the dose of a standard chest computed tomography (CT) is 8 mSv, which is comparable to 3 years' exposure to natural background radiation.

HOW TO VIEW THE FRONTAL CHEST RADIOGRAPH (POSTEROANTERIOR AND ANTEROPOSTERIOR)

The first step in reviewing chest films is orienting the radiographs correctly on the viewbox. There is nothing more embarrassing than watching a novice pontificate over a set of chest radiographs that are either upside down or reversed. *A significant part of the art and practice of medicine is just learning the jargon, lingo, routines, and rituals.* Fortunately, with the advent of digital radiography and picture and archive systems (PACS), the examinations are usually displayed correctly on computer-viewing stations.

FIGURE 2.1 The correct positioning of a chest radiograph on a viewbox. The patient's right side on the film should always be opposite the viewer's left side.

Obviously, the right (R) and left (L) markers on the film indicate the patient's right and left side, respectively. The PA film should be hung as if you are looking at the patient such that the (R) film marker is opposite your left side (Fig. 2.1). This approach applies to all frontal projection chest radiographs (either AP or PA views). Of course, the patient's head should be oriented at the top of the radiograph. The next and perhaps most critical step is making sure that the films are annotated with the correct name. Needless to say, it would be malpractice to render a film interpretation and initiate treatment on the wrong patient. Next, critique the film for quality and for positioning errors. Poor film quality will only significantly hamper your diagnostic success.

When first reviewing chest films, we suggest the observer to render an initial gestalt impression by casually glancing over the entire image for any obvious abnormality that might be readily apparent, such as an enlarged heart or a baseball-sized lung mass. *Remember always to look at all four corners of the image.* Once this is performed, we suggest reviewing the films in a logical and thoughtful manner, using a methodical approach. Unfortunately, there is no single generally accepted or standardized system for evaluating a chest radiograph, so we advise developing your own comfortable system that can be used consistently for each and every study. Remember, all commercial pilots use a standard checklist prior to takeoff, which includes making sure that there is sufficient fuel, all equipment is functionally operational, and instruments are correctly set for departure. Knowing the likelihood of human error, commercial airlines consider such checklists critical for maintaining air safety. The same principle should apply to chest film interpretations as well.

A mental checklist or system is desirable when reviewing chest radiographs. So, program your internal computer to operate with a *systematic checklist* to avoid overlooking important areas or structures, as many of the errors made in medicine are errors of omission. Experimental perception studies using retinal tracking have investigated the process of film visual interrogation for experienced and inexperienced reviewers. The arrows in Fig. 2.2A roughly approximate the visual pathway

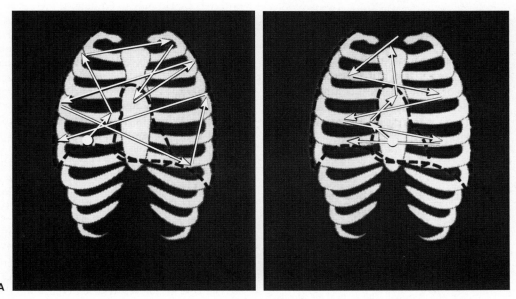

FIGURE 2.2 Illustration of a probable eye search pattern of a rookie (**A**) and by someone with a systematic approach (**B**) to a radiograph. Note that the rookie's search pattern is highly disorganized.

used by a novice viewing a chest radiograph. In practice, film review by the inexperienced is random and quite haphazard, often resulting in significant omissions. If you persist with this rookie approach, errors are inevitable! The arrows on Fig. 2.2B on the other hand, demonstrate a deliberate visual approach characteristic of experienced reviewers, making sure all regions of the film are visually inspected. Because of experience and practice, radiologists generally review radiographs using more of a generalized or gestalt approach, implementing a more circumferential and highly efficient visual pathway.

A common question relates to how long it should take to thoroughly inspect a set of chest films. While there are no correct answers, the time required to completely interrogate a film largely depends on experience. For novices, sufficient time should be around 20 seconds. In comparison, experienced reviewers can accurately review a film in a matter of seconds. It should be pointed out that excessive time spent looking at films only increases the likelihood of false-positive findings, that is, erroneously "identifying" lesions that do not exist. This phenomenon occurs for all reviewers regardless of experience. Staring at films rarely improves one's perception. One important caveat that is worth remembering is that "you only see what you know." Lack of knowledge about chest anatomy and normal radiographic findings will only limit your success in film interpretation.

The following system is suggested which can be used for a lifetime, or until you develop the requisite experience and skill to modify this approach. In developing a standardized approach, we find it useful to start at the top of the film to make sure the tracheal air column is midline. This accomplishes two missions: first, the tracheal air column should be midline and superimposed over the thoracic spine. This ensures that there is no appreciable malpositioning of the patient (Fig. 2.3). Second, deviation of the trachea implies mass effect usually by thyroid enlargement. This finding is quite common and usually

$$\frac{(AB)}{CD} = \text{Cardiothoracic}$$

FIGURE 2.4 Method for determining the cardiothoracic ratio. The cardiothoracic ratio is calculated by measuring the transverse diameter of the heart (B) and dividing by the transverse thoracic measurement CD.

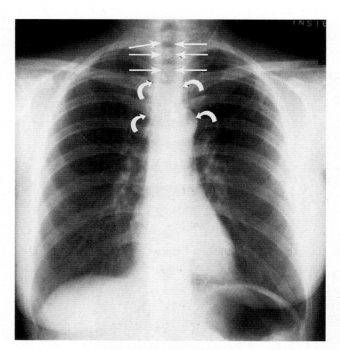

FIGURE 2.3 Chest PA radiograph. Normal. The vertical air density trachea (*straight arrows*) should always be midline. The narrow mediastinum is water density (*curved arrows*).

missed in daily practice. Next, follow the trachea inferiorly to arrive at the cardiac shadow, rendering an impression about the overall heart size. The transverse diameter of the cardiac silhouette should not exceed 50% of the transverse diameter of the thoracic cage measured or estimated at the same level. This is called the *cardiothoracic ratio* (Fig. 2.4). This measurement, however, applies only to PA films as there is considerable magnification of the cardiac silhouette on AP films. By convention, PA films are preferred since this technique has the heart closest to the film thereby limiting the degree of artificial magnification. *The greater the distance between an anatomic structure and the radiographic film, the greater the magnification.* As a useful analogy, consider the shadow cast by your hand from a light source. If we consider a flashlight as the x-ray source and the ceiling as the film, the closer the hand is to the ceiling, the more accurate the size of the shadow. Also, remember that diaphragmatic elevation as occurs commonly in shallow inspiration also tends to make the heart more horizontal and larger than it really is. With experience, cardiac size rarely requires actual determination of the cardiothoracic ratio. You should be able to quickly ascertain whether the cardiac silhouette is normal or not with just a little practice.

Next, evaluate the cardiac shape. What actually determines the cardiac shape? The convex right cardiac border is formed by the right atrial shadow, residing just superior is a vertical straight border rendered by the superior vena cava (Fig. 2.5, see Fig. 2.38A). The left ventricle constitutes the left heart border and cardiac apex. The superior left cardiac border should be concave in most cases (Fig. 2.5). The right ventricle is

Aortic arch (knob)

Main and left pulmonary
arteries

Left atrial appendage

Left ventricle

FIGURE 2.5 Chest posteroanterior (PA) radiograph. Normal. The convex right cardiac border is formed by the right atrium (*straight thin arrows*), and the *heavy arrows* indicate the location of the superior vena cava. The left cardiac and great vessels border might be considered as four skiing moguls. From cephalad to caudad the moguls are the aortic arch, the main and left pulmonary arteries, the left atrial appendage, and the left ventricle.

directly superimposed on the cardiac silhouette and is not a border-forming structure on frontal radiographs. Similarly, a normal sized left atrium is also not visible on PA or AP radiographs (Fig. 2.6). In cases of left atrial enlargement, the superior left heart border becomes convex, and in severe cases, the right lateral edge of the left atrium may become superimposed over the right atrial shadow, producing what is known as the *double-density sign* (see Fig. 2.69A). As the left ventricle enlarges, the cardiac apex moves to the down and out. As

the right atrium enlarges, the right heart border becomes protuberant (Fig. 2.7).

Next, your visual pathway should take you superiorly to the aortic arch (knob), pulmonary arteries, and the main stem bronchi. The left and right pulmonary arteries and the main stem bronchi form the hilar shadows (Fig. 2.8). On normal chest radiographs, the left hilum is more cephalad than the right hilum approximately 70% of the time and is at the same level in 30% of normal subjects. The normal right hilum should never be cephalad to the left hilum. The pulmonary arteries and their lobar branches emanate outward from the hili. The main pulmonary artery segment tends to be more prominent in the young and athletic, especially in females, but this prominence usually disappears with age. The *aortopulmonary window* is the concavity or space immediately below the aortic arch knob and just above the left pulmonary artery shadow (Fig. 2.9). Convexity of the aortopulmonary window raises the suspicion of either a mass or adenopathy occupying this space. It is important to remember that in the elderly the thoracic aorta commonly becomes tortuous or ectatic, and this should not be interpreted as abnormal.

Now your gaze should be directed to the mediastinum and evaluate it for widening; however, this may take some experience. Also, remember that on recumbent portable films the mediastinum likely will be wider in appearance than it would be

Left atrial appendage

Left atrium

Right ventricle

FIGURE 2.6 The approximate location of the left atrium and right ventricle on a normal PA or AP chest radiograph. These cardiac chambers cannot be delineated on normal studies. However, the left atrial appendage can occasionally be seen in normal hearts.

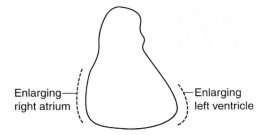

Enlarging right atrium

Enlarging left ventricle

FIGURE 2.7 Cardiac silhouette changes during right atrium and left ventricle enlargement. As the right atrium enlarges, the convex right heart border enlarges to the patient's right. As the left ventricle enlarges, the cardiac apex moves to the patient's left and downward.

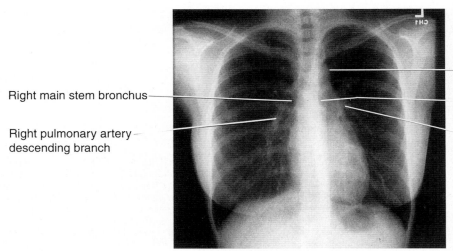

Right main stem bronchus

Right pulmonary artery descending branch

Transverse aortic arch (knob)

Left main stem bronchus

Left pulmonary artery descending branch

FIGURE 2.8   Chest PA radiograph. Normal. It is important to note that the air-filled main stem bronchi appear black, whereas the blood-filled pulmonary arteries appear white. See Table 1.1 in Chapter 1.

on an upright film. Most of the mediastinum shadow is caused by the great vessels and the vascular pedicle. The vascular pedicle extends from the thoracic inlet cephalad to the base of the heart caudally. The right border of the pedicle is the superior vena cava, and the left border is the aortic knob near the origin of the left subclavian artery (Fig. 2.3, see Fig. 2.68D). Now divide the lungs into horizontal thirds and compare the right and left lung fields for symmetry (Fig. 2.9). Next, evaluate the sharply demarcated domed diaphragms; the right hemidiaphragm should normally be about 1 to 2 cm higher than the left. This mild elevation is due to the liver, which resides immediately inferiorly. The lateral recesses of the diaphragms

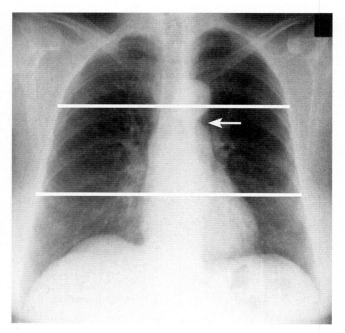

FIGURE 2.9   Chest PA radiograph. Normal. Divide the PA or AP chest radiograph into horizontal thirds and compare the right and left lung fields moving in a head-to-foot direction. Note the aortopulmonary window (*straight arrow*).

form the lateral costophrenic angles, which should be sharp and form an acute angle where the diaphragms insert laterally to the chest wall. Finally, determine the location of the gastric air bubble, which should reside immediately underneath the left hemidiaphragm on an upright film (Fig. 2.10).

Although the osseous structures are not well delineated on chest radiographs, significant abnormalities can occasionally be identified and should be detected if at all possible. As part of a routine chest film, exposure should allow the reviewer a cursory evaluation of the lower cervical spine, thoracic spine, and ribs (Figs. 2.10 and 2.11). Ribs are difficult to evaluate, so you need to trace each one visually or use your fingertip. On a PA radiograph, the horizontal portions of each rib are the posterior arcs and the anterior ribs are usually angled downward (Fig. 2.11). Portions of the shoulder girdle are usually included in the field of view and can be evaluated without much difficulty. As always, you should compare the right and left sides of the chest for symmetry.

HOW TO VIEW THE LATERAL CHEST RADIOGRAPH

Now position the lateral chest radiograph on the viewbox with the patient's head oriented to the top of the film. There is no hard-and-fast rule about the direction that the patient should be facing, but by convention it is customary to have the patient facing left (Fig. 2.12). Once again, begin the radiograph evaluation by casually viewing the entire image looking for any obvious abnormality. As on PA and AP radiographs, begin by estimating the size and shape of the cardiac shadow, which lies anteriorly in the chest cavity. On the lateral projection, the right ventricle forms the anterior border of the cardiac silhouette. The left ventricle forms the major portion of the inferior–posterior cardiac border, and the left atrium forms the superior–posterior cardiac border (see Fig. 2.12). On most lateral chest radiographs, the posterior wall of the inferior vena cava (*straight arrows*) can be seen as it enters from the abdomen in to the right atrium (Fig. 2.12). The identification of the inferior vena cava is useful to determine left

— Cervical spine

— Dorsal spine

Right hemidiaphragm —

Right costophrenic —
angle (sulcus)

— Left hemidiaphragm
— Left costophrenic angle (sulcus)

FIGURE 2.10 Chest PA radiograph. Normal. After comparing the lung fields, you next view the diaphragms, costophrenic angles, and lower dorsal spine. Note the close proximity of the gastric fundus air to the left hemidiaphragm (*arrow*). Always remember to identify the breast shadows in female patients (*curved arrows*).

ventricular size. The left ventricle is considered enlarged when the left ventricular posterior edge is 2 cm or more posterior to the inferior vena cava. The right atrium is a superimposed chamber and is not visualized on the lateral projection.

The lateral film is the best view to evaluate the hila. By drawing a vertical line down the tracheal air column, the hila can be separated into left and right. The dominant shadow ventral to your line is largely composed of the right main pulmonary artery, which should be about the size of your thumbprint. The left hilum, composed of the left pulmonary artery, resides posterior to the line and should be about one third the size of the right (Fig. 2.13). Then observe the ster-

num and search the retrosternal and retrocardiac spaces for abnormal or pathologic water or air shadows (Fig. 2.14A). On the lateral view, the retrosternal lucency primarily reflects the pneumatized upper lobes, whereas the right middle lobe and the lingular segments of the left upper lobe project over the cardiac silhouette. The lower lobes are located in the retrocardiac space overlying the spine extending inferiorly to abut the diaphragms (Fig. 2.14B). It is important to understand the pulmonary lobar spatial relationships to assist in locating pathologic pulmonary processes.

Finally, again observe the contours of the diaphragms and the posterior costophrenic angles (or sulci), which dive deep to

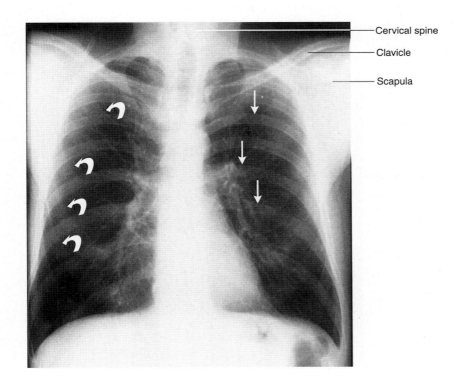

—Cervical spine

— Clavicle

— Scapula

FIGURE 2.11 Chest PA radiograph. Normal. The posterior ribs (*straight arrows*) are horizontal and anterior ribs (*curved arrows*) are angled caudad or inferiorly. All of these osseous structures must be included in your checklist as well as the shoulder girdles and cervical and dorsal spine areas.

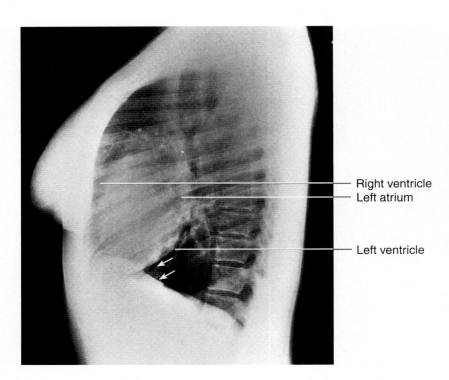

— Right ventricle
— Left atrium

— Left ventricle

FIGURE 2.12   Chest lateral radiograph. Normal. The radiograph is positioned on the viewbox with the patient facing to either your left or right. Note that the cardiac silhouette is an anterior structure and makes an excellent starting point for your evaluation. The faint vertical water density line (*straight arrows*) represents the inferior vena cava.

overlie the upper lumbar spine. The right hemidiaphragm should be slightly lower and more magnified than the left. This is important in determining the location of a small pleural effusion, which may not be apparent on the frontal film. Note that the right hemidiaphragm can be seen in its entirety, because air in the right lower lobe abuts the soft tissue density hemidiaphragm allowing a sharp interface to be formed. On the left side, only the apex and posterior portions of the hemidiaphragm are visualized. The anterior aspect of the left diaphragm, which lies adjacent to the heart and pericardial fat, becomes largely obscured due to similar densities of these structures (Fig. 2.15). This observation is an important radiological concept; *whenever two abutting objects of similar density are in direct juxtaposition, the interface or borders be-* *tween these objects is lost.* This phenomenon is known as the *silhouette_sign* and is a powerful and important radiological observation useful for detecting pathology. Because most pulmonary pathology is water or soft tissue in density, the silhouette sign facilitates the detection and location of such pathology. For example, disease processes within the left lower lobe such as pneumonia or atelectasis will obscure the border of the left hemidiaphragm (see Figs. 2.49A, B). Similarly, since the right middle lobe is located immediately adjacent to the right cardiac border, any right middle lobe process should obliterate the right cardiac border on the frontal radiograph. The same observation also holds true for disease processes within the lingular segments of the left upper lobe, which will obscure or silhouette out the left heart border.

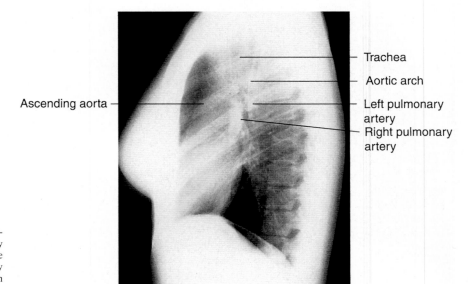

— Trachea

— Aortic arch

Ascending aorta —

— Left pulmonary artery
— Right pulmonary artery

FIGURE 2.13   Chest lateral radiograph. Normal. Note that the oval-shaped right pulmonary artery lies anterior and inferior relative to the left pulmonary artery. The left pulmonary artery crosses cephalad over the left main stem bronchus and it lies inferior to the aortic arch.

Sternum manubrium

Sternum body

Retrosternal space (upper lobes)

Dorsal vertebral body

Retrocardiac space (lower lobes)

A

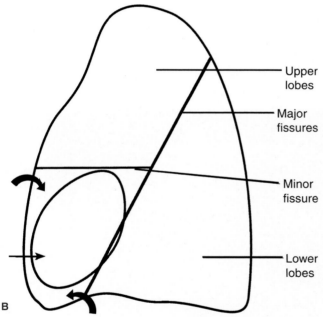

Upper
lobes

Major
fissures

Minor
fissure

Lower
lobes

B

FIGURE 2.14   A: Chest lateral radiograph. Normal. The anterior and posterior osseous structures should always be routinely viewed. The spine appears darker or more dense as you proceed caudally due to attenuation by the shoulders. **B:** Illustration of the spatial relationships of the pulmonary lobes on the lateral view. Note that the right middle lobe and the lingular segments of the left upper lobe (*curved arrows*) project over the heart (*straight arrow*). The lower lobes are primarily posterior structures. The major fissures extend up to approximately the T4 level.

ANTEROPOSTERIOR LORDOTIC CHEST

There are occasions when routine films show an equivocal or ill-defined lesion within the upper lobes that needs further characterization. In these situations, a special lordotic radiograph can be obtained which is essentially a frontal AP film, with the patient leaning backward (Fig. 2.16). This projection displaces the clavicles above the thoracic inlet and enables better visual evaluation of the lung apices. This specialized view is usually only indicated when upper lobe pathology is suspected on routine chest films.

DECUBITUS CHEST FILMS

Placing a patient on his/her side and obtaining an AP film by shooting across the x-ray table or bed produces what is known as a decubitus chest film. These examinations are primarily reserved when standard films suggest pleural disease (fluid or air) that needs to be confirmed and quantified. Decubitus films are capable of demonstrating very small pleural air or fluid collections and can be done portably on bedridden patients (Figs. 2.17A, B).

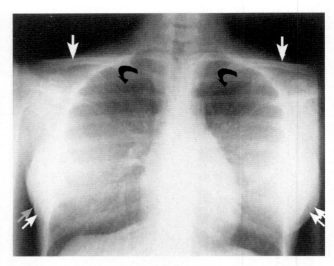

FIGURE 2.15 Chest lateral radiograph. Normal. Note that the left hemidiaphragm (*straight arrows*) is not visible anteriorly where it abuts the water density heart. On the other hand, the entire right hemidiaphragm (*curved arrows*) is visible. This is an excellent example of the silhouette sign.

FIGURE 2.16 Chest AP lordotic radiograph. Normal. This view is obtained with the patient leaning backward a few degrees. Note how the clavicles (*straight arrows*) project cephalad to the apices of both lungs allowing an improved view of the upper lobes (*curved arrows*). The scapulae project somewhat lower than on the standard AP or PA radiograph. The breasts are indicated by the *double straight arrows*.

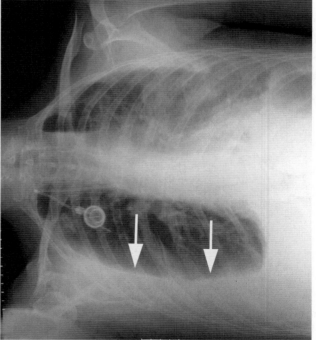

FIGURE 2.17 **A:** PA chest film shows a right pleural effusion (*arrows*). **B:** Right lateral decubitus film of same patient in figure A shows that the effusion is free-flowing and provides better quantitation of the size of the effusion.

NORMAL THORACIC SECTIONAL ANATOMY

The images in Figs. 2.18 through 2.26 demonstrate thoracic sectional anatomy by CT and magnetic resonance (MR).

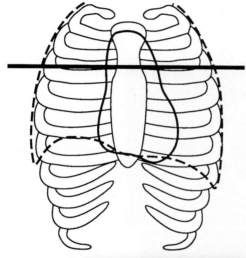

A

FIGURE 2.18 A: Approximate axial anatomic level through the aortic arch for B, C. **B:** Axial cadaver radiograph of the sectioned chest at the aortic arch level. Normal. A frozen cadaver was sectioned and then radiographed. **C:** Normal chest CT image at the aortic arch level with mediastinal windows (C).

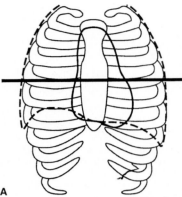

FIGURE 2.19   A: Approximate axial anatomic level through the pulmonary arteries for B–D. **B:** Axial cadaver radiograph of the sectioned chest at the level of the pulmonary arteries. Normal. **C:** Chest axial CT images at the level of the pulmonary arteries in mediastinal (**C**) windows (**D**). Normal. **D:** Chest axial MR image at the level of the pulmonary arteries. Normal.

FIGURE 2.20 **A:** Approximate axial anatomic level through the right and left atria for B–D. **B:** Axial cadaver radiograph of the sectioned chest at the level of the right and left atria. Normal. **C:** Chest axial CT images at the level of the atria in mediastinal (C) windows. Normal. **D:** Chest axial MR image at the level of the atria. Normal.

Sternum
Liver
Right ventricular cavity
Interventricular septum
Left ventricular cavity
Inferior vena cava
Esophagus
Descending aorta
Left lung

Right ventricle — Interventricular septum
Right atrium — Left ventricle
Esophagus — Coronary sinus
Aygous vein — Descending aorta
Vertebral body — Hemiazygous vein

Sternum
Right ventricular cavity
Interventricular septum
Left ventricular cavity
Liver
Esophagus
Descending aorta

FIGURE 2.21   A: Approximate axial anatomic level through the right and left ventricles for B–D. **B:** Axial cadaver radiograph of the sectioned chest at the level of the ventricles. Normal. **C:** Chest axial CT image through using a mediastinal window (**C**) Normal. **D:** Chest axial MR image at the level of the ventricles. Normal.

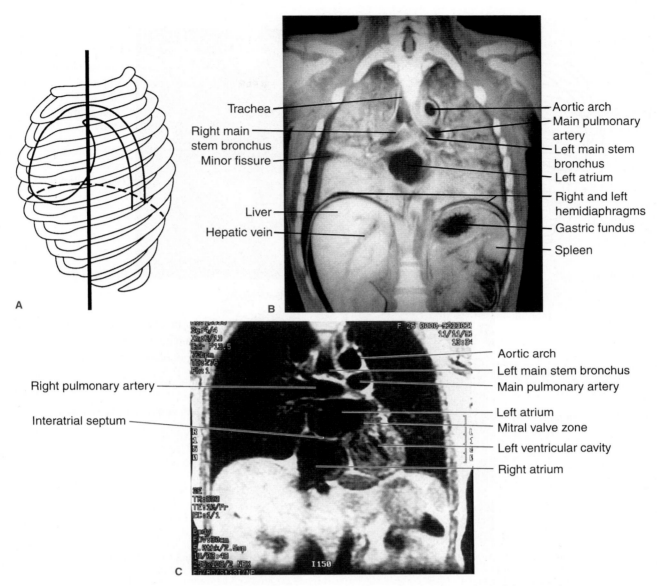

FIGURE 2.22   A: Illustration of the approximate coronal anatomic level through the left atrium for B and C. **B:** Coronal cadaver radiograph of the sectioned chest through the level of the left atrium. Normal. **C:** Chest coronal MR image through the right and left atria. Normal.

FIGURE 2.23   A: Approximate coronal anatomic level through the right atrium and left ventricle for B and C. **B:** Coronal cadaver radiograph of the sectioned chest through the level of the right atrium and left ventricle. Normal. **C:** Chest coronal MR image through the atria and left ventricle. Normal.

FIGURE 2.24   A: Illustration of the approximate coronal anatomic level through the left ventricle and the ascending aorta for B and C. **B:** Coronal cadaver radiograph of the sectioned chest through the left ventricle and the ascending aorta. Normal. Note that the convex right cardiac border is due to the right atrium (*straight arrows*). **C:** Chest coronal MR image through the left ventricle and the ascending aorta. Normal.

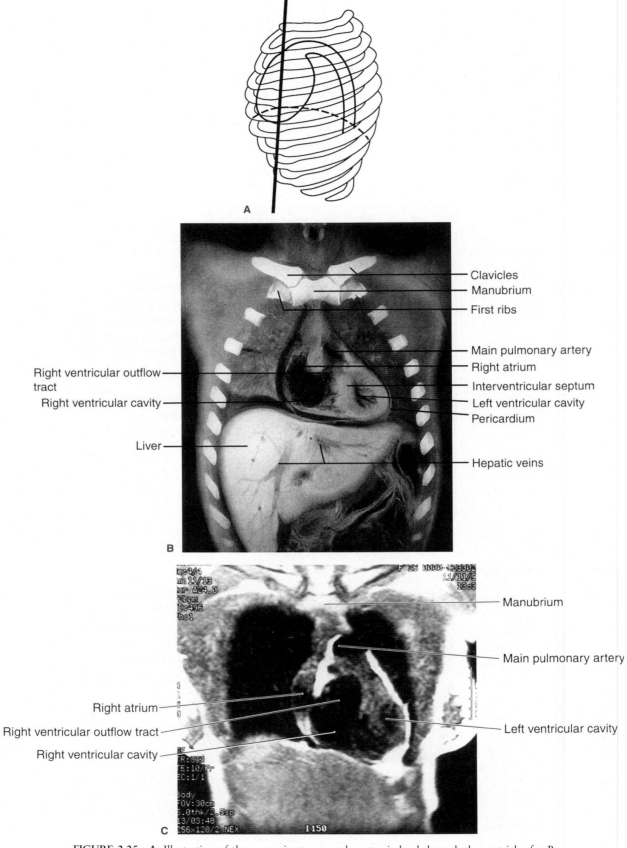

FIGURE 2.25   A: Illustration of the approximate coronal anatomic level through the ventricles for B and C. **B:** Coronal cadaver radiograph of the sectioned chest through the ventricles. Normal. **C:** Chest coronal MR image through the ventricles. Normal.

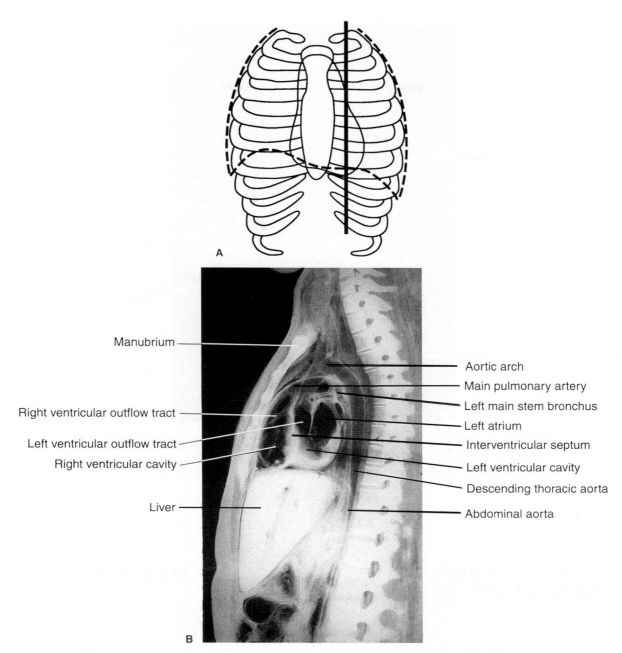

FIGURE 2.26   A: Illustration of the approximate sagittal anatomic level for B. **B:** Sagittal cadaver radiograph of the sectioned chest through the right ventricular outflow tract and the right ventricle. Normal.

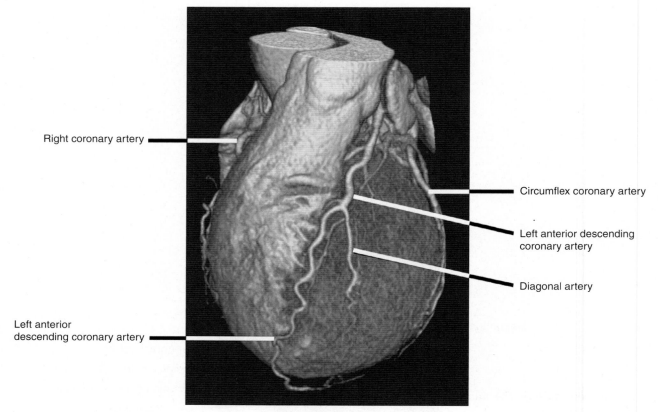

Right coronary artery

Circumflex coronary artery

Left anterior descending coronary artery

Diagonal artery

Left anterior descending coronary artery

FIGURE 2.27   Shaded surface display CT reconstructed image of the heart from a CT coronary angiogram illustrates the coronary arteries running along the left side of the heart. The left anterior descending coronary artery supplies most of the left ventricle while the circumflex artery runs in the left atrio-ventricular groove. A portion of the right coronary artery is visible along the left side of the image.

CARDIAC COMPUTED TOMOGRAPHY IMAGING

In general, computed tomography (CT) is the preferred modality for chest and pulmonary imaging primarily due to faster image acquisition, less susceptibility to artifacts than MR, and greater scanner availability. Spiral CT technology makes it possible to acquire a complete data set of the entire chest easily within one breath hold. Using standard chest CT protocols, scanners can produce contiguous 3-mm images of the entire chest usually within 15 seconds. The latest generation multislice spiral CT scanners, which possess subsecond imaging acquisition speeds are also capable of producing dynamic imaging of the beating heart with excellent spatial and temporal resolution. Using this technology, noninvasive coronary CT arteriography can be readily performed on patients with suspected coronary artery disease, negating the need in many cases for cardiac catheterization (Fig. 2.27). One significant limitation of MR for chest imaging is the lack of sufficient resolution of lung detail due to the low proton composition of lung tissue as well as potential problems of image degradation due to excessive respiratory motion.

ANOMALIES

Congenital anomalies can involve the sternum, clavicles, bronchi, lungs, heart and great vessels, and diaphragms. Anomalies which have obvious clinical manifestations are usually detected in infancy or early childhood. Other anomalies especially those involving only the skeletal system may not be apparent until revealed by radiographs obtained for unrelated reasons. While numerous chest anomalies exist, only a few will be illustrated.

Pectus excavatum, or funnel chest (Fig. 2.28), is a common and usually asymptomatic abnormality of the chest wall that can be associated with other congenital abnormalities such as Marfan's syndrome, scoliosis, and Poland's syndrome (1). Therapy which consists of surgical repair is usually performed in patients with chest pain or for cosmetic reasons. Pectus carinatum, or pigeon breast (Fig. 2.29), can be either a congenital or an acquired abnormality wherein the sternum bows anteriorly. These patients are usually asymptomatic, and corrective therapy is usually not indicated (1). The acquired form of pectus carinatum may occur in patients with untreated congenital heart disease.

Another skeletal abnormality is congenital absence of the clavicles (Fig. 2.30), which is associated with cleidocranial

FIGURE 2.28   Chest PA (**A**) and lateral (**B**) radiographs. Pectus excavatum. Note that on the PA view the cardiac silhouette is rotated and displaced to the patient's left, and the left cardiac border is straight simulating mitral valve disease. There is mild deformity of the ribs bilaterally on the PA view. The extent of the defect is best appreciated on the lateral view where the anterior ribs (*straight arrows*) project anterior to the sternum (*curved arrows*).

FIGURE 2.29   Chest PA (**A**) and lateral (**B**) radiographs. Pectus carinatum. The PA view is essentially normal with mild dorsal spine scoliosis. The exaggerated anterior bowing of the sternum (*straight arrow*) is best appreciated on the lateral view.

FIGURE 2.30 Chest AP radiograph. Cleidocranial dysostosis with bilateral absence of the clavicles. This was a routine chest radiograph in an asymptomatic 20-year-old woman.

dysostosis, a syndrome manifested by delayed or incomplete calvarial ossification, hypoplasia or aplasia of the clavicles, and many other associated osseous abnormalities (2).

Superior migration of the azygos vein up over the superior recess of the right upper lobe creates a mock vertical fissure-like opacity (Fig. 2.31, see Fig. 2.37B) which is created by indentation of both the visceral and the parietal pleural surfaces along the arc-like course of the vein as it courses inferiorly to insert normally into the superior vena cava. This azygos fissure, which is only visualized on PA radiographs as a thin curvilinear line, is a common normal variant and portends no clinical significance.

The most common thoracic aortic anomaly is a right aortic arch with a left descending thoracic aorta. In these cases, the transverse portion of the thoracic aorta crosses from right to left posterior to the esophagus to establish the descending thoracic aorta which runs in a left paraspinal location (Fig. 2.32). On the PA radiograph, the right-sided arch often appears more cephalad than a normal left-sided arch. There are five types of right aortic arch, and the classification is based on the arrangement of the arch vessels (3). Right-sided aortic arches can also be found in tetralogy of Fallot and other severe congenital heart anomalies.

Another vascular anomaly is coarctation of the aorta. Anatomically, this anomaly consists of a focal narrowing or stricture of the descending portion of the thoracic aorta. The degree of coarctation is variable, and the signs, symptoms, and physical findings vary with the location and degree of stenosis. Disparate blood pressures between the upper and lower extremities suggest the diagnosis.

The upper extremities blood pressures may be unequal if the location of the stenosis is proximal to the origin of left subclavian artery. Additional features include a systolic mur-

mur, cardiac enlargement, and pre- and poststenotic aortic dilatation depending on the location and severity of the stenosis. Often, the site of stenosis can be identified on routine chest radiographs (Fig. 2.33). Rib notching can occur along the inferior aspect of the ribs reflecting augmented collateral blood flow through dilated intercostal arteries in an attempt to bypass the stenotic segment (Fig. 2.33).

CONFUSING EXTRATHORACIC CONDITIONS

On occasion there are objects outside the thorax that can be confused with intrathoracic pathology (Figs. 2.34 to 2.36). It is important to keep such possibilities in mind at all times.

FOREIGN BODIES, LINES, AND TUBES

Another pitfall on chest radiographs that must be kept in mind is the presence of intrathoracic foreign bodies (Fig. 2.37). Some foreign bodies such as lines and tubes are intentionally placed within the thorax. It is very important to recognize the typical appearances of these commonly used lines and tubes, especially when caring for patients in acute care areas. The normal and some abnormal locations of some of these lines and tubes are demonstrated in Fig. 2.38.

POSTOPERATIVE CHEST PROBLEMS

It is important to recognize some common radiographic findings that may be present on postoperative chest images (Fig. 2.39).

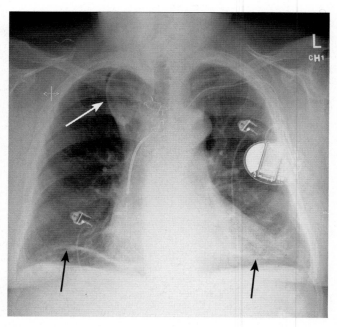

FIGURE 2.31 Chest PA radiograph. Azygos lobe. The azygos lobe is outlined with a *straight white arrow.* Also note the areas of discoid atelectasis in the lower lobes (*black arrows*) on the chest film.

FIGURE 2.32   Chest PA (**A**) and lateral (**B**) radiographs, barium swallow (**C**), and chest CT (**D**). Right-sided aortic arch and left descending thoracic aorta. This 42-year-old male smoker was suspected of having cancer of the lung. A neoplastic mass was suspected on the PA radiograph (**A**) but this proved to be an ill-defined aortic knob to the right of the midline (*straight arrows*). The right aortic arch is indenting the right side of the trachea). The right-sided aortic arch indents the posterior aspect of the trachea (*straight arrows*) on the lateral radiograph (**B**). Barium swallow (**C**) confirms a significant indentation on the posterior aspect of the barium-filled esophagus (*straight arrows*) secondary to the crossing aortic arch (*curved arrow*). The diagnosis is confirmed on chest CT (**D**) that shows the right-sided aorta (*single straight arrow*) passing posterior to the esophagus and trachea (*double straight arrows*) to reach the left side of the thorax. Again, note the indentation on the right side of the trachea (*curved arrow*) secondary to the right-sided aortic arch.

A

B

C

FIGURE 2.33   Chest PA (**A**) and lateral (**B**) radiographs. Coarctation of the aorta. The classical PA radiographic appearance is an indentation (*arrow*) involving the lateral aspect of the proximal descending aorta (**A**) and a posterior indentation (*arrow*) involving the posterior aspect of the proximal descending aorta on the lateral radiograph (**B**). These indentations represent the site of stenosis or coarctation in the proximal descending aorta. Rib notching (black/white arrows Figure A) is also evident along the inferior margins of several ribs. This notching represents collateral blood flow through dilated intercostal arteries. Figure C is an aortic angiogram which shows the classic narrowing of the upper portion of the descending thoracic aorta characteristic of coarctation (*arrow*).

FIGURE 2.34   PA chest radiograph. Hair artifacts (*straight arrows*) projecting over the upper lobes. Hair, hair braids, ponytails, and ribbons can project over the upper lobes and should not be confused with a pathologic process.

FIGURE 2.35   Chest PA (**A**) and lateral (**B**) radiographs. Bilateral breast augmentations or implants. The breast implants (*straight arrows*) are partially opaque, and the native breasts are indicated by the *curved arrows*. Note the benign postoperative calcification on both the PA and lateral views (*double straight white arrows*) in the inferior aspect of the right breast. The hyperinflated lungs are probably within limits.

FIGURE 2.36   Chest PA (**A**) and lateral (**B**) radiographs. Multiple soft tissue nodules projecting over the thorax from neurofibromatosis. Multiple subcutaneous soft tissue nodules (*arrows*) project over the thorax and must not be mistaken for pulmonary nodules.

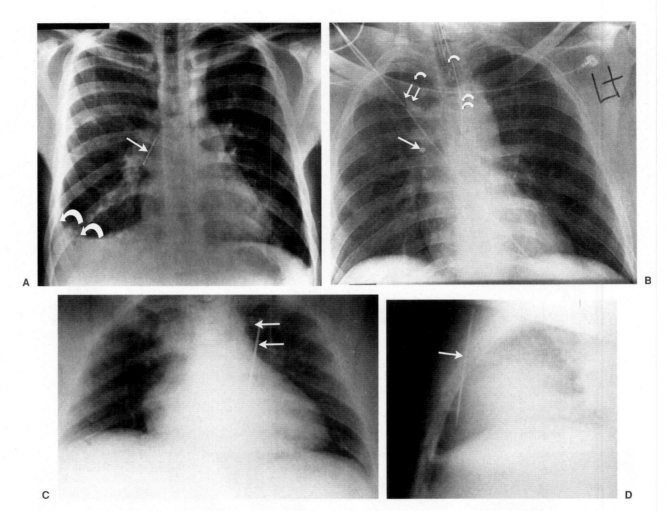

FIGURE 2.37   **A:** Chest PA. Aspirated straight pin (*straight arrow*) in the right intermediate bronchus. Note the right pleural effusion (*curved arrows*). It has been estimated that there must be at least 125 cc of pleural fluid before it is recognized on PA and AP views. **B:** Chest portable AP radiograph. Tooth fragment (*straight arrow*) in the right bronchial tree. The patient was involved in a motor vehicle accident, and a portion of a tooth was missing. The chest radiograph shows the tooth fragment projecting over the right upper bronchial tree. Note that the endotracheal tube (*single curved arrow*) lies to the patient's right of the nasogastric tube (*double curved arrows*). An azygos lobe is present, and the *double straight arrows* indicate the position of the azygos vein that is more lateral and cephalad than normal. The azygos lobe (*curved white arrow*) is visible. **C, D:** Chest AP (**C**) and lateral (**D**) radiographs. Darning needle lodged in the right ventricle. The child of this young mother accidentally stabbed her with a darning needle. Note that the needle (*straight arrows*) projects over the right ventricle region in both views. The needle was successfully removed at thoracotomy.

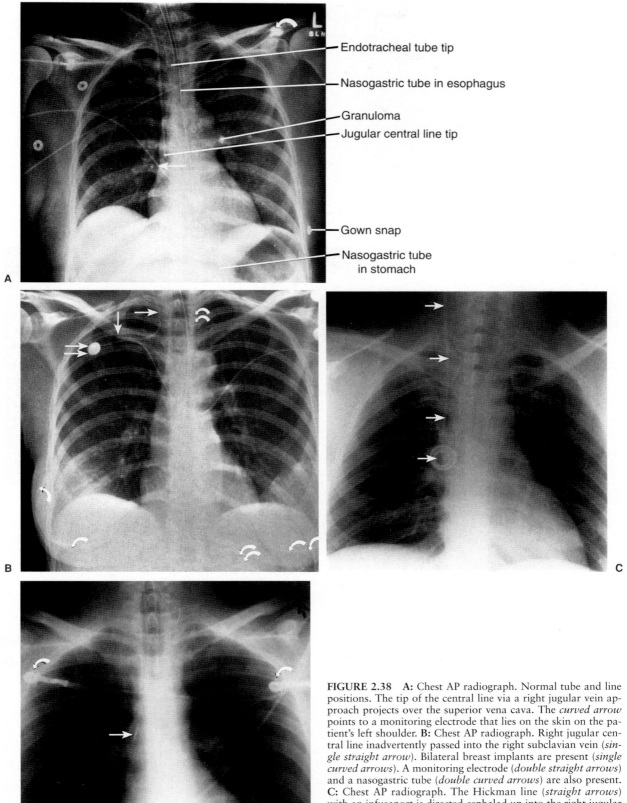

— Endotracheal tube tip

— Nasogastric tube in esophagus

— Granuloma
— Jugular central line tip

— Gown snap

— Nasogastric tube
　in stomach

FIGURE 2.38　A: Chest AP radiograph. Normal tube and line positions. The tip of the central line via a right jugular vein approach projects over the superior vena cava. The *curved arrow* points to a monitoring electrode that lies on the skin on the patient's left shoulder. **B:** Chest AP radiograph. Right jugular central line inadvertently passed into the right subclavian vein (*single straight arrow*). Bilateral breast implants are present (*single curved arrows*). A monitoring electrode (*double straight arrows*) and a nasogastric tube (*double curved arrows*) are also present. **C:** Chest AP radiograph. The Hickman line (*straight arrows*) with an infusaport is directed cephalad up into the right jugular vein rather than caudad toward the superior vena cava. The tip of the line is beyond the edge of the radiograph. **D:** Chest AP radiograph. Endotracheal tube (*arrow*) inadvertently placed in right intermediate bronchus. External monitoring electrodes are present (*curved arrows*).

Nasogastric tube

Endotracheal tube tip

Sternum wire sutures

Blood

Chest tube

Nasogastric tube

A

B

C

FIGURE 2.39 **A:** Chest AP supine radiograph. Postoperative left hemothorax. The white homogeneous density in the region of the left upper lobe represents active bleeding in the thorax 2 hours following coronary artery bypass grafting. The patient was reoperated to evacuate the blood and control the bleeding. The *straight arrows* indicate a right jugular Swan-Ganz catheter. **B, C:** Chest AP (**B**) and lateral (**C**) radiographs. Right pneumonectomy. The *straight arrows* indicate the presence of an air–fluid level in the chest cavity that is a common finding following pneumonectomy. Gradually over a period of days the right chest cavity will fill with fluid. Left lower lobe atelectasis is manifested by the retrocardiac double density (*curved arrow*). Left lower lobe atelectasis is common following thoracic surgery. There is obliteration of the right hemidiaphragm (silhouette sign) by the right pleural fluid.

Air in the Wrong Places

An important chest problem that can have significant clinical ramifications is pneumothorax (air accumulation within the pleural space). Pneumothorax most often is secondary to trauma or due to iatrogenic causes. A list of potential etiologies is shown in Table 2.1. Spontaneous pneumothorax most commonly occurs in young, thin asthenic male adults but can involve female patients as well. These patients typically present with a sudden onset of unilateral chest pain that can be accompanied by varying degrees of shortness of breath. The etiology of spontaneous pneumothoraces is likely due to rupture of small lung cysts. As is true for all pleural air collections, treatment depends on size of the pneumothorax and whether coexisting clinical symptoms such as dyspnea exist.

The definitive radiographic diagnosis of pneumothorax is made by identifying the *visceral pleura edge* (Fig. 2.40A). Figure 2.40 illustrates three cases of pneumothorax of varying sizes.

TABLE 2.1
PARTIAL LIST OF PNEUMOTHORAX ETIOLOGIES

Traumatic
1. Trauma/penetrating chest wounds
2. Iatrogenic
   a. Thoracoscopy
   b. Thoracentesis
   c. Placement of central line
   d. Artificial ventilation (barotrauma)
   e. Postthoracic surgery
   f. Transthoracic or bronchoscopic lung biopsy

Spontaneous
1. Rupture of a bleb or bullae
2. Secondary to underlying pulmonary disease (fibrosis, emphysema)
3. Secondary to pneumomediastinum

Swan-Ganz catheter
(jugular approach)

Tip endotracheal tube

Nasogastric tube

Swan-Ganz catheter
tip in right
pulmonary artery

Atelectasis

Left hemidiaphragm

Pneumothorax

Deep sulcus
sign

Endotracheal tube tip

Nasogastric tube

Jugular central line tip in
superior vena cava

FIGURE 2.40 **A:** Chest PA radiograph. Small right pneumothorax. A thoracentesis was performed to remove right pleural fluid (*straight arrow*), but it resulted in a right pneumothorax. The visceral pleura is outlined by the *curved arrows*. There is air in the pleural space (*double straight arrows*) lying between the visceral pleura and the parietal pleura or chest wall. The result is a partially collapsed or atelectatic right lung. Note that the trachea (*) is midline. **B:** Chest AP radiograph. Moderately large right pneumothorax. While on the ventilator, this patient developed right chest pain and shortness of breath. There is a moderate-sized right pneumothorax. The right lateral costophrenic sulcus or angle is very deep and lucent compared to the left, and this is called the *deep sulcus sign*. A deep sulcus sign should always make you suspicious for pneumothorax is indicative of tension. Note the double density behind the cardiac silhouette (*straight arrows*) and the associated obliteration of the left hemidiaphragm medially (*curved arrow*) representing left lower lobe atelectasis. **C:** Chest AP radiograph. Right tension pneumothorax. This patient was on the ventilator and developed right chest pain and hypotension. There is a large right pneumothorax with near complete collapse of the right lung. *Straight arrows* indicate the visceral pleural line. Note the right deep sulcus sign (*curved arrow*). The heart is displaced to the left indicating a tension pneumothorax.

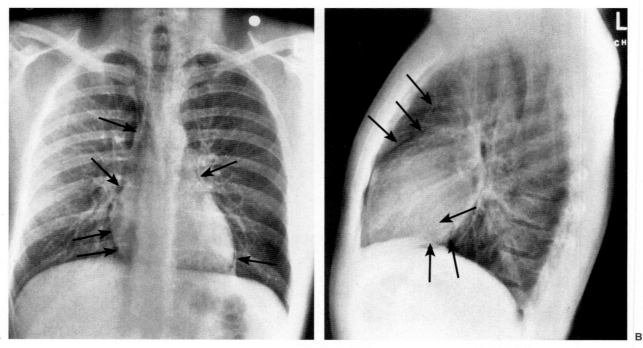

FIGURE 2.41 Chest PA (**A**) and lateral (**B**) radiographs. Pneumomediastinum. This patient had routine chest radiographs for vague chest pain, and surprisingly, the radiographs revealed mediastinal air (*straight arrows*). The etiology was never found, and the air resolved spontaneously.

Additional findings include an abnormally hyperlucent lung or hemithorax and loss of normal lung markings on the affected side. Upright or decubitus films are the most sensitive methods to document the presence of pleural air. Recumbent portable films on the other hand are notoriously insensitive for demonstrating even large pleural air collections, largely because the air resides immediately ventral to the lung and in essence becomes invisible. A *tension pneumothorax* is present when the air component within the pleural space is sufficiently large to produce mass effect upon the mediastinal structures and ipsilateral diaphragm. In these cases, the mass effect on the heart and great vessels can produce acute cardiovascular collapse due to diminished cardiac output. Acute respiratory problems are also likely to coexist due to compression of lung tissue and mass effect upon the diaphragm (see Fig. 2.40C). A tension pneumothorax is a surgical emergency requiring immediate placement of chest tube to decompress the pleural space.

Pneumomediastinum refers to air within the mediastinum (Fig. 2.41) and has a number of etiologies listed in Table 2.2.

TABLE 2.2

SOME ETIOLOGIES OF PNEUMOMEDIASTINUM

Traumatic
1. Closed chest trauma
2. Secondary to chest and neck surgery
3. Esophageal perforation
4. Tracheobronchial perforation
5. Vigorous exercise
6. Asthma
7. Ventilator induced (barotrauma)

Spontaneous
1. Bleb or bullae rupture
2. Idiopathic

Pneumomediastinum is usually accompanied by unexplained chest wall and cervical subcutaneous emphysema, which may suggest the diagnosis. The presence of air within the mediastinum is usually an ominous sign suggesting rupture of the esophagus or trachea. Cases of spontaneous pneumomediastinum can be encountered in younger adults, which eventually resolve in a few days, usually without ever identifying the source of the air.

In cases of significant chest trauma, especially those involving rib fractures, or rapid deceleration injury, lacerations or tears of lung tissue may occur. Pulmonary lacerations may be difficult to detect on routine chest radiographs but are readily apparent on CT (Fig. 2.42). Patients with pulmonary lacerations often have coexisting pneumothoraces and areas

FIGURE 2.42 Chest axial CT through the lung bases. Lung parenchymal lacerations (*straight arrows*) in the left lower lobe. The lacerations are surrounded by airspace disease (contused lung parenchyma) (*curved arrows*).

FIGURE 2.43 Chest PA (**A**) and lateral (**B**) radiographs. Esophageal hiatal hernia. The *straight arrows* indicate the large esophageal hiatal hernia that contains an air–fluid level. The chest is otherwise normal.

of pulmonary hemorrhage. Lacerations of the lung usually require no treatment and usually heal spontaneously.

Other Air Accumulations in and Around the Chest

Hiatal hernias which represent superior displacement of the stomach into the lower chest often present with a focal collec-

tion of air residing immediately posterior to the heart (Fig. 2.43) and may contain an air–fluid level if fluid is present within the stomach. Hiatal hernias are often an incidental discovery on chest films. Their presence should be noted as co-existing gastroesophageal reflux disease is likely, which may result in esophagitis and chest pain.

Infection leading to abscess formation can occur within the soft tissues of the chest wall or back (Fig. 2.44). The diagnosis is suggested when an air–fluid level is identified in the soft

FIGURE 2.44 Chest PA (**A**) and lateral (**B**) radiographs. Right axillary abscess. This patient was postoperative following a right axillary node dissection. A right axillary air–fluid level (*straight arrows*) is well visualized on both the PA and lateral views. The abscess was subsequently drained.

FIGURE 2.45   Chest PA (**A**) and lateral (**B**) radiographs. Left upper lobe lingular abscess (*straight arrows*). There is air within the abscess cavity. Infiltrates are present in the lower lung fields (*curved arrows*).

tissues of the thorax. Obtaining two orthogonal views of the chest is required to accurately locate the air collection to make sure that the lesion is not within the pleural space or lung (Fig. 2.45).

Pneumoperitoneum is a significant abnormal air accumulation in the abdomen that often can be identified on chest radiographs (Fig. 2.46). As little as a few cubic centimeters of air may be detected on upright radiographs of the lower chest and upper abdomen. Spontaneous pneumoperitoneum due to perforation of a hollow intra-abdominal viscus requires immediate surgical attention to prevent peritonitis.

FIGURE 2.46   Chest AP radiograph. Pneumoperitoneum. The patient experienced sudden onset of severe abdominal pain, and physical examination revealed a boardlike rigidity of the abdomen. The patient proved to have a perforated duodenal ulcer at surgery. The *straight arrows* indicate the free subdiaphragmatic air secondary to the perforated ulcer.

Too Much Air in the Lungs

Chronic obstructive pulmonary disease (COPD; Fig. 2.47A, B) is a significant health problem worldwide. Largely due to smoking, COPD is the fifth most common cause of death in the United States (1) and is a major factor of morbidity. The terminology surrounding lung disease is confusing and includes chronic bronchitis, emphysema, and COPD. COPD is airway obstruction without a specific known pathophysiology. Table 2.3 lists some of the COPD etiologies. Emphysema is enlargement of the airspaces distal to the terminal bronchioles without fibrosis (1). Radiographically, patients with COPD have exaggerated lung volumes with flattening of the diaphragms

TABLE 2.3
PARTIAL LIST OF COPD ETIOLOGIES
1. Cigarette smoking 2. Air pollution 3. Childhood infections 4. Heredity

FIGURE 2.47   Chest PA (**A**) and lateral (**B**) radiographs. Chronic obstructive pulmonary disease (COPD). The lungs are hyperlucent and markedly hyperinflated. The diaphragms are flat on the lateral view and nearly flat on the PA radiographs (*straight arrows*). The retrosternal airspace is overexpanded and the AP dimension of the chest is greater than normal. **C, D:** Chest PA radiograph (**C**) and axial prone chest CT (**D**). Idiopathic pulmonary fibrosis. This 79-year-old man had a long history of shortness of breath. On the PA chest radiograph (**C**), there are typical linear changes (*straight arrows*) that represent fibrosis. On CT (**D**), the fibrosis is mainly peripheral (*straight arrow*) and there is an overall honeycomb appearance to the lung parenchyma.

and increases in the anterior–posterior dimension of the chest wall (i.e., barrel chest deformity). Due to air trapping and lung destruction, the lungs typically look abnormally hyperlucent. Cysts or bullae may also be present as well, usually residing in the upper lung zone regions which is the location of the most severe lung disease occurring in COPD related to cigarette smoking.

In contrast, interstitial lung disease refers to the development of lung fibrosis. Pulmonary fibrosis, (Fig. 2.47C, D) is a disease process characterized by the development of linear or scarlike changes in the lungs with diminished lung volumes. Usually a progressive disease, the etiologies of pulmonary fibrosis are extensive and in some cases, a causative etiology cannot be firmly established without open lung biopsy.

ATELECTASIS, PULMONARY EMBOLI, AND INFECTIONS

It is important to remember that most pathologic conditions of lung such as pneumonia, tumor, infarction, and atelectasis will appear as opacities of gray on radiographs. So, *think water density or gray* when viewing radiographs and concentrate less on the black. After all, black densities in the lungs represent air contained within alveoli.

Atelectasis

Atelectasis represents the loss of pneumatization of lung tissue. Atelectasis may be minimal in size (Figs. 2.31 and 2.48) appearing as linear shadows within the lungs (discoid atelectasis) or may result in complete collapse of an entire lobe or lung (Fig. 2.49). There are five types of atelectasis: Passive atelectasis refers to airless lung arising from prolonged recumbency or shallow breathing. Compressive atelectasis refers to lung tissue which is compressed by an adjacent structure, such as a large pleural effusion. Adhesive atelectasis occurs when alveoli collapse due to insufficient surfactant such as occurring in hyaline membrane disease in neonates. Postobstructive atelectasis occurs when there is complete airway occlusion (tumor, foreign body, or mucous plug). Cicatricial or rounded atelectasis occurs when lung

TABLE 2.4
GENERAL ETIOLOGIES OF ATELECTASIS

1. Postobstructive
   a. Tumor in airway
   b. Foreign body in airway
   c. Infection
   d. Mainstem intubation
2. Postoperative
3. Extrinsic pressure
   a. Pleural fluid
   b. Pneumothorax
4. Restrictive motion
   a. Trauma
   b. Neuromuscular diseases
   c. Infections

tissue curls into a ball due to an inciting adjacent pleural abnormality. It is important to understand that atelectasis is not by itself a primary disease process but rather suggests underlying lung disease or airway abnormality (3). The general etiologies are listed in Table 2.4 and the radiographic signs are listed in Table 2.5.

Discoid atelectasis is a morphological term describing a linear opacity found on chest radiographs. It is generally believed that discoid atelectasis results from several factors including shallow tidal volumes and cough-inhibiting factors with pooling of secretions. Radiographically discoid atelectasis appears as a horizontal linear density measuring a few millimeters in width and variable in length (Fig. 2.48).

Pulmonary Emboli

Pulmonary thromboembolic disease (PE) is a very common disease with important clinical implications. Pulmonary embolic disease has a number of etiologies as shown in Table 2.6. Most cases occur in hospitalized and incapacitated patients wherein a thrombus originating in lower extremity and/or pelvic veins dislodges and passes up into the pulmonary arteries. Other potential sources of thromboembolic disease may originate from indwelling central lines, which can become infected resulting in septic pulmonary emboli (Fig. 2.50A, B).

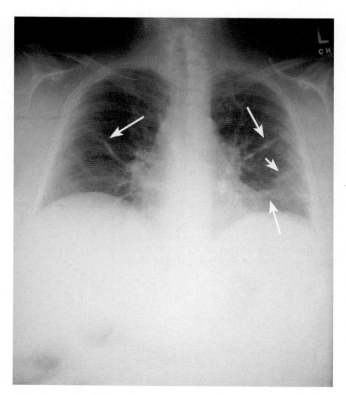

FIGURE 2.48 Chest PA radiograph. Bilateral discoid (platelike) atelectasis. The *straight arrows* indicate the typical appearance of this abnormality that is commonly found in postoperative, posttrauma, severely ill, and debilitated patients.

TABLE 2.5
RADIOGRAPHIC SIGNS OF ATELECTASIS

Primary
1. Loss of volume of involved segment, lobe, or lung
2. White-appearing consolidated lung tissue
3. Air bronchograms
4. Coaptation of bronchi and vessels

Secondary
1. Upward elevation of the hemidiaphragm
2. Mediastinal shift toward side of collapse
3. Rib becomes closer apposed
4. Indistinct hilum and hilar displacement

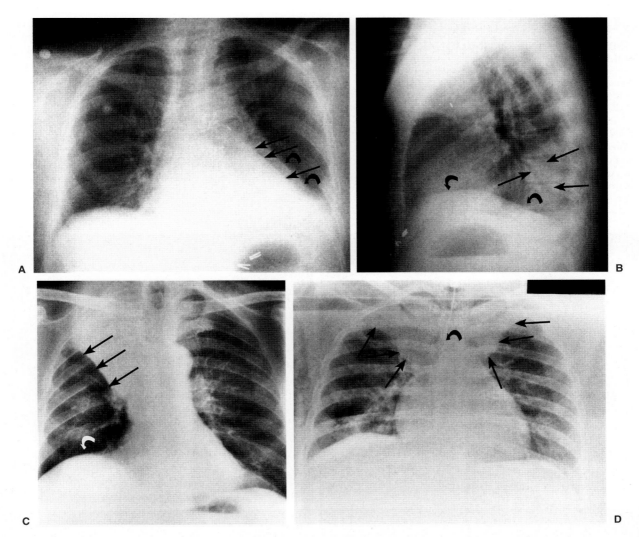

FIGURE 2.49 **A:** Chest PA radiograph. Postoperative left lower lobe atelectasis. There is a double density behind the cardiac silhouette, and the *straight arrows* indicate the edge of the atelectatic left lower lobe, whereas the *curved arrows* indicate the left cardiac border. The left hemidiaphragm is poorly visualized because the water density atelectatic left lower lobe is in juxtaposition to the left hemidiaphragm or a silhouette sign. **B:** Chest lateral radiograph. Same patient as in A. There is a positive spine sign (*straight arrows*). Remember that on the lateral view, the spine should appear darker as you proceed caudad because there is more lung in the lower thorax. When a water density disease process like atelectasis or pneumonia is present in the lower lobes, the spine will appear whiter as you proceed caudad rather than darker (spine sign). The left hemidiaphragm cannot be seen as it is silhouetted by the atelectasis in the left lower lobe, but the entire right hemidiaphragm can be seen (*curved arrow*). **C:** Chest AP radiograph. Right upper lobe atelectasis. There is consolidation of the right upper lobe reflecting atelectasis. The minor fissure is elevated indicating volume loss (*straight arrows*). The right pulmonary artery and the ascending aorta are obscured by the water density atelectasis, and the right hemidiaphragm (*curved arrow*) is elevated indicating volume loss. **D:** Chest AP radiograph. Bilateral upper lobe atelectasis (*straight arrows*). This 30-year-old woman developed bronchospasm in the operating room. Both upper lobes are airless and collapsed, and the mediastinum is silhouetted. The *curved arrow* indicates the tip of an endotracheal tube.

TABLE 2.6

COMMON ETIOLOGIES OF PULMONARY EMBOLIC DISEASE

1. Venous thromboembolism
   a. Postsurgical
   b. Bed rest
   c. Trauma
   d. Neoplasm
2. Foreign body
   a. Bone marrow post–long bone fracture
   b. Amniotic fluid
3. Septic emboli
4. Air

Depending on the size of the clot burden, PE can result in lung infarction, hemorrhage, pulmonary hypertension, and even death. Patients with acute PE usually present with sudden chest pain, shortness of breath, and occasionally hemoptysis. The radiographic signs in these patients are highly variable and range from normal radiographs to grossly abnormal examinations. Usually some radiographic abnormality is identifiable in acute cases. A CT study (*which is now considered the examination of choice*) (Fig. 2.50C) is required to establish the diagnosis. With the advent of CT, which has a sensitivity of 95% for PE, invasive pulmonary angiography has been essentially rendered obsolete.

FIGURE 2.50 **A:** Chest PA radiograph. Bilateral septic emboli secondary to an infected Hickman catheter. The chest radiograph is grossly abnormal with multiple bilateral opacities (*straight arrows*) reflecting to septic emboli. The differential diagnosis would include pneumonia, embolic disease, atelectasis, and hemorrhage. The tip of the Hickman catheter (*curved arrow*) is in the superior vena cava. **B:** Chest axial CT through the level of the left atrium in the same patient as A. Pulmonary infarcts (*straight arrows*) appear as peripheral, wedge-shaped, homogeneous opacities (infarcted lung) which are pleural based. **C, D:** Chest axial CT images through the pulmonary arteries in a different patient than A and B. Bilateral pulmonary artery thromboemboli secondary to lower extremity deep vein phlebothrombosis. This 30-year-old man developed bilateral lower extremity edema and shortness of breath following a long automobile trip. There are filling defects (*straight arrows*) in the right and left pulmonary arteries created by the thromboemboli. The curved arrow on figure C points to an area of pulmonary infarction. (*continued*)

External monitoring electrode

Metallic surgical clips

E

FIGURE 2.50 (*Continued*) **E:** Left pulmonary arteriogram. Multiple left pulmonary artery pulmonary emboli (*straight arrows*) within the left main pulmonary artery and its branches secondary to lower extremity deep vein thrombosis. This 72-year-old woman was 72 hours status postcoronary artery bypass grafting and developed shortness of breath and hypoxia. The angiographic catheter (*curved arrows*) is visible in the left pulmonary artery.

Pulmonary angiography might be indicated to establish the diagnosis of PE when CT studies are indeterminate, but this indication is considerably uncommon (Fig. 2.50D).

Pulmonary Infections

Pulmonary infections have many etiologies, some of which are listed in Table 2.7. Patients with pulmonary infections, that is, pneumonia, often present with fever, chest pain, and cough. The radiographic appearances of pneumonia are highly variable, and often it is impossible to determine the etiology of pneumonia based on the radiographic appearances alone. The radiographic findings vary from a small ill-defined infiltrate to complete unilateral or bilateral opacification of the lung tissue

(Figs. 2.51 to 2.55). Many pneumonias have associated parapneumonic pleural effusions which if secondarily infected result in a pus accumulations in the pleural space (empyema). Lung abscess, another complication of pneumonia especially with *Staphylococcus aureus*, *Streptococcus pyogenes*, and gram-negative organisms, appears as a cavitary area of lung consolidation (Fig. 2.45). Since pneumonias in general appear as water density airspace shadows, alternative diagnoses such as tumor or pulmonary hemorrhage should be considered in the differential diagnoses.

Many patients who are immunosuppressed are particularly susceptible to pulmonary infections especially from fungal and mycobacterial organisms such as tuberculosis. Despite new therapies and improved public health measures, pulmonary tuberculosis continues to be a persistent and problematic disease. Tuberculosis should always be considered as a potential pathogen especially in homeless patients or those with AIDS (Table 2.8).

TABLE 2.7

SOME GENERAL ETIOLOGIES OF PNEUMONIA

1. Infections
   a. Bacterial
   b. Viral
   c. Fungal
   d. Parasitic
2. Aspiration
3. Radiation
4. Chemical

TABLE 2.8

DIFFERENTIAL DIAGNOSIS OF PULMONARY TUBERCULOSIS

1. All other pneumonias
2. Hemorrhage
3. Emboli
4. Tumor

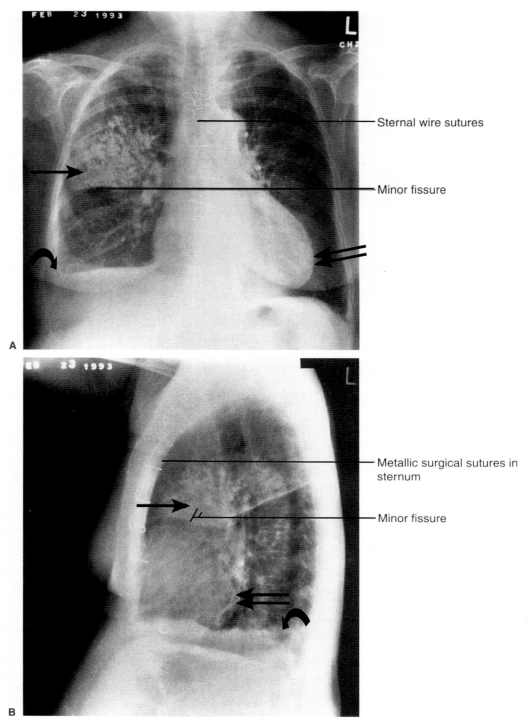

FEB 23 1993

L
CH2

Sternal wire sutures

Minor fissure

A

EB 23 1993

L

Metallic surgical sutures in sternum

Minor fissure

B

FIGURE 2.51 Chest PA (**A**) and lateral (**B**) radiographs. Right upper lobe partially confluent pneumonia (*straight arrows*). On the PA and lateral views, there is a small amount of right pleural fluid (*curved arrows*) and mild left ventricular enlargement (*double arrows*). Note that the pneumonia is located in the upper lobe above the minor fissure.

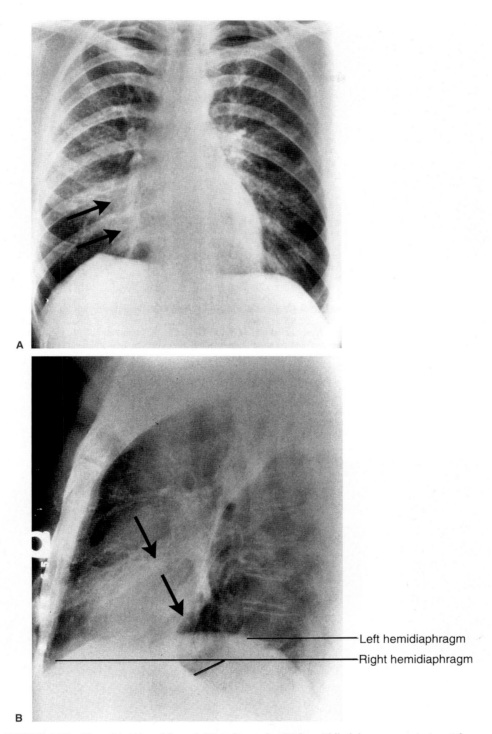

FIGURE 2.52 Chest PA (**A**) and lateral (**B**) radiographs. Right middle lobe pneumonia (*straight arrows*). On the PA radiograph, the right cardiac border is obscured (silhouette sign) as both the right middle lobe infiltrate and the right atrium are similar in density. On the lateral view, the pneumonia projects over the heart and partially silhouettes the anterior aspect of the right hemidiaphragm.

FIGURE 2.53 Chest PA (**A**) and lateral (**B**) radiographs. Left upper lobe lingular pneumonia (*straight arrows*). On the PA radiograph, the left cardiac border is not visible (silhouette sign) as both the left upper lobe lingular infiltrate and the heart are anterior water densities. Also, note that the left hemidiaphragm is clearly visible (*not silhouetted*) on the PA view. The *curved arrows* on the lateral view indicate the left major fissure, and note that the pneumonia projects over the heart.

FIGURE 2.54 Chest PA (**A**) and lateral (**B**) radiographs. Right lower lobe pneumonia (*straight arrows*). On the PA radiograph, the right cardiac border is clearly visible and the right hemidiaphragm is partially silhouetted (*double straight arrows*). These findings indicate that the infiltrate is posterior or in the right lower lobe as confirmed on the lateral radiograph (*straight arrows*). There is a positive spine sign on the lateral radiograph. Also, there are old healed left rib fracture deformities (*curved arrows*).

FIGURE 2.55   Chest PA (**A**) and lateral (**B**) radiographs. Bilateral varicella (chicken pox) pneumonia. There are diffuse nodular infiltrates throughout both lung fields. These patients are usually critically ill, and the skin lesions helped make the diagnosis.

FIGURE 2.56   **A:** Chest PA radiograph. Right upper lobe tuberculosis. The tuberculous infiltrate in the right upper lobe (*straight arrow*) is partially obscured by the right clavicle. **B:** Chest axial CT through the upper thorax showing cavitary tuberculosis in the left upper lobe in a different patient.

Patients with tuberculosis present with a variety of symptoms ranging from fatigue to fever, cough, weight loss, and hemoptysis. Chest radiographic findings vary from a poorly defined infiltrate to nodular infiltrates often with cavitation (Fig. 2.56). *Remember that the diagnosis must be confirmed by appropriate laboratory findings and cultures.*

TUMORS

Pulmonary nodules and mass lesions are commonly encountered on chest radiographs. Unfortunately, separating benignity from malignancy remains difficult as most nodules encountered have no defining characteristics. Pulmonary nodules may be smooth or spiculated, large or small, single or multiple. Once discovered, it is imperative to make every attempt to morphologically classify nodules based upon shape, size, and border definition. One approach to their diagnosis is to divide them into benign and malignant categories (Table 2.9). Spiculated nodules suggest malignancy; however, there are a host of malignant lung nodules that are smoothly marginated, particularly metastatic deposits. Multiple noncalcified nodules suggest a diagnosis of metastatic disease, especially if a primary cancer is known to exist (Fig. 2.57). Gross calcification of a lung nodule suggests a benign diagnosis, specifically granulomatous disease, and these nodules usually do not present much of a diagnostic challenge. Calcifications within granulomas are variable including solid, centrally located nidus, or laminar patterns. If there is doubt as to whether or not a nodule contains calcification, CT imaging can be used to definitively measure the density of the nodule (Fig. 2.58). When the CT density of a pulmonary nodule measures greater than 200 Hounsfield units, and the pattern of calcification composes most of the volume of the nodule, a benign entity is confirmed with no further evaluation or surveillance required. On the other hand, any noncalcified nodule necessarily requires further evaluation or surveillance for at least a 2-year period before a diagnosis of benignity can be established. A solitary noncalcified nodule which does not change in size or appearance over a 2-year period is considered benign according to conventional standard of care practices. This rule should be applied with caution, as there are exceptions, especially when the pretest probability of malignancy is high.

Approach to a Pulmonary Nodule

A logical approach to the workup of a noncalcified soft tissue density pulmonary nodule depends on a host of factors including pretest probability of malignancy, size and morphology of the nodule, and age of the patient. Clearly, there is considerable difference in the likelihood of malignancy of a smooth 1-cm nodule in a 30-year-old nonsmoker and a 2-cm spiculated nodule in a 60-year-old smoker. Other factors elevating the suspicion of malignancy include rapid nodule growth on serial examinations, pleural effusions, mediastinal adenopathy, and the presence of bone or liver lesions reflecting potential metastatic disease. The initial workup of any pulmonary nodule should always include comparison with prior films to ascertain whether the nodule is new or is growing. Once growth is confirmed either through comparison films or surveillance examinations, the nodule should be considered malignant until proven otherwise. Growth of any nodule usually necessitates surgical removal or biopsy (Fig. 2.59). As a general rule, percutaneous CT-guided biopsy of any solitary pulmonary nodule generally is not indicated since the results of biopsy will be either positive for tumor cells or nondiagnostic, that is, no tumor cells identified. If lesion cytology is positive for tumor, surgical resection is thus indicated. On the other, hand a nondiagnostic biopsy mandates that the lesion must be either surgically removed or alternatively followed with serial examinations. If the pretest probability for cancer is low and surveillance remains a reasonable course of action in light of a negative biopsy, then surveillance (and not biopsy) of the lesion would be advisable. Conversely, if the level of suspicion is so high that surgical resection will be performed regardless of the outcome of the biopsy, then surgical resection would be the best first course of action. Biopsy of any solitary nodule only adds an unnecessary intermediate step that essentially adds no value in the workup of a pulmonary nodule. The only exceptions to this rule is when a patient is not considered a surgical candidate and tissue is needed prior to instituting therapy, or if a pulmonary nodule is discovered in the setting of a known primary cancer. The decision to biopsy these cases then is warranted in an effort to determine whether the nodule is a primary lung carcinoma or a metastatic deposit.

MEDIASTINAL COMPARTMENTS AND LESIONS

The location of a mediastinal mass is very useful in arriving at a presumptive pathologic diagnosis. Knowledge of the anatomical constituents of mediastinal compartments significantly narrows the differential diagnosis (Table 2.10). Traditionally,

---

TABLE 2.9

A PARTIAL LIST FOR THE DIFFERENTIAL DIAGNOSIS OF PULMONARY MASSES

Benign
1. Granuloma (histoplasmoma, tuberculoma)
2. Adenoma
3. Hamartoma
4. Round pneumonia
5. Bronchogenic and pericardial cysts
6. Arteriovenous malformation
7. Pulmonary infarction

Malignant
1. Primary malignant tumors
   a. Squamous cell carcinoma
   b. Adenocarcinoma
   c. Small cell carcinoma
   d. Bronchoalveolar carcinoma
   e. Carcinoid
2. Lymphoma
3. Metastatic neoplasm

FIGURE 2.57   Chest PA (**A**) and lateral (**B**) radiographs. Diffuse bilateral pulmonary metastases. The metastatic lesions are not calcified and typically are variable in size. The infusaport (*straight arrows*) is used to administer medications. The tip of the infusaport catheter (*curved arrows*) projects over the superior vena cava in both views. **C:** Chest axial chest CT through the level of the ventricles. The multiple widespread metastases are variable in size.

the mediastinum can be divided into four generalized compartments: The superior compartment resides from the thoracic inlet inferiorly to a line drawn horizontally from the sternal–manubrial junction (angle of Louis). Structures residing in this compartment include the thyroid gland, esophagus, trachea, and great vessels of the head and neck, including the top of the thoracic aorta. The anterior mediastinal compartment resides from the posterior margin of the sternum back to the anterior surface of the pericardium. Structures residing in this compartment include fat, thymic gland, occasional thyroid tissue, anterior chest wall muscle and bone, lymphoid tissue,

and the ascending thoracic aorta. Therefore, it would be logical to limit the differential diagnosis of any anterior mediastinal mass to one of these anatomical constituents. A useful pneumonic for anterior mediastinal mass lesions is the "terrible Ts" which include thymoma, thyroid tumors, terrible lymphoma, and thoracic aneurysms (Figs. 2.60A, B and 2.61A, B). This differential while useful, necessarily excludes other possibilities such as chest wall sarcomas, vascular aneurysm, and fatty tumors, that is, lipomas. The middle mediastinal compartment extends from the ventral pericardium posteriorly to the ventral surface of the thoracic spine and includes a host of

FIGURE 2.58 Chest PA (**A**) and lateral (**B**) radiographs. Calcified granuloma (*straight arrows*) in the right lower lobe. The homogeneous high-density appearance of this small nodule strongly suggests calcification, which makes the diagnosis of granuloma fairly certain, and no further workup was needed. Incidentally, there is mild cardiomegaly and hyperinflation of the lungs due to chronic obstructive pulmonary disease. **C:** Chest axial CT through the left atrium level. The lesion in the right lower lobe is very dense and calcific in appearance, and the lesion measures 1016 Hounsfield units. These findings indicate a benign calcified granuloma.

FIGURE 2.59 Chest PA (**A**) and lateral (**B**) radiographs. Histoplasmoma superior segment left lower lobe (*arrows*). This noncalcified solitary nodule was seen on a routine chest radiograph on this 58-year-old asymptomatic man. The differential diagnosis of a solitary noncalcified pulmonary nodule was entertained, and malignancy could not be excluded. Thoracotomy and resection of the lesion resulted in the diagnosis of a benign histoplasmoma.

TABLE 2.10

DIFFERENTIAL DIAGNOSIS FOR MEDIASTINAL MASSES

Anterior Mediastinum
1. Thyroid and parathyroid masses
2. Thymus masses (Fig. 2.60A, B)
3. Teratoma
4. Tortuous vessels such as aneurysm of ascending aorta (Fig. 2.61A, B)
5. Lymph nodes
6. Chest wall/bone tumor

Middle Mediastinum
1. Pericardial fat pad and pericardial cyst (Fig. 2.60C, D, E)

2. Bronchogenic cyst and bronchogenic carcinoma
3. Lymph nodes/lymphoma
4. Diaphragm hernia (Morgagni)
5. Great vessel aneurysms

Posterior Mediastinum
1. Neurogenic tumors
2. Duplication cysts
3. Lymph nodes
4. Esophageal lesions including esophageal hiatal hernia (Fig. 2.43A, B)

FIGURE 2.60 Chest PA (**A**) and lateral (**B**) radiographs. Thymoma (*straight arrows*). The lesion clearly lies in the anterior mediastinum. **C, D:** Chest PA (**C**) and lateral (**D**) radiographs. Pericardial cyst (*straight arrows*). This lesion was found on a routine chest radiograph in an asymptomatic 54-year-old female patient. (*continued*)

FIGURE 2.60 (*Continued*) Figure 60E is a CT image of the cyst (*arrows*), which resides adjacent to the right heart border. These cystic masses usually are on the right side at the cardiophrenic angle. The differential diagnosis was bronchogenic cyst, Morgagni hernia, and diaphragmatic tumor. The diagnosis can sometimes be made by ultrasound or CT imaging. In this case, the diagnosis was made at thoracotomy. **F, G:** Chest PA (**F**) and lateral (**G**) radiographs. Neuroblastoma. In the PA view, the mass can be seen through the cardiac shadow (*straight arrows*). The lateral view shows the mass to be posterior in location as there is loss of definition of the lower dorsal spine vertebral bodies and a positive spine sign.

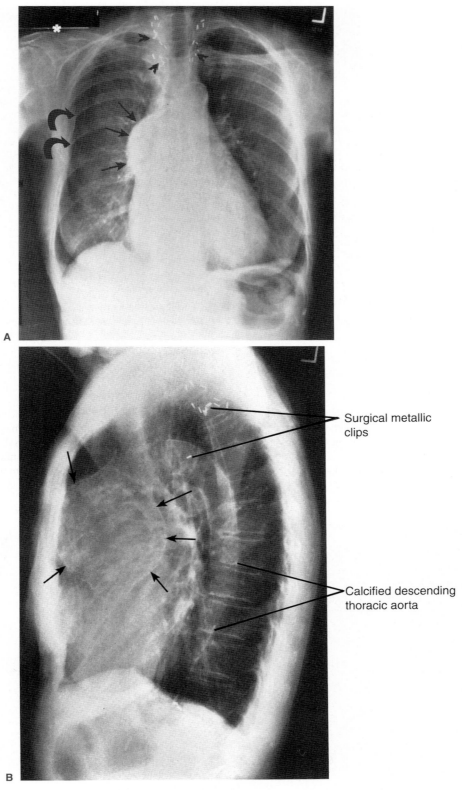

Surgical metallic
clips

Calcified descending
thoracic aorta

FIGURE 2.61   Chest PA (**A**) and lateral (**B**) radiographs. Large calcified ascending thoracic aorta aneurysm (*straight arrows*). The aneurysmal calcification is faint on both views. On the PA radiograph, the heart appears enlarged but on the lateral view it is within normal limits. Note the old healed right rib fracture deformities (*curved arrows*). The lungs are hyperinflated. Note the surgical clips (*arrowheads*) and the artifact (*) appearing on the right shoulder.

FIGURE 2.62   Chest PA radiograph. Lymphoma. This young adult male was admitted because of an abnormal white blood count. There is a large mediastinal mass (*straight arrows*) with associated bilateral hilar lymphadenopathy (*curved arrows*). The mass resides within the anterior and middle mediastinum. This is a typical appearance of lymphoma of the chest.

FIGURE 2.64   Chest AP radiograph. Carcinoma of the lung with rib destruction. The moderately sized primary carcinoma in the left upper lobe (*straight arrows*) has partially destroyed a left rib posteriorly (*curved arrow*). Note that the lungs are overexpanded, probably secondary to chronic obstructive pulmonary disease. A monitoring electrode runs across the thorax from left to right.

anatomical structures such as the heart, pericardium, aortic knob, hila, esophagus, lymph nodes, and nerves, just to name a few (Fig. 2.60C–E). The differential diagnosis when presented with a mass within the middle mediastinum is considerably extensive. The posterior mediastinum (Fig. 2.60F, G) extends from the ventral spine to the chest wall posteriorly and includes the dorsal spine vertebral bodies, spinal cord and

nerve roots, and the descending thoracic aorta (1). Fortunately, the majority of posterior mediastinal masses are related to the neuroaxis, which makes the differential quite easy. It is also important to remember that since lymphoid tissue is found in all parts of the mediastinum, lymphoma is a reasonable consideration for any mediastinal mass regardless of location (Fig. 2.62).

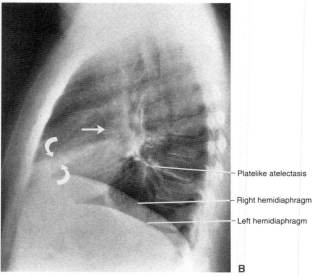

Platelike atelectasis

Right hemidiaphragm

Left hemidiaphragm

FIGURE 2.63   Chest PA (**A**) and lateral (**B**) radiographs. Right infrahilar primary neoplasm (*straight arrows*) causing right middle lobe atelectasis (*curved arrows*). The right hemidiaphragm is mildly elevated secondary to the right middle lobe atelectasis. Note on the lateral view how nicely you can see the right and left hemidiaphragms. The right hemidiaphragm can be seen in its entirety, whereas the left hemidiaphragm is silhouetted anteriorly by the heart. The *double arrows* indicate bilateral infraclavicular notching or rhomboid fossae. These fossae are a variation of normal, and they give origin to the costoclavicular or rhomboid ligaments (1).

Superior vena cava
Trachea
Esophagus
Azygos vein
Aortic arch

FIGURE 2.65 Chest PA (**A**) and lateral (**B**) radiographs and a chest axial CT image (**C**) through the level of the aortic arch. Cavitating primary squamous cell carcinoma of the left upper lobe. In Figs. A and B the large tumor mass (*curved arrows*) contains an air–fluid level secondary to tumor necrosis (*four white straight arrows*). There is a partially confluent pneumonia in the right middle lobe (*multiple black straight arrows*). On the CT (Fig. C) the air–fluid level is indicated by two straight arrows.

The detection of mediastinal masses by chest films is somewhat limited due to considerable limitations in sensitivity. Small lesions are often never visible on radiographs, requiring further imaging with CT for diagnosis. However, secondary radiographic findings that suggest the presence of a mediastinal mass include tracheal deviation, segmental or lobar atelectasis, hilar enlargement, pleural effusions, and bony destruction adjacent to a mass (Figs. 2.63 to 2.65).

CARDIAC AND GREAT VESSELS

While gross enlargement of the heart or a specific chamber implies either myocardial or valvular disease, the radiographic appearance of the heart in and by itself correlates poorly with cardiac function. More advanced imaging modalities such as echocardiography, magnetic resonance imaging, and CT provide much better anatomical and functional information from which accurate quantitative data relating to myocardial mass, ejection fraction, and valvular movement can be obtained.

Aneurysms, Enlarged Vessels, and Vascular Calcifications

Aneurysms of the thoracic aorta and branch vessels are commonly encountered acquired abnormalities due to atherosclerotic disease, infection, or connective tissue disorders such as Marfan's syndrome. Aneurysms of vessels often present as a mass lesion in any of the four mediastinal compartments as described above (Fig. 2.61). Aneurysms may also affect the pulmonary arteries commonly resulting in unilateral hilar enlargement. Physiologic aberrations of blood flow may produce enlargement of both pulmonary arterial trunks (Fig. 2.66). A

FIGURE 2.66 Chest PA radiograph. Right atrial enlargement and enlarged pulmonary arteries. The right atrium is enlarging to the patient's right side (*straight arrows*), and the pulmonary arteries are larger than normal (*curved arrows*). These changes are consistent with pulmonary hypertension.

partial list of etiologies for central pulmonary arterial enlargement is included in Table 2.11. Finally, atherosclerotic calcification of thoracic vessels occurs commonly with advancing age, usually without associated vascular aneurysm. This intimal calcification is readily apparent radiographically and should not be viewed as abnormal in patients older than 60 years of age (Fig. 2.67). Premature vascular calcification, however, may be an indication of hyperlipemic states or diabetes mellitus.

TABLE 2.11

PARTIAL DIFFERENTIAL DIAGNOSIS OF ENLARGED PULMONARY ARTERIES

High-Volume Situations
1. Left-to-right shunts
2. High cardiac output situations (anemias, thyrotoxicosis)

Peripheral Arterial Narrowing and Occlusion
1. Thromboembolic disease
2. Idiopathic pulmonary hypertension

Central Enlargement
1. Pulmonary hypertension
2. Pulmonary artery aneurysm

Pulmonary Edema

Congestive heart failure (Fig. 2.68) is an extremely important problem which is commonly encountered by nearly all health care providers. While there are many etiologies for pulmonary edema (Table 2.12), the most common cause is left ventricular failure due to ischemia or infarction, that is, congestive heart failure. Patients with frank congestive heart failure commonly present with dyspnea on exertion, orthopnea, paroxysmal nocturnal respiratory distress, weight gain, lower extremity edema, cough, and occasionally hemoptysis.

It is important to appreciate and recognize the varied radiographic presentations of congestive heart failure which are essentially predicated upon the hydrostatic effects of left ventricular dysfunction (Table 2.13). The first radiographic sign of congestive heart failure is *cephalad redistribution* of pulmonary blood flow to the upper lobes. This phenomenon of upper lobe vascular recruitment is in response to impaired oxygen exchange across the capillary–alveolar interface. On a normal upright film, the bulk of pulmonary blood flow occurs

FIGURE 2.67 Chest axial CT image through the level of the left atrium. The right coronary artery, the circumflex coronary artery, and ascending and descending aorta all contain calcifications (*straight arrows*).

Right atrium

Right ventricular outflow tract
Right coronary artery
Left ventricular outflow tract
Ascending aorta
Circumflex coronary artery
Left atrium
Descending aorta

FIGURE 2.68 Chest radiograph illustrating the stages of congestive heart failure. Figure (**A**) shows cephalad redistribution of pulmonary blood flow to the upper lobes. Notice the relative enlargement of the upper lobe vessels compared to the lower lobe vasculature. The straight arrow indicates Kerley B lines. A pacemaker is present. Figure (**B**) shows development of bilateral Kerley B lines (*arrows*) which represent fluid in the interstitium. Figure (**C**) shows classic batwing pulmonary edema in a patient in frank congestive heart failure. Figure (**D**) shows that the vascular pedicle is a transverse measurement obtained by drawing a line from the azygos vein leftward to a point where it intersects a perpendicular line drawn vertically from the left innominate artery and aortic arch. The vascular pedicle provides information about the intravascular volume, becoming wider in conditions of fluid excess or congestive heart failure. The absolute measurement is not as important as is the interval change on serial radiographs from day to day.

TABLE 2.12

ETIOLOGIES OF PULMONARY EDEMA

1. Cardiogenic (heart failure)
2. Neurogenic (head injury)
3. Increased permeability (lung injury edema)
   a. Toxic gas or smoke inhalation
   b. High-altitude sickness
   c. Aspiration
   d. Contusion
   e. Fat embolism
   f. Sepsis

TABLE 2.13

RADIOGRAPHIC FINDINGS IN PULMONARY EDEMA

1. Vascular redistribution (increase size of vessels in the upper lobes)
2. Airspace disease (batwing distribution and gravitational)
3. Kerley B lines
4. Interlobar fissure thickening
5. Pleural effusions
6. Central peribronchial cuffing
7. Vascular congestion

in the lower one third of each lung. The upper lobes vessels are usually collapsed and fairly inconspicuous. In attempt to improve oxygenation, pulmonary blood flow is diverted to the upper lobes. Radiographically, this process is manifested by enlargement of the upper lobe pulmonary arteries. The pulmonary vessels at this stage should remain sharp.

With further deterioration in cardiac function, fluid spills out into the connective tissues surrounding the pulmonary vasculature. This phenomenon produces interstitial edema or *Kerley B lines*, which are identified on chest films as small parallel linear shadows in the periphery of both lower lobes. Additionally, since interstitial fluid also surrounds the pulmonary vessels and smaller bronchi, the borders of these structures appear less sharp. This is known as *vascular congestion and peribronchial cuffing*, respectively. In cases of severe cardiac dysfunction, extravascular fluid eventually flows into the alveoli and pleural spaces. Fluid in the alveoli is radiographically depicted as bilateral symmetric air space disease usually in a perihilar or batwing distribution. This airspace disease represents true pulmonary edema. Pleural effusions are common in congestive heart failure and are usually symmetric in size (Fig. 2.17). Occasionally chest decubitus views are useful in confirming and quantifying the amount of pleural fluid.

Additional radiographic findings in congestive heart failure (or fluid overload) include widening of the vascular pedicle, which anatomically reflects excessive intravascular volume within the superior vena cava and azygos vein. The vascular pedicle width is measured from the lateral aspect of the superior vena cava at the insertion of the azygos vein horizontally to a line drawn vertically from the origin of the subclavian artery (Fig. 2.68D). In contrast, disease processes producing noncardiac pulmonary edema, that is, adult respiratory distress syndrome lack most of the features characteristic of hydrostatic edema. In these situations, pulmonary edema results directly from some form of lung injury whereby the gap junctions of capillaries and the tight junctions of alveolar epithelium become diastatic, allowing vascular fluid and all cellular constituents to pass directly into the alveoli. In these cases, there is neither vascular redistribution nor evidence of interstitial edema. Furthermore, the development of pulmonary edema with lung injury is often patchy and asymmetric at onset, eventually becoming more uniform in distribution with time. Because of the highly cellular composition of fluid, the overall course of the disease is protracted taking weeks to months to resolve. Adult respiratory distress syndrome is also associated with considerable respiratory dysfunction, poor lung compliance, and higher levels of morbidity.

Valvular Heart Disease

Significant cardiac valve disease, whether acquired or congenital, can be suspected radiographically by its hemodynamic effects. Cardiac chamber enlargement and poststenotic dilatation are incipient radiographic findings in patients with prolonged valvular dysfunction. Valvular dysfunction can be either stenosis or insufficiency. In either case, impairment of the ejection fraction eventually results in myocardial fatigue and subsequent chamber dilatation. All four cardiac valves are susceptible to disease, but the aortic and mitral valves are most commonly affected. Examples of mitral and aortic valvular disease are illustrated on Figs. 2.69 and 2.70, respectively.

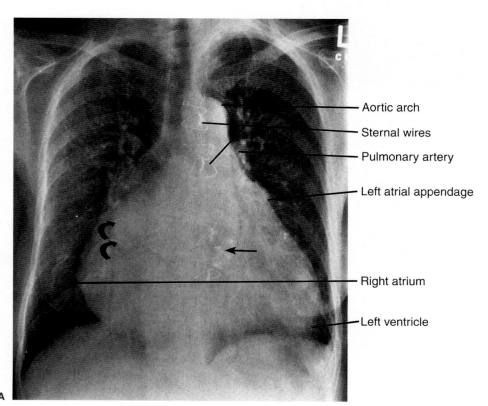

— Aortic arch
— Sternal wires
— Pulmonary artery
— Left atrial appendage
— Right atrium
—Left ventricle

FIGURE 2.69   Chest PA (**A**) and lateral (*continued*)

A

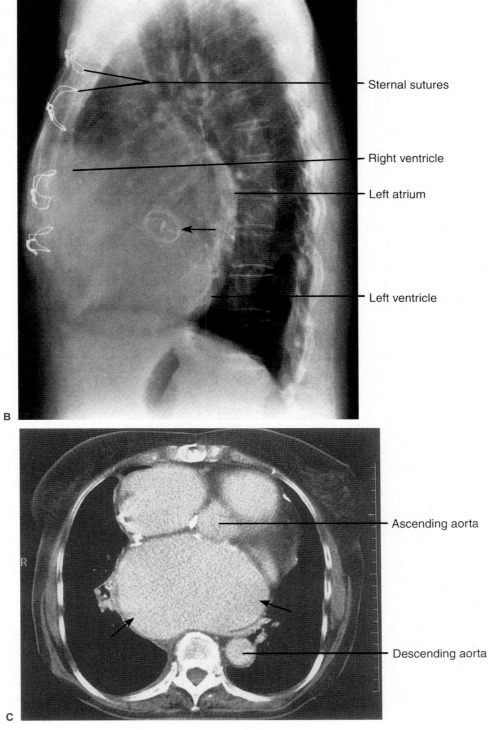

Sternal sutures

Right ventricle

Left atrium

Left ventricle

B

Ascending aorta

Descending aorta

C

FIGURE 2.69 (*Continued*) (**B**) radiographs. Severe cardiomegaly and a prosthetic mitral valve (*straight arrows*). The patient had mitral valve stenosis and regurgitation that necessitated a prosthetic mitral valve. All of the cardiac chambers are enlarged. On the PA view, the enlarged left atrium creates the double density indicated by the *curved arrows*, and the left atrial appendage is prominent along the left cardiac border. Also, on the PA view, there is right atrial and left ventricular enlargement. On the lateral view, right ventricular enlargement results in fullness of the retrosternal space. Also, on the lateral view, there is enlargement of the left atrium and ventricle. **C:** Chest axial CT image through the atrium level. Left atrial enlargement (*straight arrows*). This is a different patient from that in A and B. This patient also had mitral stenosis resulting in left atrial enlargement. (*continued*)

FIGURE 2.69   (*Continued*) **D:** Chest PA radiograph. Mitral stenosis and cardiomegaly. There is a nice demonstration of the classic moguls in mitral stenosis that are visible along the left cardiac border consisting of the aortic knob, a prominent left pulmonary artery, the enlarged left atrial appendage, and the left ventricle. Also, the double density of an enlarged left atrium (*straight arrows*) can be identified. **E:** Chest PA radiograph. Mitral annulus calcification (*straight arrows*). This patient was asymptomatic, and the calcified mitral annulus was an incidental finding on a routine chest study. There is mild cardiomegaly with mild enlargement of the left ventricle.

A   B

FIGURE 2.70   Chest PA (**A**) and lateral (**B**) radiographs. Aortic valve stenosis and regurgitation. Systolic and diastolic aortic valve murmurs were discovered during a routine physical examination. There is left ventricular enlargement (*straight arrows*) manifested by rounding of the cardiac apex on the PA view, and on the lateral view the enlarged left ventricle projects more than 2 cm posterior to the inferior vena cava). The latter finding is a fairly reliable sign for left ventricular enlargement. The ascending aorta appears dilated (*arrow heads*), and this is often found in aortic stenosis.

KEY POINTS

- PA and lateral views are the routine standard chest radiographs and every attempt should be made to acquire these projections.

- AP is the standard portable chest radiograph and should be obtained only on patients who are unable to be transported to the radiology department.

- If thoracic bone imaging is necessary, it is imperative to order the specific radiographs relating to these structures such as dedicated ribs, shoulder, or thoracic spine views.

- Position PA/AP chest radiographs on the viewbox with the right side label opposite the viewer's left. Lateral films should be viewed with the patient facing to the left.

- Develop a simple systematic approach for viewing chest radiographs to avoid errors of omission. Practice and experience are paramount in developing a "good eye." Also remember that you only see what you know. Knowledge of normal anatomy is a key to successful film interpretation.

- The cardiac transverse diameter should not exceed 50% of thoracic cage transverse diameter. This is called the *cardiothoracic ratio*.

- Cardiac size estimation is most generally accomplished by gross eyeballing and this becomes easier with experience.

- Cardiac size appears larger on the AP than the PA view because of magnification.

- The right atrium forms the convex right cardiac border and the left ventricle forms the cardiac apex on AP or PA radiographs.

- On chest radiographs, any unusual soft tissue opacity should be considered as indication of pathology.

- Excessive translucency on a chest radiograph generally indicates too much air, and its location will help make the diagnosis.

- Border definition is lost whenever two similar densities abut each other. This is known as the *silhouette sign* and represents a fundamental key observation for identifying pathologic processes within the chest.

References

1. Fraser RS, Pare JA, Fraser RG, Pare PD. *Synopsis of diseases of the chest,* 2nd ed. Philadelphia: WB Saunders, 1994.
2. Edeiken J. *Roentgen diagnosis of diseases of bone,* 4th ed. Baltimore: Williams & Wilkins, 1990.
3. Juhl JH, Crummy AB. *Paul and Juhl's essentials of radiologic imaging,* 7th ed. Philadelphia: JB Lippincott Co, 1993.

Suggested Reading

El-Khoury GY, Bergman RA, Montgomery WJ. *Sectional anatomy by MRI,* 2nd ed. New York: Churchill Livingstone, 1995.

CHAPTER 3 ■ ABDOMEN

EDMUND A. FRANKEN, JR.

Careful history and physical examination allow diagnosis of most abdominal complaints. When diagnosis remains uncertain following these procedures, an abdominal radiograph is often the first diagnostic imaging procedure requested. Recall that in women of childbearing age, consideration of possible pregnancy should precede a radiograph.

The anteroposterior (AP) radiograph (often referred from "KUB," i.e., kidney, ureter, bladder), the most frequently performed abdominal imaging study, is performed with the patient supine (Fig. 3.1A). An upright radiograph (Fig. 3.1B) is useful in searching for free intraperitoneal air and/or intestinal air–fluid levels. If the patient cannot stand, a decubitus radiograph obtained with the patient lying on either the right or, preferably, the left side (Fig. 3.1C) can be substituted.

VIEWING ABDOMINAL RADIOGRAPHS

Step 1 is to position the radiograph correctly on the viewbox, with the film R (right side) marker opposite the viewer's left side and the patient's head toward the top of the film. On the AP upright radiograph, there should be a sign indicating an upright view, usually an arrow near the R or L marker, pointing toward the patient's head. Similarly, decubitus radiographs should be clearly labeled as such and should note which side is up or down.

Step 2 is to glance at the entire radiograph in a relaxed manner to allow an obvious abnormality to jump out at you.

When you do discover an abnormality, do not terminate your subsequent search.

Step 3 is to evaluate the radiograph systematically. Any system or checklist will suffice. Table 3.1 will work, until you develop your own. First, locate the water density liver and spleen silhouettes. One clue to locating liver and spleen edges is the presence of bowel gas in the right and left upper abdominal quadrants. Such bowel gas permits an indirect estimate of the location of the hepatic and splenic borders, because the gas is located at the lower edges of the liver and spleen. With a little experience, you will recognize a normal-sized liver. When the liver shadow extends to the iliac crest, it is usually enlarged. Also with more experience, you will readily detect an enlarged spleen (splenomegaly; Fig. 3.2).

In the normal radiograph, psoas muscle margins are usually visible. A nonvisible psoas margin should alert you to a possible abnormality adjacent to that structure. As your eyes drift toward the renal shadows, evaluate their size, shape, and position. The renal silhouettes are visible because they are water density structures (gray) surrounded by variable amounts of retroperitoneal fat (black). You should attempt to locate the upper and lower renal poles as well as their medial and lateral borders. If the renal long axis is not parallel with the psoas muscle margin, you should consider a mass or other water density abnormality in the kidney or the retroperitoneum. Always look for calcifications (white) in the abdomen, especially in the region of the kidneys, ureters, urinary bladder, and the gallbladder (discussed later).

The term *Aunt Minnie*, coined by the late Dr. Ben Felson, refers to the unmistakable and unforgettable appearance of

FIGURE 3.1   A: Patient positioning for an AP supine abdomen radiograph. This examination is performed with the patient supine, either on a radiographic table or in bed (using a portable x-ray unit). **B:** Patient positioning for an AP upright abdomen radiograph. This examination is usually accomplished in the radiology department, with the patient standing. **C:** Patient positioning for a left lateral decubitus abdomen radiograph. The patient's arms are positioned comfortably out of the way.

FIGURE 3.2 Abdomen AP supine radiograph. Splenomegaly. The water density spleen is enlarged (*straight arrows*), and the inferior margin projects just above the left hip (*double straight arrows*). The large spleen has displaced the intestinal gas into the right abdomen. The liver size is normal (*L*, liver). Incidentally noted are phleboliths (*curved arrows*), small intravenous stones secondary to calcified thrombi.

FIGURE 3.3 Abdomen AP supine radiograph. Normal. The psoas muscles (*straight arrows*) and the right kidney (*curved arrows*) are visible. The left renal silhouette is obliterated by intestinal gas. It is common to have intestinal gas and contents obliterating the renal shadows. (*L*, liver; *S*, spleen).

your Aunt Minnie, or Uncle Al, or any other family character. A radiologic Aunt Minnie describes an image appearance so classic that, once you see it, you never forget it. The following abdominal radiographic Aunt Minnies (Figs. 3.3 to 3.9) are commonly encountered. File them away in your visual–cerebral computer, and your ability to recognize them will make you a star in the eyes of your colleagues, teachers, and patients.

Now, evaluate the bowel gas pattern (see the next section). Last but not least, look at the bones systematically, beginning with the visible ribs and spine (Fig. 3.10). Study the pedicles of the lower dorsal and lumbar spine, proceeding from head

to foot. They resemble automobile headlights on an AP radiograph. A missing pedicle indicates a destructive process, such as metastatic disease. Evaluate all visible bones, including the pelvis, hips, and femurs, for their overall density and any abnormalities.

Use a similar search system for the AP upright abdominal radiograph while being especially alert for free air beneath the diaphragms. Free intraperitoneal air is usually visualized only on an upright radiograph, because only this position allows free air to rise to the subdiaphragmatic regions.

TABLE 3.1

ROUTINE FOR EVALUATING ABDOMINAL RADIOGRAPHS

1. Once-over glance
2. Liver and spleen
3. Psoas shadows
4. Renal contours and position
5. Abdominal calcifications
6. Intestinal gas pattern
7. Bones

EVALUATING THE INTESTINAL AIR OR GAS PATTERN

Intestinal gas (black) provides a natural contrast medium that can be useful for detecting abdominal disease. When evaluating the intestinal gas pattern, ask yourself several important questions. Is the bowel gas pattern normal? Remember that there is normally some air or gas in the stomach, small intestine, colon, and rectum. With experience, you will begin to recognize abnormal amounts of air in the gastrointestinal (GI) tract. This is similar to recognizing a normal heart on a chest radiograph. If the gas pattern is not normal, ask more questions. Is there too much or too little air? Is the air in the wrong place?

FIGURE 3.4 Abdomen AP supine radiograph. Classic appearance of tablets or pills (*straight arrows*) in the GI tract. All the tablets are the same size and shape with homogeneous density. (Not all tablets or pills can be visualized on a radiograph.)

FIGURE 3.5 Abdomen AP supine radiograph. Metal coins (*straight arrows*) in the left trouser pocket. The patient was not completely disrobed prior to obtaining the radiographs. Note the degenerative or osteoarthritic changes in the lower lumbar spine (*curved arrows*).

FIGURE 3.6   Abdomen AP supine radiograph. An umbrella-shaped inferior vena cava filter (*straight arrow*), placed in the inferior vena cava by angiographic technique, entraps venous thromboemboli originating in the lower extremities and pelvis.

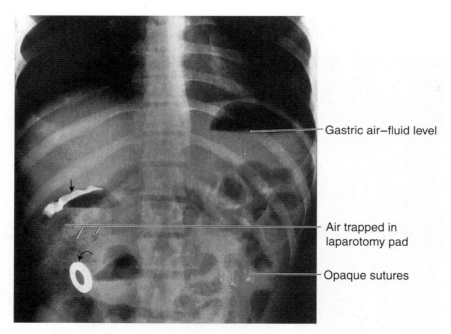

FIGURE 3.7   Abdomen AP upright radiograph. Surgical laparotomy pad in a postoperative abdomen. The radiograph was obtained when the patient experienced severe postoperative abdominal pain and distention. The *straight arrow* indicates the opaque strip in the laparotomy pad, and the *curved arrow* indicates the metallic ring attached to the laparotomy pad. Note the mottled black appearance of the air trapped in the laparotomy pad. The air–fluid level in the gastric fundus gives a clue to the upright position of the patient.

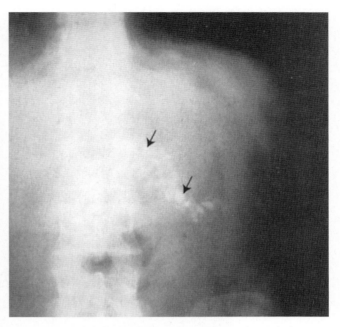

FIGURE 3.9 Abdomen AP supine radiograph. Calcifications (*straight arrows*) in the body and tail of the pancreas owing to chronic pancreatitis.

FIGURE 3.8 Abdomen AP supine radiograph. Cholelithiasis (gallstones). The calcified calculi (*straight arrows*) are faceted. Surgical metallic clips (*curved arrows*) are secondary to previous abdominal surgery.

FIGURE 3.10 Abdomen AP supine radiograph. Normal. Representative vertebral pedicles are shown by *straight arrows*. The water density urinary bladder is shown by *curved arrows*.

Colon splenic flexure

Transverse colon

Small intestine

Ascending colon

Surgical skin clips

Sigmoid colon air

Rectal air

FIGURE 3.11   A: Abdomen AP supine radiograph. Postoperative adynamic ileus. Air is present through-out the entire GI tract, including the rectum (not shown). Note the haustrations in the transverse colon. **B:** Lower abdomen AP supine radiograph 24 hours later in the same patient. A considerable amount of intestinal air has moved into the rectum and sigmoid colon, confirming the diagnosis of adynamic ileus.

Too Much Bowel Gas

Here, where differential diagnosis includes adynamic ileus and bowel obstruction, we need a systematic approach to arrive at the correct diagnosis. In adynamic ileus (also referred to as *paralytic ileus* or just *ileus*), there is too much bowel gas in the entire GI tract, including the small and large intestines (Fig. 3.11A, B). Adynamic ileus may arise from intra-abdominal cases or as a reflex phenomenon from disease elsewhere. The multiple etiologies are listed in Table 3.2. If you identify comparable amounts of gas in the small and large intestines and in the rectum, this generally indicates adynamic ileus. Air in the rectum may be a key differential point.

TABLE 3.2

ADYNAMIC ILEUS—MAJOR CAUSES

Intra-abdominal
- Postoperative or posttraumatic
- Postinflammatory: pancreatitis, enteritis, colitis
- Pain-related: renal colic, epidural disease

Extra-abdominal
- Septicemia
- Metabolic disease: hyperkalemia, uremia
- Medications (especially narcotics)
- Prolonged bed rest

FIGURE 3.12 Abdominal radiograph. Small bowel obstruction. There are many dilated loops of small bowel in the midabdomen. They are identified as small bowel by their position, semihorizontal orientation, and valvulae conniventes traversing the entire transverse diameter. There is a small amount of residual barium in a collapsed descending colon (*arrows*). Incidentally noted are the nasogastric and abdominal drainage tubes. (Courtesy of Bruce Brown, M.D.)

In intestinal obstruction, another reason for too much bowel gas, there is usually air-filled, dilated intestine proximal to the point of obstruction and little or no air distal to the obstruction (Fig. 3.12). In both ileus and obstruction, often the dilated small and large bowels containing too much air will have air–fluid levels noted on upright and decubitus radiographs.

If a diagnosis of obstruction versus adynamic ileus is not readily apparent, it is necessary to obtain additional studies to arrive at the correct diagnosis. These include barium studies, computed tomography (CT) (Fig. 3.13), and ultrasound (US). Note the relative ease of identifying small versus large bowel using CT.

If you diagnose intestinal obstruction, you next need to determine the location of the obstruction. Is the obstruction in the small or large bowel? In small bowel obstruction, there are loops of dilated small bowel proximal to the obstruction site and little or no gas in the colon or the rectum. In large bowel obstruction, there is dilated colon proximal to the obstruction site but little or no air distally and minimal air in the rectum.

Sometimes it is difficult to differentiate dilated small from large bowel. One way is to identify the valvulae conniventes and colon haustra. *Valvulae conniventes* are regularly spaced, thin mucosal folds that extend across the entire small bowel lumen (Fig. 3.12). On the other hand, the colon can usually be identified by the somewhat irregularly spaced transverse

bands, called *colon septa* or *haustral folds*, that do not extend completely across the colon lumen (Fig. 3.11).

Sigmoid volvulus is a dramatic clinical event that occurs predominantly in elderly patients with a long history of constipation. The chronic constipation results in a redundant sigmoid mesentery that has the potential to twist on itself like a garden hose. If twisting occurs, there is complete or partial obstruction, and an abdominal radiograph shows a dramatically dilated sigmoid colon. Barium enema is confirmatory, with complete obstruction to the retrograde flow of barium at the site of the twist (Fig. 3.14). The obstruction can often be relieved by gently passing a sigmoidoscope past the point of the obstruction or twist.

Too Little Bowel Gas

When the abdominal radiographs show a paucity or absence of bowel gas, the differential diagnosis listed in Table 3.3 should be entertained.

FIGURE 3.13 Abdominal axial CT. Small bowel obstruction. **A:** Here are many dilated loops of small bowel, some of which contain barium. The only colon visualized (*arrow*) in the left lower abdomen is tiny. (The aortic image (*curved arrows*) shows a segment of calcified intima, indicating previous aortic dissection.) **B:** CT at the level of the pelvis confirms the dilated small bowel extending into the pelvis (the rectum is surgically absent). (Courtesy of Gerald Decker, M.D.)

FIGURE 3.14 Sigmoid volvulus **A:** Abdominal radiograph. The air-filled, obstructed sigmoid colon (*arrows*) arises from the pelvis. **B:** Barium enema. Contrast introduced per rectum shows obstruction and a twist (*arrow*) at the sigmoid colon. (Courtesy of Bruce Brown, M.D.)

TOO LITTLE BOWEL GAS

- Enlarged abdominal organs
- Intra-abdominal tumor
- Fluid-filled intestines
- Gastroenteritis
- Neurological deficit (with reduced swallowing)

TABLE 3.4

ABDOMINAL AIR OR GAS IN THE WRONG PLACE

- Pneumoperitoneum from ruptured intestines: ulcer, trauma, cancer, enteritis
- Abscess
- Pneumatosis intestinalis

Gas in the Wrong Places

There are several situations in which air is found outside of the intestinal lumen (Table 3.4). Free air in the peritoneal cavity results from any process that perforates the intestinal tract. AP supine and upright abdominal radiographs should be performed if there is clinical suspicion of gut perforation. The upright position allows free intraperitoneal air to rise to the subdiaphragmatic regions of the abdomen (Fig. 3.15). If the upright view is not possible owing to the patient's condition, a decubitus radiograph will suffice. On a decubitus radiograph, the air rises to the nondependent portion of the peritoneal cavity (Fig. 3.16). Either technique has the potential to identify as little as 2 cc of free intraperitoneal air, as long as the patient is in the upright or decubitus position approximately 5 minutes prior to the radiograph.

Another example of air in the wrong place is pneumatosis intestinalis (Fig. 3.17). Causes of this are listed in Table 3.5. Gas-filled abscesses can be found in any location, including the abdomen (Fig. 3.18).

GASTROINTESTINAL CONTRAST STUDIES

For inspection of the mucosal surface of the esophagus, stomach, and duodenum, endoscopy is often preferred. To evaluate the gut lumen and wall, traditional radiologic GI contrast studies are accurate, safe, and less expensive than the endoscopic studies and enjoy excellent patient acceptance. These studies consist of fluoroscopy and radiographs obtained following introduction of barium sulfate (metallic density or white) and/or air (black) into the GI tract.

Upper Gastrointestinal Series

For an upper GI series, the patient swallows liquid barium, often combined with gas-producing crystals, under fluoroscopy

TABLE 3.5

PNEUMATOSIS INTESTINALIS

- Bowel ischemia
- Steroid and immunosuppressive therapy
- Proximal to intestinal obstruction
- Collagen diseases
- Neonatal necrotizing enterocolitis
- Benign idiopathic pneumatosis

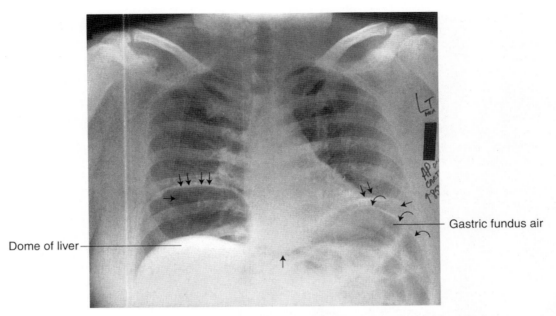

Dome of liver⎯

⎯ Gastric fundus air

FIGURE 3.15　Chest AP upright radiograph. Free intraperitoneal air. The right and left hemidiaphragms (*double arrows*) are elevated owing to bilateral subdiaphragmatic air (*single straight arrows*). The black zone between the right hemidiaphragm and the dome of the liver represents free intraperitoneal air. On the left, there is air in the gastric fundus as well as free air surrounding the gastric fundus, allowing visualization of both sides of the stomach wall (*curved arrows*). When you see both sides of the gut wall, this represents free intraperitoneal air (Rigler's sign).

⎯ Liver

⎯ Small intestine (valvulae conniventes)

⎯ Nasogastric tube

FIGURE 3.16　Abdomen left lateral decubitus radiograph (left side down). Free intraperitoneal air in a patient with small bowel obstruction and perforation. The free intraperitoneal air (*straight arrow*) is between the right rib cage and the liver. The dilated small bowel contains multiple air–fluid levels (*curved arrows*).

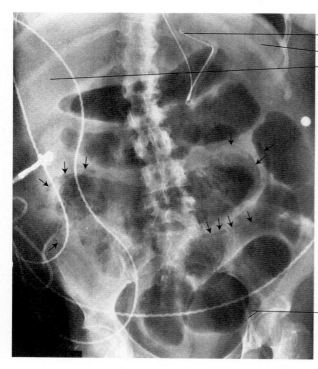

— Nasogastric tube
— Spleen
— Liver

— Femoral line

FIGURE 3.17   Abdomen AP supine radiograph. Pneumatosis intestinalis (air in the bowel wall). There is widespread bubbly air within the small intestine walls (*arrows*).

Gallblader —

— Liver

— Common bile duct

— Small intestine

FIGURE 3.18   Abdomen AP supine radiograph. Right subdiaphragmatic abscess. The black areas along the right lateral aspect of the liver represent air in the abscess cavity (*straight arrows*). Incidentally noted is contrast material in the common bile duct, gallbladder, and small bowel, injected during an endoscopic retrograde cholangiopancreatography (ERCP). Some of the contrast spilled into the small intestine. The filling defect (*curved arrow*) in the gallbladder is probably a calculus.

FIGURE 3.19 Normal upper GI series. Barium filled stomach and duodenum. The patient is in the prone position. Gas (*short arrow*) is seen in the gastric fundus, a peristaltic wave (*long arrows*) crosses the gastric antrum, the pylorus (*curved arrows*) separates the duodenal bulb and stomach.

to visualize the esophagus, stomach, and small intestine (Fig. 3.19). When both barium and air are used, the process is referred to as a double-contrast study. When barium is used alone, it is a single-contrast study. Preparation for an upper GI series consists simply of nothing by mouth (*non per os* [NPO]) for 8 to 12 hours prior to the study. When perforation of the upper GI tract is suspected, water-soluble contrast media is used.

Antegrade Small Bowel Examination

The usual small bowel examination is performed after an upper GI series by having the patient drink additional barium. Serial radiographs of the abdomen are performed at 15- to 30-minute intervals thereafter to evaluate the small bowel as barium passes through (Fig. 3.20). Fluoroscopy is commonly used as a supplement to study the terminal ileum when barium begins to enter the colon or to further investigate abnormalities seen on the serial radiographs.

Enteroclysis

Enteroclysis is a focused examination of the small intestine, wherein air and barium sulfate are introduced directly into the small intestine via a nasointestinal tube. Under fluoroscopy, the tip of the tube is placed just beyond the duodenal–jejunal junction and contrast is injected (Fig. 3.21). Advantages of this procedure are that the small bowel can be distended and the stomach and duodenum do not obstruct visualization. The main disadvantages are the discomfort associated with a nasal tube and the radiation exposure.

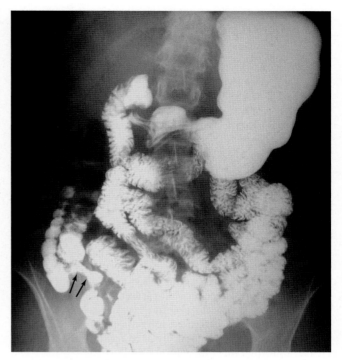

FIGURE 3.20 Normal antegrade small bowel examination. Barium was administered by mouth, and this radiograph was done about 30 minutes later. Note the barium-filled stomach, duodenal C-loop, feathered jejunum in the upper abdomen, and relatively formless mucosa of the ileum in the lower and right abdomen. The terminal ileum (*arrows*) entering the cecum can be identified. (Courtesy of Bruce Brown, M.D.)

Retrograde Small Bowel Examination

On occasion, especially when disease of the terminal ileum is suspected and previous examinations are nondiagnostic, barium can be refluxed from a filled colon into the ileum. Although

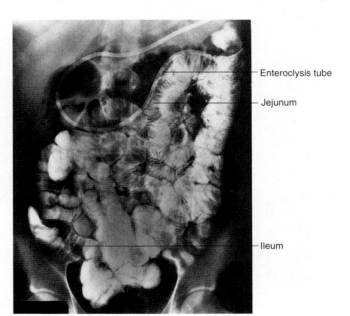

FIGURE 3.21 Small bowel enteroclysis. Normal. The nasointestinal tube has been positioned just beyond the duodenal–jejunal junction. Barium fills the entire small bowel.

the procedure is useful, there is considerable patient discomfort, alleviated slightly by antispasmodic agents.

Barium Enema

Introduction of barium sulfate and/or air into the colon via a rectal tube is called a lower GI series or barium enema. For this study, it is important to have a clean colon; this is best accomplished with laxatives and large amounts of orally ingested fluids. Barium and often air are administered via a rectal tube under fluoroscopic observation. When both air and barium are used, it is called a double-contrast study (Fig. 3.22), whereas barium alone is a single-contrast study. A properly performed barium enema has minimal associated discomfort. The double-contrast study is preferred to evaluate intraluminal and mucosal diseases, such as small ulcers and polyps. Again, if colon perforation is suspected, a water-soluble contrast medium is used.

Colonoscopy, an expensive alternative to colon barium studies, can directly visualize the mucosa. However, it requires conscious sedation because of patient discomfort. Virtual colonoscopy is an examination of the entire colon using multidetector CT and a dedicated software program so that the colon is displayed throughout its length with stacked images created to form a three-dimensional (3-D) picture of the colon at each level. The examination is usually performed after administration of an agent that tags fecal material, which can then be subtracted from the viewed images. Before the examination begins, the colon is insufflated with air so that the images resemble the interior view of the colon as would be seen by endoscopy. Virtual colonoscopy has the ability to discover almost all colon cancer (Fig. 3.23) as well as larger polyps (Fig. 3.24) (which are premalignant). The examination takes

FIGURE 3.22   Barium–air contrast colon examination. The entire colon is filled with barium and air. Films are made in prone, supine, and both decubitus positions so that different parts of the colon can be visualized with the air-contrast techniques. (Courtesy of Bruce Brown, M.D.)

FIGURE 3.23 "Apple core" invasive cancer discovered on virtual colonoscopy. **A:** The virtual colonoscopy image shows a large endoluminal mass (*straight arrows*), associated with narrowing of the colon lumen (*curved arrows*). **B:** Coronal CT reconstruction of the colonoscopic image. The tumor (*arrows*) is noted on both sides of the colon lumen and extrudes into the pericolic space. (Courtesy of J.G. Fletcher, M.D.)

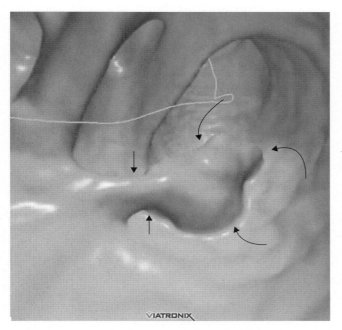

FIGURE 3.24 Virtual colonoscopy. Colon polyp detected in virtual colonoscopy. The stalk (*short arrows*) and the polyp (*curved arrows*) are readily apparent. (Courtesy of Wei Chang, M.D.)

but a few minutes and does not require the sedation and analgesics required for optical colon endoscopy. As experience with the technique has increased, it seems more accurate than barium enema techniques and perhaps as good as optical colonoscopy. Its disadvantages are the use of radiation and probably reduced detectability of flat mucosal lesions. It is much less expensive than optical colonoscopy. At the time of this writing, indication for its use as a substitute for screening optical colonoscopy is imprecise, but considerable improvement of the technique is anticipated.

STUDY OF GALLBLADDER AND BILIARY TRACT

In years past, the oral cholecystogram was performed to visualize the gallbladder following the oral ingestion of special iodinated compounds that are excreted into the biliary system and subsequently concentrated in the gallbladder. The study is seldom performed now because of the greater accuracy of US. With US, one can examine the liver and biliary tract as well as the gallbladder. CT and magnetic resonance imaging (MRI) are needed in certain situations to complement US.

In endoscopic retrograde cholangiopancreatography (ERCP), the endoscopist passes a fiberoptic scope under fluoroscopic control antegrade through the esophagus, stomach, and duodenum and retrograde into the common bile duct. The pancreatic ducts can also be cannulated. Contrast media can be injected into any of these structures and appropriate radiographs obtained (Fig. 3.25). ERCP is usually performed when less-invasive studies (CT, US, MRI, or contrast studies) are indeterminate or nondiagnostic or as part of a therapeutic endoscopic procedure.

URINARY TRACT EXAMINATIONS

The first methodology to examine the urinary tract directly (about 1900–present) was to inject radiopaque material directly into the bladder or other urinary structures (retrograde cystography or pyelography) at the time of cystoscopy. It was later discovered that intravenous contrast material that is excreted by the kidneys could be given with relative safety; excretory urography (EU) was developed shortly thereafter. Other names given for the EU are intravenous urogram and intravenous pyelogram. Multislice CT has now evolved as the new standard, CT urography (CTU). A multifaceted radiologic approach to genitourinary (GU) problems is now possible, with supplemental US and MRI examination.

EU with traditional radiographs, although still a useful technique, is performed much less frequently in the investigation of GU disease than is CTU, principally because the renal parenchyma, pelvicalyceal system, ureter, and bladder can be more accurately visualized with multislice techniques. US remains a valuable technique to complement radiographic investigation.

Excretory Urography and Computed Tomography Urography

Both EU and CTU involve the administration of an intravenous contrast medium that is excreted by the kidneys. In CTU the contrast medium is delivered in bolus fashion to

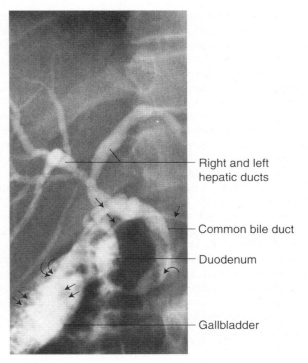

Right and left hepatic ducts

Common bile duct

Duodenum

Gallbladder

FIGURE 3.25 Endoscopic retrograde cholangiopancreatography (ERCP). Cholelithiasis and choledocholithiasis. The gallbladder is filled with calculi (*double straight arrows*), and there is a large calculus in the distal common bile duct (*curved arrow*). A nasobiliary drain (*straight single arrows*) is in place with the tip (*double curved arrows*) in the gallbladder.

maximize renal parenchymal visualization. In EU one recognizes the urinary structures as seen through overlying bowel gas, soft tissue, and so on. In CTU, multidetector CT is utilized, permitting visualization of urinary structures without overlying structures. A further advantage is the ability to reconstruct images in any plane—axial, coronal, and sagittal. A final advantage of CTU is a reconstruction technique so that the urinary tract is viewed in 3-D with all other structures subtracted.

Disadvantages of CTU include a higher patient radiation dose (about double) and additional cost. 3-D reconstruction requires image manipulation by a specially trained technologist. Thus, the EU remains an accepted technique for most children, for many follow-up studies, and at sites without multidetector CT. Both types of examinations are featured in this chapter.

Excretory urography (EU) and CT urography (CTU) do not require special patient preparation, merely abstaining from food and liquids for several hours before contrast administration.

The timing of EU and CTU radiographs can be varied, depending upon the patient's clinical problems. Nevertheless, both techniques usually require examination during the nephrographic phase (for visualization of the renal cortex), followed by image(s) of the pelvicalyceal system and bladder, which are opacified later. Delayed films can be obtained for hours, or even days, in situations such as ureteral obstruction or renal failure.

Viewing an Excretory Urogram or Computed Tomography Urogram

An EU study begins with a preliminary or scout radiograph that includes the entire abdomen. You can evaluate this preliminary radiograph using the same system as described previously. The radiographs obtained immediately following intravenous contrast media demonstrate the nephrogram phase wherein the contrast media is located in the renal capillaries, glomeruli, and proximal convoluted tubules (Fig. 3.26A). Compare the nephrograms for symmetry, as size discrepancy is suspicious for unilateral renal disease.

Next, evaluate the later postcontrast injection radiographs, at which times the contrast media is normally present in the calyces, renal pelves, portions of the ureters, and urinary bladder (Fig. 3.26B). Normal calyces are sharp in outline, with various numbers and geometry. Oblique, prone, and abdominal compression radiographs are often obtained to better display portions of the urinary tract.

The CTU is evaluated for the same factors as the EU, albeit in different fashion. A computed abdominal radiograph is performed, followed by axial scans of the abdomen before, immediately after, and at a later time following the bolus of contrast material (Fig. 3.27). In special situations (e.g., study of renal donor), immediate postcontrast scans can be obtained to visualize renal arteries and later the veins. As in the EU, pay attention to size and symmetry of the kidneys, pelvicalyceal systems, and bladder.

Other Urinary Tract Examinations

Direct injection of contrast material into the bladder or ureter (retrograde pyelogram) is of value when a detailed view of a portion of the ureter or pelvicalyceal system is necessary. It is often an adjunct to endoscopy.

Vesicoureteral reflux, a condition in which bladder urine refluxes in retrograde fashion into the ureters, is a common phenomenon of children but infrequent in adults. It can be associated with urinary tract infection. With the voiding cystourethrogram, contrast medium is introduced via urethral catheter into the bladder. Subsequent fluoroscopy and filming allow one to identify and quantitate vesicoureteral reflux if present (Fig. 3.28). At the completion of the study, the patient voids, with the voiding sequence recorded in some imaging form. This allows detection of urethral abnormalities, which can produce bladder obstruction and secondary vesicoureteral reflux. Cystography and retrograde urethrography are examinations usually performed to detect urinary extravasation in trauma cases.

ABDOMINAL ULTRASOUND

Ultrasound (US), being a different modality from x-rays, shows abdominal organs in a different fashion. There are roughly three patterns of reflected US:

1. No reflection of the sound wave. Almost all of the sound passes through the area. This is termed sonolucent and is traditionally viewed as black on images. Fluid, such as in ascites or abdominal cysts, is sonolucent.
2. Reflection of some and transmission of some sound. Solid organs, such as the kidney or liver, are examples. US waves are reflected, particularly at boundaries of organs of differing echogenicity, such as the boundary between the liver and kidney.
3. Reflection of all sound. Bone, other calcifications, and air in the gut are examples. One can make use of this by noting such shadowing and the absence of echoes distal to a lesion to help diagnose gallstones and like abnormalities.

There are two major problems in learning to read US images:

1. It requires one to think differently. You are looking at differences in transmission and reflection of US rather than transmitted x-rays.
2. Orientation of the image. This is the chief stumbling block. One may consider the US image as representing a roughly pie-shaped wedge of tissues, less than 1 cm thick, below the US transducer.

Even experienced radiologists and clinicians have considerable difficulty figuring out the nature of the US image if they did not perform the study. Orientation must be provided by the person who performed the scan. In most situations, there is a relatively fixed method of performing abdominal US. In general, one evaluates each area of interest in at least two dimensions, typically axial (transverse) and longitudinal (sagittal). For technical reasons, the direction of the scan beam shows the anatomy best if it is perpendicular to the organ of interest. As few abdominal organs are 100% oriented anterior–posterior or medial–lateral, the scanned images are, to varying degrees, oblique.

Probably the best method to be introduced to US is to attend an imaging session with a knowledgeable mentor who discusses the anatomy as it is being scanned. Combined with this, learn the usual routines for US scanning in your institution and

FIGURE 3.26   Abdomen AP EU. Normal. **A:** There are symmetric nephrograms 1 minute postinjection of contrast media. The renal outlines (*straight arrows*) are clearly defined owing to the presence of the contrast media within the kidneys. **B:** Note that it is possible to see the calyces, infundibula, renal pelves, portions of ureters, and urinary bladder on this 15-minute radiograph.

FIGURE 3.27 Normal CT urogram in a potential renal donor. **A:** Preliminary scout image of the abdomen is normal except for benign small calcifications (*arrows*) in the pelvis. **B:** Scout image with superimposed lines indicating the many axial slices performed to create the image data. **C:** One slice of the nonenhanced scan of the abdomen before administration of contrast. No abnormalities of the kidneys or other areas are noted. **D:** Coronal CT images after contrast administration shows aorta, single bilateral renal arteries (*arrows*), and normal size kidneys. **E:** Axial scan early after contrast demonstrates well demarcation of renal cortex and medulla. (*continued*)

FIGURE 3.27 (*Continued*) **F:** Coronal reconstruction at the same time as E. **G:** Later reconstructed coronal image showing normal kidneys, ureters, and bladder. **H:** Coronal image of the urinary tract viewed from posterior showing entry of the ureters into the bladder (*arrows*). **I:** Later coronal image showing both renal veins (*arrows*) as well as arterial structures.

FIGURE 3.28 Cystourethrogram. Vesicoureteral reflux. Contrast introduced via urethral catheter into the bladder fills the bladder and refluxes into the left ureter.

try to figure out how each image was performed. Conventionally, images are labeled as to the method by which they are done, for example, kidney—transverse.

There are many abdominal applications of US related to its widespread availability and cost (it is about half the cost of CT and about one third that of MRI). Ultrasonography is valuable in the workup of diseases involving the liver, biliary tract, kidneys, abdominal aorta, and abdominal masses. It is particularly useful in defining fluid versus solid (e.g., cyst versus solid mass) as well as in imaging fluid-filled structures, such as the gallbladder, urinary bladder, and renal pelvis. The various abdominal organs and pathologic processes have their own characteristic echo patterns, as shown in Fig 3.29.

Obstetric and gynecologic US is particularly important because of the absence of significant biological risk to the fetus or maternal genital structures. In obstetric US, the fetus is surrounded by amniotic fluid, making visualization easier (Fig. 3.30). In addition, one can use real-time US images to evaluate the beating heart. For gynecological examinations, both transabdominal (Fig. 3.31) and transvaginal techniques are used. Transvaginal imaging has the technical advantage of eliminating echoes from the abdominal wall from the area of interest, allowing better definition of genital organs (Fig. 3.32).

Diagnostic US of the prostate has been disappointing, as it is relatively insensitive to identifying abnormalities of this organ. In the scrotum, US is superb. It localizes the site of disease (e.g., testis versus epididymis) and often allows specific diagnosis of the abnormality present (Fig. 3.33). Correct diag-

nosis of epididymitis versus testicular torsion versus orchitis is possible, separating those who need surgery from those who require only medical treatment. Hydrocele and varicocele are easily identified with US. Identification of testicular tumors is good, although identifying tumor type is less reliable.

COMPUTED TOMOGRAPHY AND MAGNETIC RESONANCE IMAGING OF THE ABDOMEN

Both CT and MRI are useful in the diagnosis and management of abdominal disease. CT is usually the favored procedure because of its wide availability and lower cost. Patient motion is seldom a problem in CT but is a frequent occurrence in MRI. Both techniques have the ability to produce images in any dimension (axial, sagittal, coronal, or oblique).

Except in emergencies, the patient for CT has usually fasted for several hours. In most cases (suspected renal disease is the usual exception), a dilute contrast material (such as barium or iodine containing) is given orally before the study begins to demarcate the GI tract. This allows one to identify bowel loops, distinguishing them from masses and solid organs.

Immediately before (or sometimes during) abdominal CT, contrast material is injected intravenously to allow identification of arteries and veins (the enhanced CT). The intravenous contrast is excreted by the kidneys so that the kidneys (and later the urinary collecting systems and bladder) will be opacified (see CTU).

A relatively new examination is the positron emission tomography (PET)-CT (see nuclear medicine). A special machine combines CT and PET scanning so that the patient is not moved between examinations. Software programs fuse the CT and PET images into a single image. The advantage is to combine the PET-increased sensitivity of small tumors with the improved anatomical localization of CT.

The abdominal MRI examination is tailored to the suspected abnormality, the technical details being beyond the scope of this discussion. Intravenous contrast agents, such as gadolinium, which can change the MR signal in many organs and diseases, are frequently given as part of the MR study.

How to Read Abdominal Computed Tomography and Magnetic Resonance Imaging

Reading cross-sectional images of the abdomen is not particularly difficult for the neophyte radiologist *if* one's anatomical knowledge is adequate. You will find the system for axial images described herein to be time-consuming but rewarding. First, arrange the images in order, from top (toward the head) to bottom. In many circumstances, that is already done for you electronically. Next, look at all the images (using the cine mode if available) in gestalt fashion to discover any obvious abnormalities. Then, look at each organ individually, from top to bottom (i.e., all CT slices containing the organ of interest). In each organ, evaluate the size and shape of each area of reduced or increased density. Do this for visible lung, liver, gallbladder, spleen, pancreas, adrenals, both kidneys and ureters,

Liver

Right kidney cortex

Right kidney upper collecting system

FIGURE 3.29 A: Longitudinal (sagittal) abdominal sonogram. Normal liver and right kidney echo patterns. The *cross marks* indicate the longitudinal (sagittal) liver dimension. The right kidney borders are demarcated by the *straight arrows* and the right hemidiaphragm by the *curved arrows*. **B:** Transverse (axial) abdominal sonogram. Normal spleen echo pattern. The side-to-side spleen dimension lies between the *X marks*, and the cephalocaudal dimension lies between the *crosses*. The left hemidiaphragm is indicated by the *curved arrow* (S, spleen). Note the labels on the images (A, Rt long; B, Lt trans spl). Such labels are helpful in orienting the images for the observer.

9-week fetus

Amniotic fluid

Placenta

Uterine wall

Parietal bone

Posterior skull

Amniotic fluid
Anterior skull

Parietal bone

A

B

C

FIGURE 3.30 Obstetric sonograms **A:** Study in a 9-week fetus. The *caliper markers* indicating crown to rump distance confirm the 9-week gestation. **B:** Skull of a fetus near term. The *white dotted lines* outline the skull, and the biparietal diameter confirms the fetal age. The cerebral ventricles are vaguely seen within the skull. **C:** Twin pregnancy. The uterine wall is marked by the *arrowheads*. Each fetus (*straight arrows*) is surrounded by amniotic fluid (*curved arrows*). There are separate sacs.

FIGURE 3.31 A: Transabdominal midline longitudinal (sagittal) sonogram. Normal uterus (*straight arrows*). The urine-filled bladder is essentially echo free and thus serves as an acoustic window to the pelvis. Notice the characteristic homogeneous echo pattern of the normal uterus. The endometrial stripe (*curved arrow*) represents the layers that line the endometrial cavity. The presence of the endometrial stripe indicates the absence of an intrauterine pregnancy or other intrauterine mass (*B*, urinary bladder; *V*, vagina). **B:** Transabdominal transverse (axial) sonogram. Normal uterus. The uterine fundus is outlined by the *straight arrows*; the endometrial stripe (*curved arrow*) appears smaller on the transverse image. **C:** Transabdominal right longitudinal (sagittal) sonogram. Normal right ovary (*straight arrows*). **D:** Transabdominal left longitudinal (sagittal) sonogram. Normal left ovary (*straight arrows*).

A

Ovarian follicles

B

Ovarian follicles

Iliac vessel

FIGURE 3.32 Transvaginal sonograms of the right (**A**) and left (**B**) ovaries. The dimensions of the ovaries are indicated by the X *marks* and *crosses*. Note the better definition of the ovaries, so that follicles are visible, when compared with the transabdominal images (Fig. 3-31).

the bladder, and genitals. Evaluate the stomach, duodenum, small bowel, colon/appendix, and mesentery. Study the retroperitoneum from top to bottom—aorta, vena cava, and mesenteric vessels, also looking for adenopathy or other masses. Check the peritoneal cavity for fluid or masses. Look at the vertebrae (and spinal cord within) and bony pelvis. Finally, concentrate on the abdominal wall, hips, and adjacent soft tissues. Thoroughness leads to success in reading abdom-

inal CT scans. The same methodology applies to evaluation of coronal and sagittal images.

The same system can also be applied to abdominal MRI, but—unfortunately for the nonradiologist—there are usually many more images, often with oblique planes and several pulse sequences, often later supplemented with intravenous magnetic contrast material. Normal abdominal CT and MRI anatomy is illustrated in Figs. 3.34 to 3.45.

FIGURE 3.33 Transverse scrotal sonogram. The left testis is normal. The right testis is enlarged, has reduced echogenicity, and shows streaky, black linear echodensities. These findings indicate orchitis. (Courtesy of Monzer Abu-Yousef, M.D.)

FIGURE 3.34   A: Illustration of the approximate axial anatomic level through the liver and spleen for B and C. **B:** Abdomen axial CT image through the liver and spleen. Normal. **C:** Abdomen axial MR image through the liver and spleen. Normal.

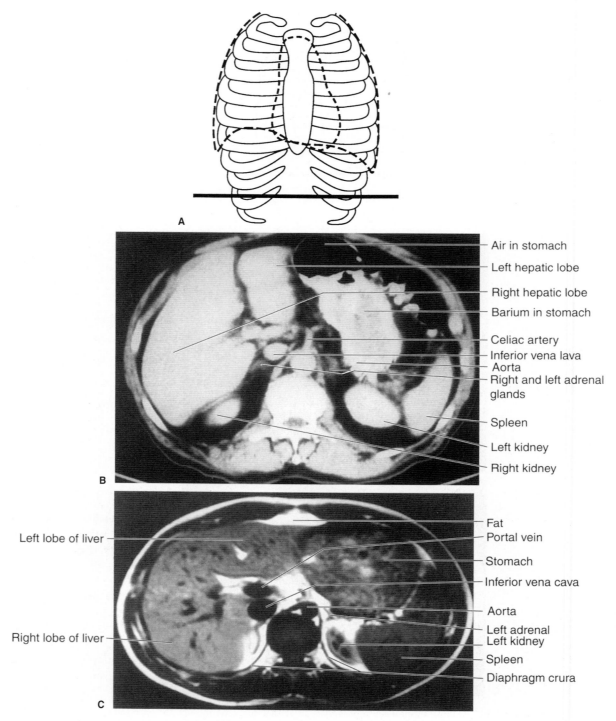

FIGURE 3.35 **A:** Illustration of the approximate axial anatomic level through the liver and spleen for B and C. This level is just caudad to the level in Fig. 3.34. **B:** Abdomen axial CT image through the liver and spleen. Normal. **C:** Abdomen axial MR image through the liver and spleen. Normal.

Superior mesenteric
vein-portal vein
confluence

Stomach air
Right hepatic lobe
Duodenum second
portion
Pancreas head and
body
Superior mesenteric
artery
Aorta
Pancreas tail
Diaphragm crura
Inferior vena cava
Psoas muscle
Right and left kidneys

Fat
Liver
Gastric body
Pancreas body
Splenic vein
Celiac artery
Aorta
Spleen
Left kidney

FIGURE 3.36 **A:** Illustration of the approximate axial anatomic level through the pancreas for B and C. **B:** Abdomen axial CT image through the pancreas level. Normal. **C:** Abdomen axial MR image through the pancreas level. Normal.

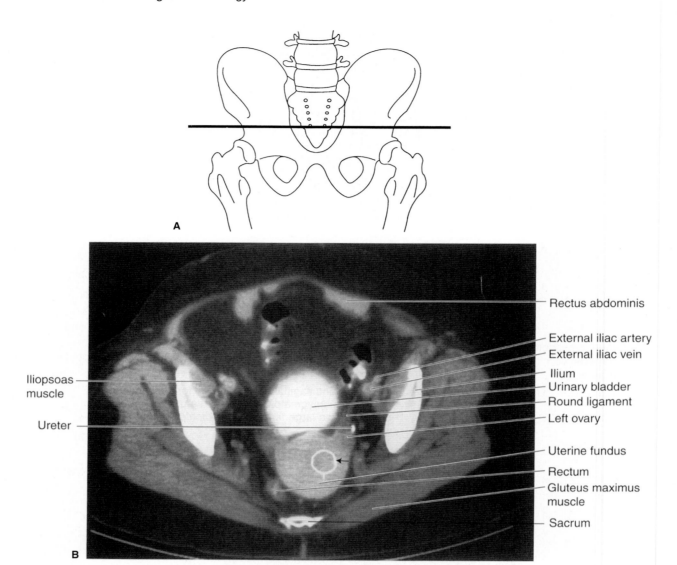

Rectus abdominis

External iliac artery
External iliac vein
Ilium
Urinary bladder
Round ligament
Left ovary

Uterine fundus
Rectum
Gluteus maximus muscle
Sacrum

Iliopsoas muscle

Ureter

FIGURE 3.37   A: Illustration of the approximate axial anatomic level for B. **B:** Female pelvis axial CT image through the uterus after intravenous contrast media. Normal. The white metallic density ring (*straight arrow*) that projects over the uterus is merely a region of interest cursor for measuring tissue density.

Sartorius muscle

Rectus femoris
muscle

Tensor fascia lata
muscle

Iliopsoas muscle

Levator ani
muscle

Pubic symphysis

Pubic bone

Pectineus muscle

Prostate gland
Prostatic urethra

Femur

Rectum

Ischiorectal fossa

Ischial tuberosity

Gluteus maximus
muscle

FIGURE 3.38   A: Illustration of the approximate axial anatomic level for B. **B:** Male pelvis axial T2 MR
image at the level of the pubic symphysis and prostate. Normal.

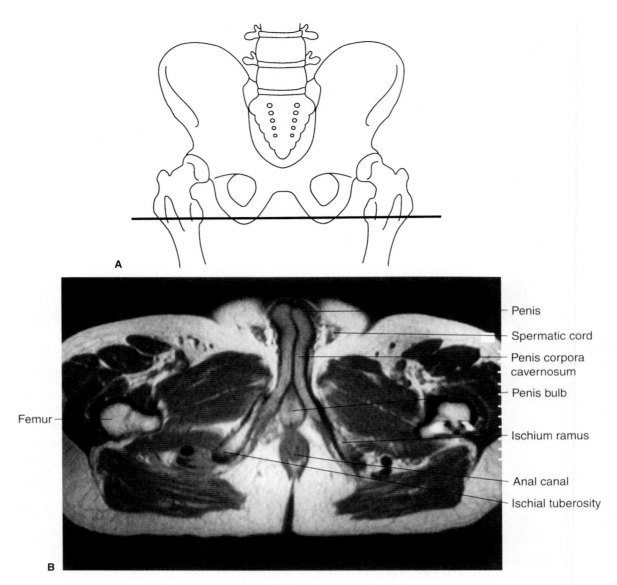

FIGURE 3.39   A: Illustration of the approximate axial anatomic level for B. **B:** Male pelvis axial T2 MR image at the level of the penile structures. Normal.

FIGURE 3.40 Female pelvis axial T2 MR image. Same anatomic level as Fig. 3.38 (R, rectum; U, uterine wall; E, endometrial cavity; C, cervix; O, ovary.) (Courtesy of Alan Stolpen, M.D.)

FIGURE 3.41 Female pelvis axial T2 MR image. Same anatomic level as Fig. 3.39. (Courtesy of Alan Stolpen, M.D.)

Right kidney

Aorta
Liver
Diaphragm crura
Spleen
Left kidney medulla
Left kidney cortex
Perinephric fat
Left psoas muscle

Ilium
Sacroiliac joint
Sacrum

FIGURE 3.42   A: Illustration of the approximate coronal anatomic level through the kidneys for B. **B:** Abdomen coronal MR image through the kidneys. Normal.

Liver

Abdominal aorta
Inferior vena cava

Transversus abdominis muscle
External oblique muscle
Internal oblique muscle
Left iliac artery
Right iliac artery
Right iliac vein

FIGURE 3.43   A: Illustration of the approximate coronal anatomic level through the aorta and inferior vena cava for B. **B:** Abdomen coronal MR image through the abdominal aorta and inferior vena cava. Normal.

FIGURE 3.44   A: Illustration of the approximate midline sagittal anatomic level for B. **B:** Male pelvis midline sagittal T2 MR image at the level of the urinary bladder and pubic symphysis. Normal.

FIGURE 3.45   A: Illustration of the approximate coronal anatomic level for B. **B:** Male pelvis coronal T1 MR image through the pubic symphysis. Normal.

FIGURE 3.46 Magnetic resonance angiography of the upper abdomen. This MR image clearly defines the celiac (*straight arrows*) and superior mesenteric (*curved arrows*) arteries and their branches. The origins of the renal arteries (*open arrows*) from the aorta are noted. (Courtesy of Alan Stolpen, M.D.)

ANGIOGRAPHY

Aortography (catheter injection into the abdominal aorta) and selective arteriography of individual vessels in the abdomen are sometimes performed for diagnostic reasons, particularly in trauma or with GI hemorrhage. With rapid CT imaging, visualization of the arteries and/or veins can be obtained using this modality after intravenous contrast material, thus avoiding the necessity for placing an intra-aortic catheter.

Recall that moving tissue, such as intravascular blood, has less MRI signal than surrounding tissue. Various technical manipulations are possible using this phenomenon, with or without the addition of magnetic contrast material, to allow excellent visualization of almost all of the major abdominal vessels without direct aortic catheterization (Figs. 3.46 and 3.47). The choice of CT angiography versus MR angiography is largely dependent on the expertise of the radiologist and the type of equipment available at individual institutions.

Conventional angiography was used in the past to delineate tumors of the solid organs. CT and MRI are now more effective and less invasive methods for characterizing masses.

IMAGING FEATURES OF GASTROINTESTINAL ABNORMALITIES USING TRADITIONAL CONTRAST RADIOGRAPHS

The gut, being a hollow organ extending from the mouth to the anus, has a basic structure and radiographic appearance throughout. If contrast material (barium) fills the gut, one obtains information about the lumen and gut wall. Visualization of the mucosal surface is improved by double-contrast techniques, as barium coating the mucosal surface contrasts with the intraluminal air. Thus, there are only a few basic patterns

FIGURE 3.47 Magnetic resonance angiography of the aorta and its branches in a patient with arteriosclerosis. The right iliac artery is occluded at its origin (*arrow*). Both renal arteries (*curved arrows*) are intact. The inferior vena cava (*curved arrows*) can be seen. (Courtesy of Alan Stolpen, M.D.)

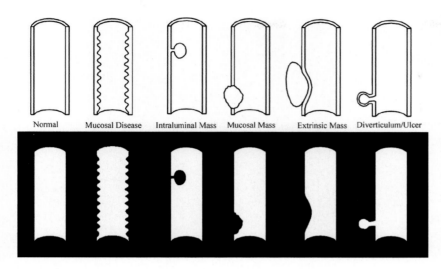

Normal   Mucosal Disease   Intraluminal Mass   Mucosal Mass   Extrinsic Mass   Diverticulum/Ulcer

FIGURE 3.48 Types of GI abnormalities (above) and their radiographic appearance (below).

that are much alike within the esophagus, stomach, and small or large bowel (Fig. 3.48). They are the following:

1. Intraluminal lesion. Examples include a polyp, foreign body, or exophytic tumor.
2. Mucosal diseases. Examples include inflammation of the mucosa and adjacent musculature, indicative of enteritis.
3. Mural lesion. The abnormality is in the bowel wall (with or without concomitant mucosal involvement). Examples include tumor, transmucosal inflammation, and edema. If the abnormality encircles the bowel wall (as is often seen in colon cancer), a napkin-ring appearance results.
4. Extrinsic lesions. Here, both the bowel wall and lumen are displaced by an extrinsic force. Examples include enlarged mesenteric nodes adjacent to the gut.
5. Extraluminal projections beyond the bowel lumen. Typical abnormalities are ulcerations and diverticula.

Symptoms arising from esophageal disease include heartburn and dysphagia (difficulty swallowing). In gastroesophageal reflux disease, common in elderly patients, heartburn and later dysphagia occur, owing to reflux of gastric contents into the esophagus, with resultant esophagitis and eventual stricture. Hiatal hernias often accompany gastroesophageal reflux. The barium esophagram easily detects hiatal hernia and stricture (Fig. 3.49). The esophagram is less sensitive in the diagnosis of esophagitis when compared with endoscopy. Esophageal cancer typically has an intraluminal and an intramural component with abnormal mucosa and narrowing of the esophageal lumen (Fig. 3.50). Esophagography is useful in studying motility disorders of the esophagus.

The majority of upper GI series are performed to detect peptic ulcer disease in either the stomach or duodenum. Clearly protruding from the lumen, ulcers are most easily seen on double-contrast examinations (Fig. 3.51). If seen *en face*, the ulcer crater appears as a glob of increased density as barium fills the ulcer crater and the lumen is filled with air (Fig. 3.52). Often, mucosal folds radiate toward the ulcer crater, aiding in its detection. With recurrent disease, deformity of the adjacent bowel, particularly in the duodenum, accompanies the ulcer.

Gastric tumors are uncommon in North America. Polyps (Fig. 3.53) are seen in the elderly. Stomach cancer usually appears as an ulcerated, irregular mucosal mass, often accompanied by concentric narrowing of the adjacent stomach.

Localized small bowel disease in North America is most often Crohn disease, which produces inflammation with mucosal ulcerations and thickening of the bowel wall (Fig. 3.54). Other localized lesions and primary small bowel tumors are rare.

A wide variety of metabolic, immune, and other disorders can involve the entire small bowel. The classic example is sprue (gluten hypersensitivity) with associated small bowel dilatation. Dilution of barium and prominence of the mucosal folds are also noted.

Barium enema studies are useful in the workup of inflammatory colon disease. Ulcerative colitis begins in the rectum and extends a variable distance proximally (Fig. 3.55). The

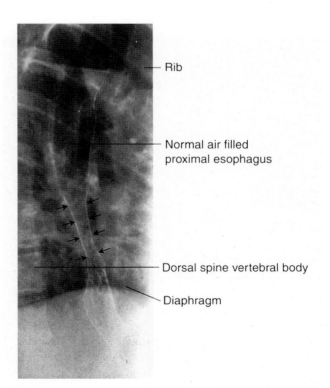

— Rib

— Normal air filled proximal esophagus

— Dorsal spine vertebral body

— Diaphragm

FIGURE 3.49 Double-contrast esophagram. Distal esophageal stricture. The smooth, long, tapered appearance of the narrowed distal esophagus (*straight arrows*) is typical of a benign stricture owing to reflux of gastric contents into the esophagus.

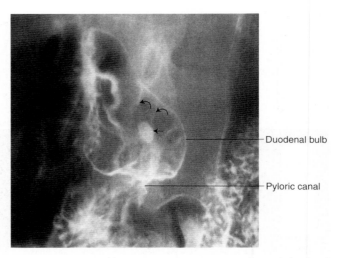

FIGURE 3.52   Double-contrast upper GI series. Central duodenal bulb ulcer (*arrow*). The duodenal mucosal folds (*curved arrows*) radiate toward the ulcer crater.

FIGURE 3.50   Barium contrast esophagram. Carcinoma of the esophagus. The cancer produces a narrowed segment with irregular mucosa and ulceration. The proximal esophagus is dilated but otherwise normal.

mucosal surface shows tiny ulcerations in a uniform nature throughout the affected area, often accompanied by loss of haustrations (the lead pipe colon). Crohn disease affecting the colon (Fig. 3.56) often spares the rectum, skip lesions are common, and deeper ulcerations occur.

The barium enema, particularly with double-contrast technique, is valuable in detecting colon polyps as well as colon cancer. Intraluminal polyps (Fig. 3.57) are more easily detected than those that are sessile (along the colon wall). Evolution of polyps into colon cancer does occur; the larger the polyp, the greater the chance the histology will show a malignant change. There are approximately 150,000 new cases of carcinoma in the colon and rectum reported each year in the United States. Early detection of this disease improves survival dramatically. As colon cancer progresses in size, it often surrounds the bowel lumen in a fashion described as an apple core or napkin ring (Fig. 3.58). Large advanced cancers are evident on abdominal CT (Fig. 3.59).

There are a number of syndromes characterized by multiple colonic polyps, sometimes with additional polyps of the

FIGURE 3.51   Gastric ulcer, upper GI series. The lesser curvature ulcer (*arrows*) protrudes from the stomach lumen.

FIGURE 3.53   Double-contrast upper GI series. Gastric polyp. The stalk (*curved arrow*) of the benign polyp (*straight arrows*) is clearly visible.

FIGURE 3.54 Crohn disease of the ileum. Antegrade small bowel examination. The affected small bowel (*arrows*) is narrowed; the adjacent space between small bowel loops indicates bowel wall thickening.

FIGURE 3.56 Crohn disease of the colon. Barium enema. The rectum, sigmoid, and ascending colon are normal. The descending and transverse colon are slightly narrowed, and the mucosa is nodular with small ulcerations (*arrows*) extending from the colon lumen.

FIGURE 3.55 Ulcerative colitis. Barium enema. The entire colon, except the cecum, is uniformly narrowed, the mucosal surface is irregular, and the overall configuration suggests a lead pipe appearance.

FIGURE 3.57 Barium enema showing villous adenoma with focal carcinoma in the polyp mucosa. A large, lobulated mass fills the lumen of the sigmoid colon.

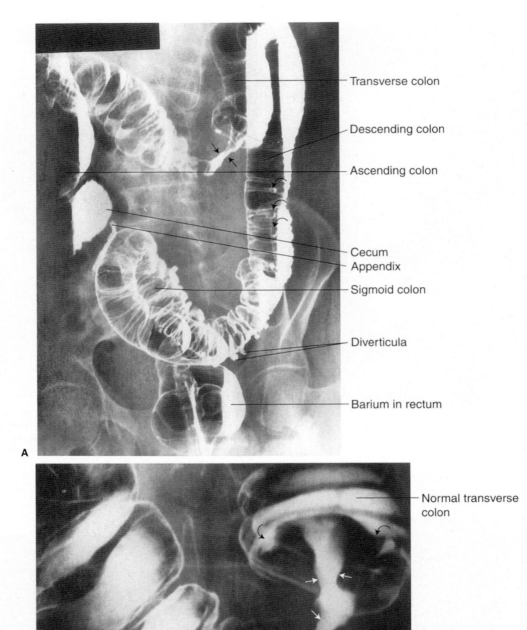

FIGURE 3.58 **A:** Adenocarcinoma of the transverse colon. Double-contrast colon examination. Note the classic apple core appearance of the colon cancer. The core represents the patent portion of the bowel lumen (*straight arrows*). Diverticula of the descending colon are seen *en face*. **B:** Close-up view of the tumor mass in A. Note the irregular mucosa of the narrowed lumen of the apple core lesion (*straight arrows*). The mass creates a shouldering (*curved arrows*) deformity in the neighboring transverse colon both proximally and distally.

FIGURE 3.59   Lower abdomen axial CT image. The *white arrow*s outline a large cecal neoplasm. The *curved arrow* show an air–fluid level within the tumor mass secondary to necrosis.

FIGURE 3.61   Normal appendix. Abdominal CT. The appendix is the wormlike, barium-filled density (*arrows*) in the right lower quadrant. (Courtesy of Bruce Brown, M.D.)

small bowel or stomach. Prominent among these is familial polyposis of the colon, which is characterized by multiple adenomas, all with malignant potential (Fig. 3.60).

As noted earlier, polyps and tumors of the colon may be identified with virtual colonoscopy (Figs. 3.23 and 3.24).

Acute appendicitis is the most common surgical disease of the abdomen. If clinical history and physical examination are

strongly suggestive of appendicitis, further imaging examinations are not needed, as the accuracy of clinical findings approaches 90%. Plain films of the abdomen are not particularly helpful in the diagnosis of appendicitis, unless a calcified appendicolith is noted. Imaging studies are most valuable in those individuals with low to moderate probability of a positive diagnosis (Fig. 3.61). In children, careful US examination performed by a skilled radiologist is frequently the study of choice; CT is sometimes difficult because of the small amount of periappendiceal fat in this age group. In adults, multislice CT of the right lower quadrant, with or without the use of contrast material, is recommended. The abnormal appendix can be identified in most cases as a small tubular structure with distended lumen, thickening of the periappendiceal wall, and inflammation of adjacent fat (Fig. 3.62). One can usually diagnose perforation of the appendix by changes adjacent to the organ.

FIGURE 3.60   Familial polyposis of the colon. Double-contrast barium enema. There are innumerable tiny polyps throughout the colon.

FIGURE 3.62   Abdominal CT transverse view of appendix. Appendicitis with perforation. A calcified appendicolith is in the lumen of the appendix (*arrow*). There is gas in the appendiceal wall and periappendiceal fluid. (Courtesy of Bruce Brown, M.D.)

FIGURE 3.63   Unilateral ureteropelvic junction obstruction abdominal sonogram. The echo-free renal pelvis and associated calyces (*arrows*) are dilated. Renal–cortical borders are outlined by *curved arrows*. (Courtesy of Monzer Abu-Yousef, M.D.)

FIGURE 3.65   Abdomen AP EU. Pelvic kidney (simple ectopia). The left kidney is situated in the pelvis, just cephalad to the urinary bladder. The upper collecting system of the pelvic kidney is indicated by the *straight arrow*. Note the foreshortened left ureter (*curved arrow*) and the normal right ureter (*double curved arrows*).

IMAGING FEATURES OF GENITOURINARY ABNORMALITIES

Certain anomalies obstruct the flow of urine, producing proximal obstruction. Congenital ureteropelvic junction (UPJ) obstructions can sometimes be diagnosed *in utero*; less severe cases do not present until later in life. The UPJ obstruction can be unilateral or bilateral. US is an excellent technique for following UPJ obstruction, showing the amount of pelvicalyceal dilatation and its effect on the renal parenchyma (Fig. 3.63). Congenital vesicoureteral junction obstruction is less frequent but usually bilateral (Fig. 3.64).

Embryologically, the kidneys develop in the pelvis and migrate cephalad into the abdomen. The kidney that fails to migrate cephalad into the abdomen is called a pelvic kidney, sacral kidney, or simple ectopia (Fig. 3.65). In a horseshoe kidney, the lower poles of the right and left kidneys are connected by a bridge, or isthmus, of renal tissue (Fig. 3.66).

Ureterocele (Fig. 3.67) refers to a dilated intramural ureteral segment that protrudes into the bladder, simulating a cobra's head. Ureteroceles result from either congenital or

FIGURE 3.64   Unilateral vesicoureteral obstruction. **A:** Coronal CT. The left kidney is normal, but a urine-filled sac surrounded by renal cortex (*arrows*) is seen on the left. **B:** Later coronal CT shows the dilated right renal pelvis (*curved arrows*) and ureter (*straight arrows*) extending to the bladder (*arrowhead*). (Courtesy of Andrew Wu, M.D.)

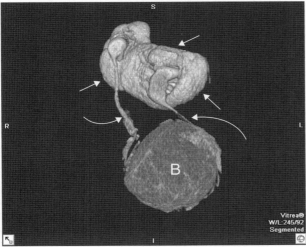

FIGURE 3.66 Horseshoe kidney. **A:** The excretory urogram shows the lower pole calyces closer to the midline than those of the upper poles. **B:** 3-D reconstruction of A shows the fused kidneys (*white arrows*), both ureters (*curved arrows*), and bladder (B).

TABLE 3.6

MASSES IN THE RENAL PELVIS

- Stones
- Tumor
- Mycetoma (fungus ball)
- Blood clot
- Necrotic renal papillae

acquired stenosis at the ureteral orifice and can cause partial ureteral obstruction.

Bladder diverticula are generally acquired but on occasion are congenital (Fig. 3.68).

Urolithiasis is one of the most common urologic problems encountered in the everyday practice of medicine. Most ureteral stones are less than 1 cm in diameter, and approximately 75% of acutely symptomatic stones are located in the distal third of the ureter. Approximately 90% of all GU calculi are radiopaque on plain film.

Some radiopaque renal calculi actually fill all or part of an upper collecting system and are called staghorn calculi (Fig. 3.69). When such calculi are bilateral, their appearance should not be mistaken for contrast media in the upper collecting systems. Although EU has been used to diagnose urolithiasis (it is valuable in quantitating the degree of ureteral obstruction), it is considerably less sensitive than CT. Current protocol for patients with suspected ureteral stones calls for multislice CT through the regions of the kidneys and ureters without intravenous contrast material, usually followed by repeat examination with contrast material (Fig. 3.70). Obviously, calculi can occur at any location in the urinary tract. The differential diagnosis for a renal pelvis filling (nonradiopaque) defect is listed in Table 3.6.

Multiple unilateral or bilateral interstitial renal calcifications are referred to as nephrocalcinosis. Nephrolithiasis, or

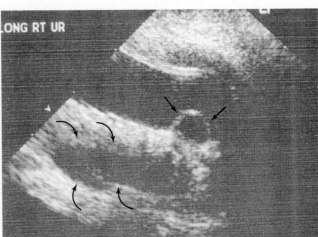

FIGURE 3.67 **A:** Pelvis AP EU. Ureterocele. Note the cobra head appearance (*straight arrows*) of the ureterocele. The left ureter is moderately dilated. **B:** Ureterocele, pelvic US. The wall of the ureterocele (*arrows*) is visualized by echo-free urine in the bladder and within the ureterocele. A dilated ureter (*curved arrows*) is noted posterior to the bladder.

FIGURE 3.68 Cystogram. Bladder diverticulum (*straight arrow*). There are unilateral pins traversing a left hip fracture (*curved arrow*).

calcification in the renal tubules, occurs with metabolic abnormalities (hypercalcemia) or with congenitally dilated collecting tubules (medullary sponge kidney). The US and CT appearances (Fig. 3.71) are pathognomic—another Aunt Minnie.

Therapeutic US has become a useful tool for breaking up calculi. This is called extracorporeal sound wave lithotripsy (Fig. 3.72). The fragmented calculi usually pass spontaneously without surgical intervention.

FIGURE 3.69 AP supine abdomen. Bilateral renal staghorn calculi. The calculi (*straight arrows*) closely resemble contrast media in upper collecting systems, demonstrating the importance of the preliminary radiograph. Incidentally noted is a left pelvic phlebolith (*curved arrow*).

GU infections are a common occurrence in medicine and usually do not require diagnostic imaging procedures. In children, especially males, with documented urinary infection, study for vesicoureteral reflux is recommended (Fig. 3.28), and US study of the kidneys is often of value. Severity of infection ranges from mild cystitis to perinephric abscess. Acute pyelonephritis usually causes renal enlargement, which may be focal (Fig. 3.73); with atrophic pyelonephritis, the kidney may shrink.

Renal cysts may be single, multiple, unilateral, or bilateral. These lesions are usually asymptomatic and often are an incidental finding on abdominal imaging performed for other reasons. Although cysts are of no clinical significance, they must be evaluated closely to distinguish them from solid tumors. This is easily done with US (Fig. 3.74) or CT (Fig. 3.75) as the water density and sharp borders of cysts are apparent. Other benign renal tumors are uncommon.

Malignant renal tumors are solid masses. Approximately 90% are renal cell carcinomas. Patients with renal cell carcinomas may present with gross or microscopic hematuria, pain, or other symptoms. US (Fig. 3.76) determines the solid nature of the mass. CT and/or MRI is the proven method of diagnosis. EU is less sensitive and accurate. The radiologic features of primary renal malignancies are shown in Table 3.8, and some examples of these tumors are shown in Figs. 3.76 to 3.79.

Malignant tumors of the urothelium occur in the renal pelvis, ureter, or bladder. As they often cause urinary obstruction, ureteral opacification displays them best (Figs. 3.80 to 3.82).

Extrinsic malignancies, such as retroperitoneal tumors, can displace or obstruct the ureter and kidneys (Fig. 3.83). Primary and secondary neoplasms can also involve the ureter and the bladder (Fig. 3.84).

Prostatic cancer is the most common neoplasm of elderly males. Neither CT nor MRI is of particular value of screening for this malignancy, but both are beneficial in staging the disease. Specifically, MRI evaluates the possibility of spread of the tumor beyond the prostate capsule, and both CT and MRI allow demonstration of pelvic lymph node metastasis (Fig. 3.85).

FIGURE 3.70   Renal calculus coronal. **A:** Axial and **B:** coronal CT without contrast material. The stone (*arrows*) lies in a lower pole calyx of the right kidney. **C:** On reconstructed CT urogram the stone (*arrow*) is more difficult to recognize. (Courtesy of Andrew Wu, M.D.)

FIGURE 3.71   Nephrolithiasis. **A:** Longitudinal US. **B:** Axial CT. These are extensive calcifications in the pyramid (not the calyces) of the kidneys. (Courtesy of Simon Kao, M.D.)

Descending colon

Transverse colon

Fragments of the calculus in the renal pelvis

Ascending colon

Fragments of the calculus in the ureter

Point of ureteral obstruction

FIGURE 3.72   **A:** Abdomen AP radiograph. Solitary radiopaque calculus in the right renal pelvis (*straight arrow*). **B:** Abdomen AP radiograph 24 hours post–extracorporeal sound wave lithotripsy. The obstructed ureter is filled with multiple small fragments of the calculus, referred to as "steinstrasse" (or "stone street"). The colon is air-filled and dilated (adynamic ileus) owing to pain of renal colic.

FIGURE 3.73 Sagittal sonogram of right kidney. Segmental pyelonephritis. Note the increased echogenicity of the upper pole. The foci of decreased lucency in both upper and lower poles are the renal pyramids. (Courtesy of Monzer Abu-Yousef, M.D.)

FIGURE 3.74 Transverse and longitudinal sonograms of the right kidney. Renal cyst of the upper pole. The cyst is echolucent, has sharp borders, and shows posterior enhancement. (Courtesy of Monzer Abu-Yousef, M.D.)

Abdominal aorta calcification

Normal left kidney

FIGURE 3.75 Abdomen axial CT image through the kidneys after intravenous contrast media. Right renal cyst. The cyst has sharp, smooth margins (*straight arrows*) and a low tissue density when compared with the remainder of the right kidney (*curved arrow*).

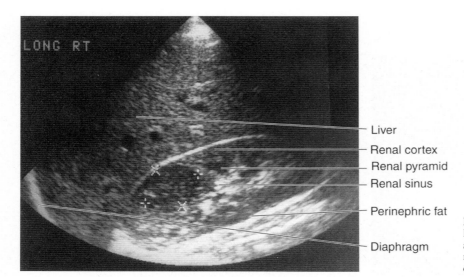

— Liver

— Renal cortex

— Renal pyramid

— Renal sinus

— Perinephric fat

— Diaphragm

FIGURE 3.76 Renal cell carcinoma. Right renal longitudinal sonogram. The electronic caliper *X marks* and *crosses* delineate an upper pole renal mass. The numerous internal echoes (hyperechoic) within the mass indicatez that it is solid.

— Normal right kidney

— Normal portion left kidney

FIGURE 3.77 Abdomen axial CT. Left renal cell carcinoma (*straight arrows*). The mass lesion is solid, and its border with the normal kidney (*curved arrow*) is poorly defined.

FIGURE 3.78 Renal cell carcinoma (*arrows*) left kidney and benign cyst (*arrow*) right kidney. CT. Note the smooth borders and spherical shape of the cyst versus the irregular border of the cancer.

— Inferior vena cava

Aorta

FIGURE 3.79 Abdomen axial T2 MR image. There is a large left renal cell carcinoma (*arrows*).

A   B

FIGURE 3.80 Transitional cell carcinoma of the left renal pelvis. **A:** Coronal CT without contrast material. A soft tissue mass (*arrows*) fills the central left renal pelvis (compare the right and left renal pelves). **B:** Axial CT with contrast. The upper pole tumor (*arrows*) replaces contrast across the posterior kidney.

FIGURE 3.81 Left retrograde pyelogram. A partially obstructing ureteral carcinoma (*straight arrows*) has resulted in a dilated proximal ureter (*double straight arrows*). A cystoscope is in the bladder.

FIGURE 3.82 Transitional cell bladder cancer. **A:** Axial and **B:** Coronal CT. The bladder (*arrows*) is filled with polypoid masses surrounded by nonradiopaque urine.

Gastric air–fluid (contrast media) level

Inferior vena cava
Aorta

Retroperitoneal fat

FIGURE 3.83 Abdomen axial CT image. Lymphoma. The tumor (*small black* and *short open arrows*) involves lymph nodes in the retroperitoneum and surrounds the enhanced aorta and inferior vena cava. The arrow labeled **1** indicates the inferior aspect of the liver.

FIGURE 3.84 Left retrograde pyelogram. Encasement of the distal left ureter by cancer of the cervix has resulted in stricture and partial obstruction of the distal left ureter (*straight arrow*). The left ureter proximal to the stricture is dilated (*curved arrows*). The cystoscope and retrograde catheter (*arrowheads*) can be seen.

FIGURE 3.85 Coronal prostate MRI in an elderly man with prostate cancer extending into adjacent tissue. Bladder = B, prostatic urethra (*curved arrows*), prostatic capsule (*small arrows*), cancer spread beyond capsule (*arrowheads*). The spreading cancer is low signal as compared to the rest of the prostate and the capsule cannot be identified in the region of the cancer. (Courtesy of Eve Clark, M.D.)

— Fetal skull

— Fetal face

— Fetal spine

— Fetal femur

FIGURE 3.86 Abdomen AP radiograph. Third-trimester intrauterine pregnancy in a breech presentation.

OBSTETRIC AND GYNECOLOGICAL IMAGING

There is seldom a need today for abdominal plain films in the diagnosis of pregnancy; however, when such a study is done (for necessity or by accident; Fig. 3.86), the risk of damage to the fetus from radiation is extremely low. Here is another Aunt Minnie—a radiograph showing an intrauterine contraceptive device (Fig. 3.87).

Routine US evaluation of the pregnant woman and her fetus, a standard practice in the developed world, is of considerable value in obstetrics. Fetal maturation, major anomalies, placental assessment, and many associated maternal conditions can be evaluated (Figs. 3.88 and 3.89). Ectopic (tubal) pregnancy is readily diagnosed with US (Fig. 3.90).

Uterine anomalies and tubal diseases affecting fertility are often studied with hysterosalpingography. In this examination, contrast material is injected into the cervix, outlining the uterine cavity and fallopian tubes (Fig. 3.91). In the normal

FIGURE 3.87 Pelvis AP radiograph. Intrauterine contraceptive device. The *straight arrow* indicates the normal position and appearance of the intrauterine contraceptive device.

FIGURE 3.88 Transabdominal transverse obstetrical sonogram. Twin pregnancy. The twin fetuses (*straight arrows*) are located in separate sacs and are surrounded by amniotic fluid (*curved arrows*). The uterine wall is indicated by *arrowheads*.

— Urinary bladder

— Placenta previa

— Region of cervix internal os

FIGURE 3.89 Transabdominal longitudinal (sagittal) sonogram. Placenta previa. The sonogram shows the placenta covering the internal cervical os, thus precluding vaginal delivery.

FIGURE 3.90 Transabdominal oblique sonogram. Ectopic pregnancy. The *large arrow* indicates a hyperechoic, blood-filled uterus. The *small arrow* indicates the gestational sac in the right fallopian tube (B, urinary bladder).

— Isthmus of fallopian tube

— Ampulla of fallopian tube

— Peritoneal contrast media spill

— Fimbriated portion of the fallopian tube

FIGURE 3.91 Hysterosalpingogram. Normal uterus (*straight arrow*) and fallopian tubes. Contrast media injected into the uterus via a cervical cannula (*curved arrows*) spills into the peritoneal space, indicating fallopian tube patency.

FIGURE 3.92 Coronal (**A**) and axial (**B**) pelvic MRI. Uterine didelphys, demonstrating two separate uteri (*arrows*) with their endometrial cavities, two uterine cervices, and two vaginas (*curved arrows*). (Courtesy of Alan Stolpen, M.D.)

woman, contrast spills into the peritoneal cavity. Uterine anomalies can be detected with US, CT, and MRI (Fig. 3.92). Infected fallopian tubes typically fill with pus (pyosalpinx) and have characteristic US features (Fig. 3.93).

Benign uterine fibroids (leiomyomatosis), the most common gynecologic tumor, can (if calcified) be recognized by their classic appearance in the abdominal radiograph (Fig. 3.94). They are often seen on other imaging modalities (Figs. 3.95 and 3.96).

Imaging has, to date, played a minor role in evaluating carcinoma of the endometrium. MRI may be useful in staging cervical cancer (Fig. 3.97).

Detectability of ovarian tumors is much better with imaging studies than with physical examination. Tumors are seldom diagnosed on plain film unless they are huge or have typical features (Fig. 3.98). Both benign and malignant neoplasms have characteristic features on US, CT, and MRI. As in the kidney, US separates solid and cystic (usually benign) masses (Fig. 3.99).

FIGURE 3.93   Coronal transvaginal sonogram. Hydro(pyo)salpinx. The fluid collection has some internal echoes; its configuration is oval with a smaller oval communication (*arrow*) at the apex; this establishes the fallopian tube as the locale of the abnormality. (Courtesy of Monzer Abu-Yousef, M.D.)

FIGURE 3.94   Pelvic radiograph. The calcified uterine fibroids (*arrows*) are an Aunt Minnie.

FIGURE 3.95   Transabdominal longitudinal (sagittal) sonogram. The uterus is outlined by the *black straight arrows*. The electronic caliper *X marks* and *crosses* outline two large fibroids. The many internal echoes within the masses indicate that they are solid.

— Lumbar spine
  vertebral body

— Lumbar intervertebral
  disc

— Sacrum

— Urinary bladder

— Coccyx

— Rectum
— Vagina

— Pubis bone

— Anal canal

FIGURE 3.96 Pelvis midline sagittal T1 MR image. The enlarged uterus is outlined by *straight arrows*. Two large fibroids are indicated by the *curved arrows*.

FIGURE 3.97 Sagittal pelvic MR image. Cervical carcinoma. There is abrupt transition of normal uterine mucosa at the tumor margin (*arrows*). Inferiorly, the tumor is more infiltrative. (Courtesy of Alan Stolpen, M.D.)

FIGURE 3.98 Pelvic radiograph. Bilateral ovarian teratoma. Each tumor contains teeth (*arrows*) and substantial intratumor fat (*curved arrows*) allowing the tumors to be better visualized. (Courtesy of Alan Stolpen, M.D.)

FIGURE 3.99 Transabdominal sagittal sonogram. Mucinous cystadenoma of the left ovary. The ovarian mass has only a few internal echoes and demonstrates posterior enhancement typical of a cyst.

ACCESSORY DIGESTIVE ORGANS—IMAGING

Almost all imaging modalities can be used for the evaluation of liver disease. In general, the plain film is relatively insensitive, although it will show calcifications or gas in the liver. Evaluation for hepatomegaly is probably best by CT or nuclear medicine scans, although US examinations are also useful. MRI of liver disease is usually reserved for circumstances in which a definitive diagnosis is not possible with another modality.

Cirrhosis in North America is most often related to chronic alcoholism or as a complication of hepatitis. The severity of cirrhosis is primarily evaluated by physical examination and laboratory tests, but imaging is often useful. Early changes include hepatomegaly with fatty infiltration of the liver, easily detected on CT (Fig. 3.100). As cirrhosis progresses, there is diminution in the size of the liver and development of heterogeneous density of the liver parenchyma with a knobby surface related to coexisting scarring and regeneration of liver nodules (Fig. 3.101). Changes of portal hypertension (splenomegaly, ascites, and dilated portal veins and tributaries) can be found in severe disease. Portal venous flow may be reduced or even reversed in severe cirrhosis, and secondary hepatic venous occlusion can occur. These can be delineated with Doppler US examination (Fig. 3.102).

The liver is the most common site for metastases from intra-abdominal organs and often from tumors elsewhere in the body (lung and breast). Metastatic tumors in the liver are found 10 to 20 times more often than primary malignant tumors. Often, the hepatic metastatic disease is the first clinical indication of tumor. Imaging of metastatic liver disease is best done with CT using intravenous contrast material. Metastatic lesions are most often of reduced density when compared with the liver parenchyma (Fig. 3.103).

FIGURE 3.100 Axial abdominal CT. Fatty liver (not in a cirrhotic patient). The *large black arrow* indicates the fatty changes. The *small black arrow* indicates vessels within the fat. The *open arrow* indicates a normal enhanced liver.

FIGURE 3.101 Axial abdominal CT. Cirrhosis. The liver margins (open area) are nodular. There are scattered fatty changes (*arrowhead*) and ascites (*short black arrow*). Both lobes (*long two-headed arrow*) are involved.

FIGURE 3.103 Abdomen axial CT. Right and left hepatic lobe metastases. The metastases (*straight arrows*) appear hypodense compared with the enhanced normal liver. Liver enhancement was accomplished by intravenous injection of contrast media.

Benign primary tumors of the liver include hepatic cysts and cavernous hemangiomas, both are incidental findings and of no clinical significance. Larger hemangiomas or others with bizarre features may require MRI to be separated from malignant lesions (Fig. 3.104). Primary hepatoma occurs primarily in patients with preexisting liver disease. Hepatoma is less dense than normal liver parenchyma and has ill-defined margins. CT and MRI are useful for defining hepatic anatomy to determine resectability of tumors.

There are many methods to image biliary tract abnormalities. US is the workhorse. Gallstones are the most common abnormalities of the gallbladder. About 10% of stones are calcified and visible on plain films (Fig. 3.8). Ultrasonography is effective in detecting gallstones, as the highly echogenic stones are surrounded by echo-free bile. Failure to propagate the sound wave distally causes shadowing (Fig. 3.105). The common bile duct is also studied during gallbladder examinations.

Acute cholecystitis can be confirmed, if US shows gallstones, with thickening of the gallbladder wall and localized tenderness. In ambiguous cases, radionuclide cholescintigraphy is performed. In acute cholecystitis, there is obstruction of the cystic duct so that radioactive material secreted from the liver fills the biliary tract, including the common duct but not the gallbladder (see Chapter 9).

In distal obstruction, such as with common duct stones or pancreatic tumors, the proximal biliary tract dilates. Recent technical developments in MRI allow the evaluation of the biliary tract and pancreatic duct noninvasively. MRI offers spectacular imaging of biliary obstruction (Fig. 3.106).

FIGURE 3.102 Hepatic venous Doppler US in a cirrhotic patient. The study shows patent hepatic veins (*arrows*) converging. The up-and-down Doppler signal indicates normal venous flow. (Courtesy of Monzer Abu-Yousef, M.D.)

FIGURE 3.104 Axial MRI. Liver hemangioma. This study performed after intravenous administration of gadolinium shows a high signal mass (*arrows*) with bright walls characteristic of a hemangioma. (Courtesy of Alan Stolpen, M.D.)

Gallbladder wall
Gallbladder lumen
Liver

FIGURE 3.105 Longitudinal decubitus sonogram. Cholelithiasis. Note how the dense gallstones (calculi, *curved arrows*) cast acoustic shadows (between the *straight arrows*) because the sound waves are unable to penetrate or traverse the dense calculi. This is similar to a shadow cast by a tree or building.

Splenomegaly is sometimes evident on the abdominal radiograph (Fig. 3.3) but is more reliably evaluated by US or CT. There are measurements available to separate the normal-sized from the enlarged spleen, although considerable overlap exists. Perhaps this is an appropriate time to again quote Ben Felson, "A radiologist with a ruler in his hand is a dangerous person."

Pancreatitis occurs as a complication of alcoholism, biliary tract disease, and sometimes trauma. Although the inflamed pancreas sometimes appears normal on US or CT examination (Fig. 3.107A), more often there is diffuse or localized swelling of the gland and inhomogenicity of US signal and CT as well as adjacent fluid (Fig. 3.108). An important complication of acute pancreatitis is pseudocyst formation. The large, frequently multiloculated cysts are visible on either US or CT (Fig. 3.108).

In pancreatic carcinoma, clinical manifestations are infrequent before metastases have occurred. Both US and CT are useful for detecting pancreatic neoplasms as well as for staging the extent of metastatic disease. Tumor involvement of the celiac or superior mesenteric vessels makes resection impossible (Fig. 3.109).

Abscess can occur anywhere in the abdomen—in a solid organ such as the liver or loculated anywhere in the peritoneal cavity (Fig. 3.110). CT is probably the best modality to detect and locate an intra-abdominal abscess. Percutaneous drainage with CT guidance is often possible.

Abdominal aortic aneurysm is a common malady, particularly of the elderly. Calcification of the wall of the aneurysm is occasionally seen on plain films or the aneurysm detected incidentally on CT (Fig. 3.110). Abdominal US detects abdominal aneurysms, often when they are relatively small. In such circumstances, serial US examinations to evaluate the progression of disease may ultimately determine the need for repair. In larger aneurysms, extensive thrombosis occurs (Fig. 3.111). Dissection of an aneurysm occurs as a complication of atherosclerosis or other disease of the aortic wall. Here, blood dissects into the vessel media, producing a false channel and compromising the true lumen. As dissection progresses, there is hemorrhage into the retroperitoneum with shock and substantial mortality. CT (Fig. 3.111C) is a valuable method of diagnosing and staging this disease.

SPECIAL PROBLEMS IN ABDOMINAL IMAGING

Trauma

In all age groups, trauma is the most common cause of preventable disease. Major types of abdominal trauma include motor vehicle accidents, falls, and assault. Imaging studies are important in the evaluation of abdominal trauma as clinical evaluation is unreliable.

The first decision in dealing with a trauma victim is, "Is there any clinical evidence of abdominal abnormality?" Unless there is at least some clinical suspicion (e.g., abdominal pain, contusion, or guarding), the likelihood of finding significant disease with special studies is very low.

FIGURE 3.106 MRI cholangiopancreatogram. The common bile duct (*arrow*) and its proximal branches are dilated owing to obstruction (*curved arrows*) from pancreatic carcinoma. The pancreatic duct (*open arrows*), gallbladder, and duodenal lumen are also visualized. (Courtesy of E. Scott Pretorius, M.D.)

A

B

FIGURE 3.107   A: Transverse abdominal sonogram. Normal pancreas. The pancreas (*arrows*) is posterior to the liver (L) and anterior to the splenic vein (*curved arrows*). *Crosses* are in place to measure transverse pancreatic diameter. (Courtesy of Monzer Abu-Yousef, M.D.) **B:** Abdominal CT. Traumatic pancreatitis. The pancreatic body and tail (*arrows*) are enlarged and of uneven density. The mass (*curved arrows*) in the region of the pancreatic head is a hematoma.

FIGURE 3.108   Pancreatic pseudocyst. Abdominal CT. The hypodense pseudocyst (*arrows*) replaces the body and tail of the pancreas. (Courtesy of Bruce Brown, M.D.)

FIGURE 3.109   Abdominal CT. Pancreatic carcinoma. The pancreatic head and body (*arrows*) are normal. There is a poorly marginated hypodense mass (*curved arrows*) in the pancreatic tail. Several hypodense metastases (*open arrows*) are noted in the liver.

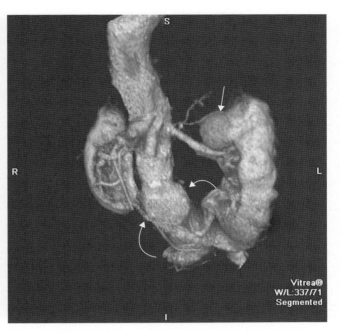

FIGURE 3.110   Abdominal aneurysm and renal cell carcinoma. CT angiogram. The cancer (*straight arrows*) extends from the superior pole of the left kidney. The abdominal aneurysm (*curved arrows*) is evident by the convexity of the aorta distal to the renal arteries.

FIGURE 3.111   **A:** Transverse and **B:** longitudinal sonograms. Abdominal aortic aneurysm. Thrombus extends from the aortic wall, restricting blood flow to the midportion (outlined by *markers*) of the aorta.

— Abdominal wall, three
   muscle layers

— Right and left kidneys

— Psoas muscle

— Quadratus lumborum
   muscle

FIGURE 3.111 (*Continued*) **C:** Axial abdominal CT. The *straight arrow* indicates the patent central lumen with thrombus (*curved arrow*) peripherally. The aortic wall (*double straight arrows*) is partially calcified.

If there is concern about abdominal injury, minimal imaging examination includes plain film with supplemental horizontal beam film (upright, decubitus, lateral). Although not a particularly sensitive examination, it is useful for orientation in subsequent studies and allows diagnosis of pneumoperitoneum, massive intraperitoneal fluid, or large soft tissue masses. Contrast studies of the gut, particularly with barium, are less sensitive than other imaging modalities, can cause significant imaging artifacts, and play no major role in acute trauma. EU is seldom performed because it is considerably less sensitive than other modalities. US, although useful in diagnosing large amounts of intraperitoneal fluid, is less sensitive than CT. Angiography plays a minor role, unless there is strong suspicion for vascular injury (e.g., a cold leg after pelvic trauma); it may have a therapeutic role in trauma patients, such as those with embolization of a bleeding spleen.

Focused assessment with sonography for trauma (FAST) has been suggested as a screening tool in abdominal trauma. The FAST scan is a US examination, usually performed in the trauma suite by an operator with basic US training. Although highly touted at the time of its introduction, current reports of its accuracy are very variable. Although specificity for diagnosis of hemoperitoneum is good, false-negative events (missing significant trauma) are quite common.

CT, particularly with multislice equipment, is the study of choice for evaluating abdominal trauma. With current equipment, the examination can be completed in less than 1 minute. Previously, most radiologists regarded patient hemodynamic stability necessary before CT could be performed. With the rapid procedure time available today, some compromise in the degree of stability is possible. Most examinations are done with administration of intravenous material. Oral contrast is customarily not given, because of the time involved for it to pass through the gut and its lesser value in diagnosis, unless bowel or pancreatic injury is suspected.

Hemoperitoneum from any source can be identified on CT, and the amount of blood can be quantified (Fig. 3.112). Multiple organ injuries are common; the liver, spleen, and kidney are affected more than other structures. Injuries to these organs are diagnosed with an accuracy of well over 95%. CT detects both the type and the severity of injury, an aid in determining which patients need immediate surgery versus nonoperative treatment (Figs. 3.112 to 3.114).

Gastrointestinal Bleeding

In acute GI bleeding, a major concern is to decide whether the source of blood loss is from the upper or lower GI tract. Statistically, about two thirds of patients have upper GI bleeding. Some common causes are listed in Table 3.7. Clinical clues are hematemesis, seen in bleeding from the upper GI tract, and hematochezia, from the colon. Melena can occur in either group but is more often associated with upper GI bleed.

Endoscopy is the procedure of choice for evaluating upper GI bleeding. It allows better localization than imaging examinations, and endoscopic treatment of the bleeding site is often possible. Imaging studies are used when bleeding is so massive that endoscopy is not practical. In these circumstances, angiography is often diagnostic and can be used therapeutically to occlude sites of bleeding (Fig. 3.115). Multislice CT can be valuable for acute bleeding, but barium is seldom indicated. For acute lower GI bleeding, proctosigmoidoscopy is the first procedure, followed by angiography, if needed.

FIGURE 3.112 Abdominal CT. Hemoperitoneum, owing to liver laceration in a child. **A:** An irregular laceration (*arrows*) is seen in the hepatic parenchyma. Blood (*curved arrows*) surrounds the borders of the liver and spleen. **B:** In the pelvis, blood fills the peritoneal cavity, outlining the infantile uterus (*arrows*).

FIGURE 3.113 Abdominal CT after intravenous contrast material. Splenic laceration. The anterior portion of the spleen (*arrows*) has irregular density and does not opacify. Hemoperitoneum is evident by the hypodense fluid at the margins of the liver (*curved arrows*).

222.0mm
0.0D
(255,273)

0.50s/10mm
+10.00mm/r

R

FIGURE 3.114 Abdominal CT after intravenous contrast material. Left kidney, traumatic laceration. Renal density is irregular anteriorly (*arrows*), indicating renal parenchyma admixed with blood.

In chronic GI bleeding, nuclear medicine studies are more sensitive than other imaging studies. Either technetium-labeled sulfur colloid or red cells can be used. These examinations allow detection of active bleeding as low as 0.05 to 0.1 cc per minute, and the examination can be done in less than an hour. Technical reasons favor one over the other in specific situations.

Acute Abdomen

A rough definition of *acute abdomen* is a situation involving a patient with acute abdominal pain and related signs wherein emergency surgery is being considered. Some common causes are listed in Table 3.8. In years past, exploratory surgery in the acute abdomen was often necessary, causing considerable morbidity and often unnecessary surgery. Imaging allows discrimination of nonsurgical disease (e.g., acute regional enteritis) versus diseases requiring surgery. It is of considerable value in delineation of the type of surgical disease—for instance, appendicitis versus ectopic pregnancy.

Traditionally, abdominal plain film and horizontal beam film are performed in all but those with the most urgent abdominal disease. Evaluation of the gas pattern and detection of pneumoperitoneum are its strong points. US is of value in certain situations, especially for gynecologic diagnosis; CT is generally more accurate in other areas.

Multislice CT is performed in most patients with acute abdomen, except those in whom clinical diagnosis is certain without imaging. These cases are done with the use of intravenous contrast (exception: suspected urolithiasis). Oral contrast and rectal contrast use have their proponents in the patient with acute abdomen, but others point out their disadvantages, particularly the increased time involved in the study.

The technique of CT examination is somewhat modified by the likely diagnosis suspected. Some common surgical causes of acute abdomen diagnosable on CT include appendicitis, bowel obstruction, urolithiasis, bowel perforation (most often peptic ulcer), gynecologic disease, pancreatitis, and aortic aneurysm. Less frequent causes include small bowel and colon disease, ischemic gut disease, and infections of solid organs.

TABLE 3.7

ETIOLOGY OF GASTROINTESTINAL BLEEDING

Esophagus, stomach, duodenum ■ Varices with portal hypertension ■ Peptic ulcer
Small bowel ■ Duplication ■ Mesenteric vascular disease ■ Meckel's diverticulum
Colon ■ Angiodysplasia ■ Polyp or tumor ■ Colitis

TABLE 3.8

COMMON CAUSES OF ACUTE ABDOMEN

Medical	Surgical
Chest disease—pneumonia, infarct, pleurisy	Appendicitis
	Cholecystitis
Cardiac disease—myocardial infarct, pericarditis	Bowel perforation
	Intestinal obstruction
Mesenteric adenitis	Pancreatitis
Ileitis, colitis	Mesenteric vascular ischemia
Renal colic	Salpingitis
Drugs	Ectopic pregnancy
Metabolic disease	Leaking abdominal aneurysm

FIGURE 3.115 **A:** Selective angiogram opacities of hepatic (*arrowheads*) and gastroduodenal (*curved arrows*) arteries. Bleeding duodenal ulcer. Contrast material (*straight arrows*) extravasates into the duodenal lumen, indicating an actively bleeding ulcer. **B:** Coils were introduced into the gastroduodenal artery. The follow-up angiogram shows the coils (*arrows*) in place with occlusion of the gastroduodenal artery. There was immediate cessation of the gastrointestinal bleeding. (Courtesy of Shiliang Sun, M.D.)

KEY POINTS

- Imaging evaluation of the abdomen usually begins with an AP supine abdominal radiograph. This is particularly helpful in evaluating the gas pattern.
- Small bowel obstruction is characterized by dilated small bowel proximally with collapsed colon and minimal rectal gas.
- In adynamic ileus, there is proportional dilatation of both small and large bowels with gas throughout the gut.
- If bowel perforation is suspected, it is critical to perform horizontal beam films (upright, decubitus, or cross-table lateral) inasmuch as little as 2 cc of free intraperitoneal air can be identified.
- Contrast studies of the gut remain a valuable method to detect intraluminal and mural diseases such as tumors, mucosal disease, and ulcerations. They are particularly useful in the small bowel, where endoscopy is technically difficult.
- US is the primary imaging modality for obstetrics and useful for detecting gallstones, renal and gynecologic disease, and abdominal aortic abnormalities.
- Abdominal CT is the method of choice for detection, localization, and characterization of tumors.
- CT diagnosis of appendicitis is very reliable, with direct visualization of the inflamed appendix in most cases.
- CTU and US are the methods of choice for most urinary tract abnormalities. EU offers less information.
- CT is the study of choice in evaluating the trauma patient.
- MRI is useful in a variety of special situations in the abdomen.

Suggested Readings

Brant WE, Helms CA. *The Brant and Helms solution: fundamentals of diagnostic radiology,* 3rd ed. Philadelphia: Lippincott Williams & Wilkins, 2006.

Dillman JR, Caoili EM, Cohan RH. Multi-detector CT urography: a one-step renal and urinary tract imaging modality. Abdom Imaging 2007;32: 519–529.

Gore RM, Levine MS. *Textbook of gastrointestinal radiology,* 3rd ed. Philadelphia: WB Saunders, 2008.

Haaga JR, Lanzieri CV, Gilkeson RC, eds. *CT and MR imaging of the whole body,* 5th ed. St. Louis, MO: Mosby, 2008.

CHAPTER 4 ■ PEDIATRIC IMAGING

WILBUR L. SMITH

NORMAL

Children are not merely small adults. Sure, the body parts (hearts, eyes, noses) are the same, but the fact that children are growing and changing subjects them to different diseases as well as to different structural appearances. Chest radiographs of young children, for instance, feature that ubiquitous but often misdiagnosed anterior mediastinal mass, the thymus (Fig. 4.1). This organ, important in the immune response, usually becomes inconspicuous by age 5 or so; however, its involution is extremely variable, and it is not uncommon to find thymic remnants on chest computed tomography (CT) scans up to age 20 years (Figs. 4.2 and 4.3). The thymus is a living piece of tissue that changes its configuration in a number of ways. In response to stress, it may shrink. When indented by the ribs, it may form a wavy border; in pathologic conditions, such as a pneumomediastinum, it may even be displaced superiorly and laterally over the lung fields (Figs. 4.4 to 4.6). The first rule in looking at children's radiographs is to expect change and variation and consider those factors before inventing a disorder that isn't real.

In general, congenital abnormalities are much more likely to present as clinical problems in neonates than they are in adults. Another way to look at it is if you got to adulthood without a congenital anomaly bothering you, it is likely that you will carry that anomaly to your grave. When you deal with an abnormal abdomen in a neonate, a congenital anomaly is extremely likely; in a 4-year-old it is somewhat likely; and in a 15-year-old it is less likely. If you play by the 99% rule in an 80-year-old, you probably shouldn't even think of congenital abnormalities as the cause of an acute abdomen. Having said this, I know that everyone will be able to find the unusual case of a congenital defect causing grief to an 80-year-old, but remember that's the zebra, not the horse!

Abdominal radiographs of neonates are very different from those of adults, whereas radiographs of older children and teenagers begin to have a lot of similarities with those of adults.

Abdominal films of neonates are especially discrepant because of a number of physiologic factors. First and foremost, neonates swallow a tremendous amount of air during their relatively inefficient breathing and eating. It is, therefore, not at all unusual to find many loops of small bowel in the plain film of a normal neonate (Fig. 4.7), whereas in an adult or older child it is unusual to see so much small bowel gas (Fig. 4.8). In fact, it is abnormal to see a gasless abdomen in a neonate! Such a finding usually means that the infant is so obtunded that it cannot swallow air, that there is a discontinuity of the gastrointestinal (GI) tract preventing air from entering the bowel, or that the infant is septic or otherwise critically ill (Fig. 4.9). All of this air in the small bowel makes the interpretation of the films difficult as far as determining bowel distention. The best rule to remember is that the bowel loops of a normal neonate are thin walled and lie in close proximity to each other. The appearance of thick-walled bowel or marked separation of the bowel loops suggests an abnormal intra-abdominal process (Fig. 4.10). Comparison of Figs. 4.7 and 4.10 illustrates this point.

The haustra of the colon are notoriously variable in their development and do not become prominent until about 6 months of age. For this reason, trying to differentiate large from small bowel on the plain radiographs of a neonate's abdomen is fraught with difficulty. Occasionally, you can get lucky and be reasonably certain in differentiation; however, most of the time it isn't even worth guessing. This makes the determination of whether there is rectal gas or not even more critical. The vast majority of newborns will have gas all the way through their GI tract by 24 hours after birth. If there is any doubt as to whether a child has rectal gas or has obstruction, the prone cross-table lateral film is invaluable in making this distinction (Fig. 4.11). Remember: if you are looking for distal gas in an infant in whom you are considering bowel obstruction, go right for the rectum! (Table 4.1).

Another big difference between neonates and older children or adults is the presence of the belly button. This necessary structure and the appurtenances appended to it make for

FIGURE 4.1 The large superior mediastinal mass that bulges both to the right and to the left is the thymus in this normal 3-month-old infant.

FIGURE 4.2 This teenager has a clearly visible thymic edge (*arrows*) on chest radiograph. Visualization of the thymus in normal teenagers is an unusual, but not rare, finding.

FIGURE 4.3 Chest CT of a 16-year-old patient shows a large thymus anterior to the opacified vessels. Note how the left lobe of the thymus (T) sticks out to abut the lung (*arrows*).

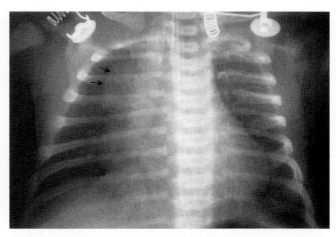

FIGURE 4.4 The large anterior mediastinal mass with the irregular margin (*arrows*) is the thymus. The thymic wave sign or undulating thymic border occurs because the costal cartilages are made of more firm tissue than the thymus; therefore, the thymus itself is indented. This is a normal finding.

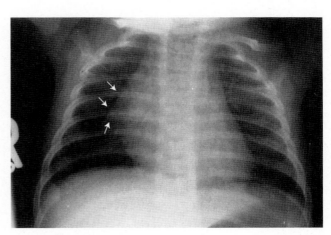

FIGURE 4.5 The so-called thymic sail sign shows the sharp edge of the thymus, somewhat like a boat sail, projected against the lung.

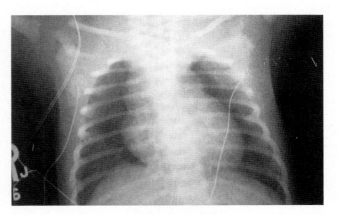

FIGURE 4.6 The large superior mediastinal mass in this otherwise well-term neonate is the thymus. If you call anything in the anterior superior mediastinum of a neonate normal thymus, you will be right 99% of the time.

FIGURE 4.7 This abdominal film shows the bowel gas pattern of a normal newborn baby. Notice that there are a number of nondistended bowel loops with considerable small bowel gas. The loops lie next to each other and are thin walled. This is a good visual picture to remember for the normal bowel gas appearance of a neonate. Older children do not have this much gas, and adults have very little small bowel gas, visible on plain films. Contrast this with Fig. 4.9, a baby with sepsis and some bowel wall edema.

FIGURE 4.9 Gasless abdomen in a very ill baby. There is almost always some gas in the stomach but very little gas distal. This is abnormal and can occur as a result of the baby being too ill to swallow or a systemic illness. In this case, the baby was immobilized so that he would not fight the ventilator and this gasless abdomen resulted. Normally, babies should have gas in both large and small bowels.

FIGURE 4.8 This plain film of the abdomen was obtained on a normal child with constipation. There is gas in the colon and stomach but very little gas in the small bowel. Contrast this to the appearance of Fig. 4.7, the neonate, where there is normally considerable small bowel gas.

FIGURE 4.10 Contrast the abdominal plain film in this critically ill and septic neonate with the normal bubbly pattern of bowel gas shown in Fig. 4.7. The loops of bowel are separated, and some of the bowel shows evidence of a moderate degree of dilation. These findings are nonspecific and can be seen in any severely ill infant. In this case, sepsis caused abnormal bowel motility in this abnormal appearing radiograph.

FIGURE 4.11 A prone cross-lateral view of the abdomen can often be helpful in showing whether or not gas is present in the rectum. Remember that because you cannot tell large bowel from small bowel in neonates, it is important to identify the rectum when you are trying to look for distal gas. Rectal gas is usually identified in the hollow of the sacrum, as in this infant.

some weird shadows on abdominal films of babies. Many an unsuspecting physician has called an umbilical clamp a bone or a foreign body (Fig. 4.12). The umbilicus itself protrudes much farther in a neonate than in an adult. Any coin-shaped lesion in the lower midabdomen of a neonate should be considered the umbilical remnant until proven otherwise. A good clue is that, owing to the air surrounding the protruding umbilical stump, the edges of the umbilicus are very sharply defined, particularly the inferior edge (Fig. 4.13).

In this chapter I will discuss some of the common radiographic diagnoses of children, first neonates, then the older child. The intent is not to be comprehensive, as there are 1000-page tomes for that; rather, this is intended to show practical imaging approaches to common diagnoses.

NEONATAL CHEST

The newborn's chest radiograph is a complex study with a substantial number of differences from that of an adult (Fig. 4.14). All babies have to change from an intrauterine environment where their lungs are fluid filled to one where they are breathing air. This transformation, which must occur within moments of birth, involves interaction of the pulmonary lymphatics, capillary vessels, and chest compression. This normal biologic process is not always smooth. In fact, many babies, if not all, have some very short-lived tachypnea in the first minute or two after being born, owing to the vagaries of clearing their normal *in utero* lung fluid. The physiologic phenomenon is reflected as the pleural effusions and streaky densities seen in the lungs on radiographs taken shortly after birth.

In an insignificant number of babies, it takes longer than a few moments to clear all of the *in utero* lung fluid. This condition has been aptly termed *transient tachypnea of the newborn* (TTN; Fig. 4.15). TTN should resolve clinically and radiographically within 24 hours, leaving behind a normal chest. In the first hours of life, however, this picture leads to a great clinical quandary because the radiograph of the neonate with TTN is indistinguishable from the radiograph of early neonatal pneumonia. There are a few clues, such as the presence of a large pleural effusion, which favors pneumonia; however, a definitive distinction can never be made. Here is a classic health care conundrum. TTN is much more common

FIGURE 4.12 A newborn infant who has just begun to swallow air. Notice the nasogastric tube marking the stomach. The oblong structure to the left of the spine (*arrows*) almost looks like a bone of some sort; however, it is clearly attached to the umbilical stump (*arrowhead*) and in fact represents an umbilical cord clamp superimposed on the abdominal film.

TABLE 4.1

CAUSES OF BOWEL OBSTRUCTION IN THE NEONATE

Atresia
Malrotation
Hernia
Meconium ileus
Hirschsprung's disease
Bowel duplications

FIGURE 4.15 Chest film of a 4-hour-old baby shows bilateral streaky densities whose distribution is asymmetric. Note that the lungs are also very hyperinflated. All this cleared within 24 hours, and the findings were due to transient tachypnea of the newborn. On this film alone, however, you cannot exclude pneumonia. It is necessary to have the follow-up film to confirm the diagnosis of transient tachypnea.

FIGURE 4.13 This baby undergoing an upper GI has a circular, bowel-filled mass in the lower midabdomen. The mass projects slightly to the left because the baby is in an oblique position (*arrows*). Note the very sharp margin, indicating that the mass protrudes off the abdominal wall. Anytime you see an extremely sharp border on a plain film of the abdomen, there has to be either air or fat surrounding that structure. In this case, air surrounds the structure because the umbilicus protrudes out from the abdominal wall. This is a typical umbilical hernia.

outcome is great, it alters the treatment choice when diagnosis is ambiguous. In other words, if you cannot tell, but the patient might die if you don't treat, overtreating is acceptable.

There are other neonatal lung diseases that exhibit radiographs showing bilateral streaky densities. TTN is the prototype for this appearance; however, neonatal pneumonia, neonatal venous stasis, and neonatal congestive heart failure can be mimicked. A few points of differentiation are possible. A large pleural effusion usually favors pneumonia and specifically *reactive* pneumonia, owing to group B streptococcal infection (Fig. 4.16). Most neonatal pneumonias are acquired during the birth process so that these pneumonias start small and tend to get dramatically worse over the first few days of life. If the streaky densities are associated with marked overaeration of the lungs, one might think of meconium aspiration. This disorder occurs when the newborns release their sphincters, spilling meconium into the amniotic fluid. This

than neonatal pneumonia; however, conventional diagnostic tests cannot separate the two. The outcome of an untreated neonatal pneumonia is dire, so what do you do? Most prudent physicians bite the bullet and treat, knowing that in many instances the antibiotics are unnecessary. This situation demonstrates the principle that if the perceived severity of possible

FIGURE 4.14 A normal newborn infant's chest. Notice the very different appearance from an adult chest. First, the heart and thymus are much larger than the cardiomediastinal silhouette of an adult. If you measure the heart and thymus (cardiothymic structures) and compare them to the diameter of the chest, often a baby's cardiothymic ratio will exceed 60% of the chest diameter. This is still normal. Notice also that the bones are very different, with a number of growth plates and other variants owing to infant development.

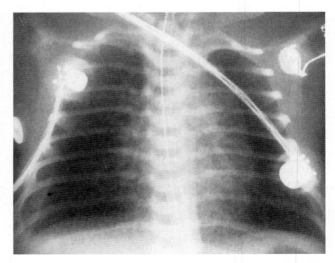

FIGURE 4.16 A very ill newborn with the streaky density pattern in both lungs and a large pleural effusion (*arrow*) on the right. Pneumonia plus a pleural effusion usually means group B streptococcal infection in neonates.

FIGURE 4.17 The anterior–posterior radiograph (**A**) and lateral radiograph (**B**) of a 1-day-old infant with severe meconium aspiration, showing marked hyperinflation of the lungs and bilateral streaky densities in both lung fields consistent with meconium aspiration. Notice on the lateral view (**B**) how flat the diaphragms are and how prominent the anterior–posterior diameter of the chest is. Meconium aspiration is highly associated with air-block phenomenon.

sphincter release, a response to stress, usually occurs *in utero* and the meconium is aspirated as the child begins to try to breathe. This is a particularly nasty pneumonia because the meconium is both irritating and viscous so that it obstructs the airways as well as causing the reactive pneumonia. One of the tips for diagnosing meconium aspiration is the massive hyperinflation of the lungs usually seen on the chest film (Fig. 4.17).

Babies can get congestive heart failure for a number of reasons, some of which involve intrinsic heart disease and many of which do not (Fig. 4.18). Arrhythmias, anemia, and arteriovenous shunts can cause high-output failure that is indistinguishable by chest film from the failure caused by intrinsic heart lesions such as hypoplastic left heart. The best clue that the streaky density pattern you are looking at on the chest film owing to heart disease is cardiomegaly. Beyond that, it is difficult to be more precise. The most important thing is to remember heart failure in your differential diagnosis.

HYALINE MEMBRANE DISEASE (AKA SURFACTANT DEFICIENCY DISEASE)

A common disorder of neonates is hyaline membrane disease (HMD). Here the clinical information helps a lot, as most of these infants are premature and most do not have respiratory distress immediately after birth. The other good news is that the radiographs are virtually diagnostic in the vast majority of cases (Fig. 4.19). The HMD radiograph shows four characteristic features: (a) diffuse granularity, (b) uniform disease, (c) air bronchograms, and (d) a relatively small lung volume. Not all radiographs will show all of these features, but most will have at least three.

HMD occurs owing to a lack of the lipid chemical surfactant that is synthesized by the alveolar lining cells of term infants.

These type 2 alveolar lining cells develop and mature during the third trimester of pregnancy; therefore, they are deficient among premature infants. Surfactant works by lowering the surface tension of the alveoli, allowing them to remain expanded. A simple analogy is that of a child's bubble pipe. You have to add soap to the water in the pipe to change the surface tension or you cannot blow many bubbles! If the surfactant is not present in the neonate's lung, the bubbles (alveoli) collapse. There you have it: The radiology of HMD is predominantly the radiology of profound atelectasis on an alveolar rather than a segmental level. In fact, some of the more forward-thinking clinicians propose changing the name of this disease to surfactant deficiency disorder.

SURGICAL CONDITIONS

Pediatric surgical disease of the chest of a neonate can be roughly defined as anything that needs prompt intervention (Table 4.2). By this definition, for example, a tension pneumothorax needing treatment with a chest tube is surgical disease. In assessing the newborn child's chest radiograph when surgical disease is suspected, you must take two steps. First, identify which side is the more abnormal (most surgical conditions are unilateral). Second, determine the direction of shift of the mediastinum. This is best done by looking at the trachea, but the position of the heart and thymus can also be secondary clues (Fig. 4.20). As a general (99%) rule, surgical conditions will displace the mediastinum *away* from the more abnormal side. For example, in the instance of a diaphragmatic hernia (a condition owing to an *in utero* defect that allows the abdominal contents to protrude into the chest), the heart and mediastinum are clearly shifted away from the side of the hernia by the mass of the protruding guts (Fig. 4.21). Therefore, if you look at the radiograph and decide that the

Vein

Posterior cerebral
branch

FIGURE 4.18 A: Cardiomegaly with pulmonary congestion in a child with congestive heart failure. The findings are nonspecific, and failure can occur due to multiple causes. **B:** A lateral arteriogram of the head of the baby shown in A shows the carotid artery branches (*arrows*) connecting to a large venous sinus, creating an arterial venous fistula. This condition is called a vein of Galen aneurysm. The baby is in high-output congestive heart failure.

FIGURE 4.19   Classic radiograph of a patient with hyaline membrane disease. Note that the lungs are relatively small in volume.

TABLE 4.2

COMMON SURGICAL CHEST CONDITIONS IN NEONATES

Pneumothorax
Diaphragmatic hernia
Lobar emphysema
Cystic adenomatoid malformation
Pleural effusions (large)

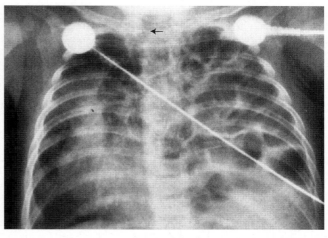

FIGURE 4.21 Bubbly material fills the left chest, displacing the heart and mediastinum far to the right. These bubbles actually are air-filled bowel. Notice the trachea area. Position of the trachea is the single best indicator of mediastinal displacement.

FIGURE 4.20 A very ill neonate. Note that the bubbly mass in the left lung base causes the heart and mediastinum to be shifted from left to right. First you decide which lung is abnormal (in this case, clearly the left). If the heart and mediastinum are shifted away from the abnormal lung, it is almost always surgical disease of the chest. Incidentally, the mass in this case is a cystic adenomatoid malformation, a benign tumor of the lung caused by abnormal budding of the foregut.

side with the bowel in the chest is the abnormal side, and then look at the mediastinal position, you can readily deduce that this is a surgical condition and an emergency.

When you are deciding on the more abnormal lung in neonates, remember that birth is a time of transition. In our example of a diaphragmatic hernia, *in utero* the bowel is filled with fluid. It isn't until the infant begins to breathe and swallow air that the gut assumes its normal postnatal air-filled condition. Therefore, the first film in a neonate may show a fluid density filling the chest, but within a few moments the normal swallowing of air results in replacement of this fluid density by the bubbly appearance of air-filled bowel.

In some conditions this transition to an air-filled mass can be even further delayed until 2 or 3 days after birth. This usually occurs in situations in which the connection between the lung and the tracheobronchial tree is abnormal, and it can take a considerable period of time, up to several days, for the normal *in utero* lung fluid to empty out and the air to fill the lung anomaly. A good example of this is lobar emphysema, a condition whereby the tracheobronchial airway connects abnormally to a lobe of the lung, allowing air to flow in but not out. The lobe, therefore, hyperinflates, becoming a tumor in the chest. Babies don't breathe air *in utero*; their lungs are fluid filled. Right after birth, this abnormally connected lobe is full of lung fluid as is the rest of the lung. The same mechanics that do not allow air to escape freely also do not allow the fluid to escape freely; therefore, it takes a long time for turnover of the fluid to take place, and the initial chest film looks like a solid (water) density mass with mediastinal displacement (Fig. 4.22). In a sense, it doesn't make

FIGURE 4.22 **A:** A neonatal chest film shows mediastinal shift from left to right and a partially opaque fluid density in the left upper lobe. This is a patient with congenital lobar emphysema and only partial emptying of the fluid from the emphysematous lobe. **B:** The same patient at age 11 months demonstrates findings more typical of lobar emphysema with the markedly hyperinflated upper lobe herniated across the midline (*arrows*). The principle for surgical disease remains valid; mediastinal shift away from the abnormal side needs rapid intervention.

any difference because criteria one and two for diagnosing a surgical condition are met no matter what the status of the mass; however, it's always nice to make a precise diagnosis.

ESOPHAGEAL ATRESIA

Our discussion so far has focused on lung disease, but of course there are other significant organs in the pediatric chest, including the heart and the esophagus. Esophageal abnormalities that are of importance in children are usually related to esophageal atresia. The most common form of esophageal atresia is a blind-ending proximal esophagus with a fistula extending from the trachea or left main stem bronchus to a blind distal esophagus. Inhaled air travels through the fistula and into the rest of the GI tract; therefore, the initial films can look superficially normal. The clues are that the GI tract is more distended by air than usual and the proximal esophageal pouch is very dilated. Clinicians become alerted to this condition when the child chokes on feedings and the pediatrician cannot pass a nasogastric tube into the stomach (Fig. 4.23).

There are two less prevalent but still frequent variants of esophageal abnormalities. The first is esophageal atresia without fistula, in which case the abdomen is gasless because the infant cannot swallow any air to displace the fluid that is in the abdomen *in utero* (Fig. 4.24). Such infants are usually

FIGURE 4.23   This very ill infant choked on being fed his first bottle. The chest radiograph shows a very dense right upper lobe infiltrate because of aspiration pneumonia. Note that the nasogastric tube won't go any farther than the upper esophagus (*arrows*). A surgical clip was placed to identify the site of the tracheoesophageal fistula as this infant was too ill to undergo primary repair of the esophageal atresia; a first-step procedure, ligating and dividing the fistula, was undertaken to protect his lungs. Survival of children with tracheoesophageal fistula correlates directly with the amount of lung disease owing to aspiration.

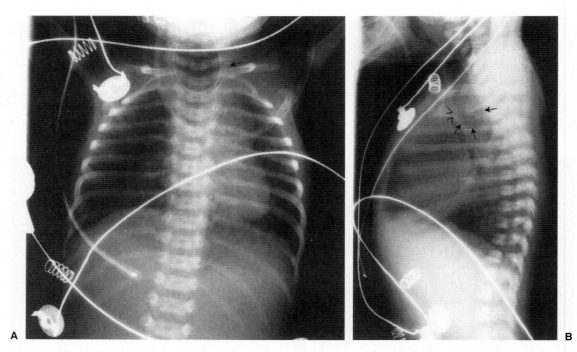

FIGURE 4.24   **A:** A typical radiograph of a child with esophageal atresia. Note the nasogastric tube (*arrow*) coiled in the upper esophagus. There are two major differences between this film and that of the child shown in Fig. 4.23. First, this child has not gotten aspiration pneumonia because this abnormality was recognized earlier and the child was not fed. Second, note that there is no gas in the abdomen. Patients with tracheoesophageal fistula always have the very distended stomach as each breath pumps air into that organ. The absence of gas in the abdomen makes the diagnosis of esophageal atresia without fistula. **B:** This lateral view of the same patient shows the very dilated proximal esophagus (*arrows*). Note that the dilated esophageal pouch displaces the airway anteriorly (*arrowheads*). These infants will often have abnormalities of the airway that accompany the abnormalities of the esophagus.

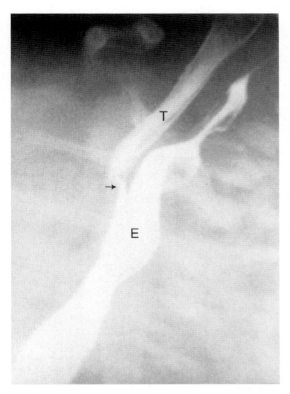

FIGURE 4.25   A barium esophagram on a baby with recurrent pneumonia shows a connection between the esophagus (E) and the trachea (T), a so-called H-type tracheal–esophageal fistula. This abnormality can sometimes be extremely difficult to detect.

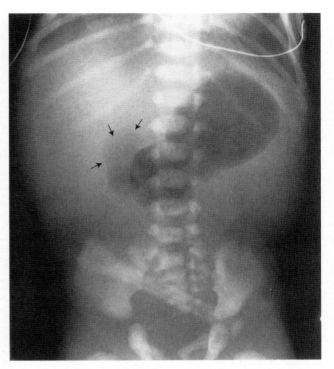

FIGURE 4.26   A newborn infant with marked abdominal distention. Note that the gas goes no farther than the very dilated duodenal bulb (*arrows*). This is characteristic of the so-called double-bubble sign of duodenal atresia. Whenever you see a patient with duodenal atresia, think of the very frequent associations of Down syndrome and congenital heart disease and the less frequent association of esophageal atresia.

FIGURE 4.27   This infant had a moderate degree of abdominal distention at birth, which progressed to a worrisome abdominal distention within 6 hours. Note that there is no gas in the rectum and that only two dilated loops of bowel are identified, predominantly in the upper abdomen and to the left of the spine. These films are most consistent with abdominal obstruction very high in the bowel but distal to the duodenum. This is an example of surgically proven jejunal atresia.

quite ill and need emergent surgery. The second variant is tracheoesophageal fistula without esophageal atresia. This so-called H-type fistula can be a difficult diagnosis. The nasogastric tube test is normal so that the diagnosis is not readily apparent to the clinician. The child usually presents frequent pneumonias because each time the infant eats, some of the material goes into the lung. Whenever you have an infant with frequent and recurrent pneumonia, this entity, along with cystic fibrosis, needs to be considered (Fig. 4.25). A barium esophagram is necessary to confirm the diagnosis.

CONGENITAL BOWEL ABNORMALITIES

Bowel Atresia

In babies, the commonest cause of bowel obstruction is atresia of the bowel. Atresia occurs owing to a number of complex intrauterine processes, most of which involve vascular supply to the wall of the bowel. Radiographs of the atresia vary tremendously according to the level at which the atresia occurs; however, they have common features. First, there is no gas distal to the level of the atresia, and second, the bowel proximal to the atresia is disproportionately dilated. Beyond that, it is just a matter of looking at the radiograph to try to guess how far down the bowel you can go before you encounter the atresia (Figs. 4.26 to 4.28). As a general rule to

A

B

FIGURE 4.28   A: Abdominal radiograph of a 1-day-old baby with abdominal distention shows evidence of multiple dilated bowel loops and no gas in the rectum. The findings are consistent with an ileal atresia. **B:** A decubitus view of the same infant illustrated in A shows multiple air–fluid levels. The presence of air–fluid levels is sometimes valuable in distinguishing ileal atresia from meconium ileus. Air–fluid levels favor ileal atresia. Incidentally, note our old friend, the cord clamp.

help you establish the level, remember that the duodenal bulb is located in the right upper quadrant of the abdomen; therefore, if you have a dilated stomach and loop only in the right upper quadrant, duodenal atresia is likely. The jejunum is predominantly in the upper abdomen and predominantly on the left side, whereas the ileum is in the right lower quadrant. If you see many dilated bowel loops and particularly large loops preponderantly to the right of the spine, it is probably an ileal atresia, whereas if the loops are confined to the upper abdomen and predominantly to the left, it is probably jejunal atresia. These are 70:30 rules, so don't get too preoccupied with them; on the other hand, they can be very helpful.

FIGURE 4.29 A newborn infant with a very distended abdomen. Note the bubbly appearance (*arrows*) in the right lower quadrant of the abdomen. These bubbles coupled with a paucity of gas in the rectum are characteristic of meconium ileus. The vast majority of babies with meconium ileus will also have cystic fibrosis.

Meconium Ileus

Meconium ileus is a condition that mimics a distal bowel atresia and that deserves special note because of its prevalence in the white population. In meconium ileus, the contents of the bowel (meconium) are abnormal, becoming thick and viscous due to the lack of digestive enzymes. This material compacts in the ileum to cause a complete obstruction. One could think of it as analogous to filling a pipe with tar. Technically, this is not an atresia; however, it mimics an atresia because the bowel is completely obstructed by intraluminal content. There are a few signs that can be used to distinguish meconium ileus from ileal atresia. The meconium ileus usually entraps some air so that one sees a bubbly appearance at the level of the meconium-filled bowel (Fig. 4.29). Also, the meconium is so thick and tar-like that it does not form air–fluid levels with the swallowed intestinal gas. This is in contradistinction to an ileal atresia, whereby the fluid intraluminal contents of the bowel interact with the swallowed gas to form multiple air–fluid levels.

No discussion of intestinal obstruction in neonates would be complete without mention of microcolon. *Microcolon* is another term for the small lumen colon that is encountered in babies with distal intestinal obstruction, usually either meconium ileus or ileal atresia. Babies' colons dilate because of the presence of intraluminal content, that is, meconium. This meconium is formed *in utero* by sloughing of the cells and mucus from the GI tract. If there is enough downstream bowel from

an obstruction (e.g., in the instance of duodenal atresia), there will be enough cells and mucus sloughed to form meconium and the colon will have this meconium content. If, however, the obstruction is low so that there is not enough bowel distal to the obstruction to form meconium, then one gets an unused or microcolon. Microcolon is, therefore, a common sign of distal bowel obstruction (Fig. 4.30). You can obviously be fooled, because diseases like Hirschsprung's disease, in which the lumen is intact but the colon does not transport meconium normally, occasionally give you a microcolon. Again, the 99% rule prevails that microcolon means distal obstruction.

Hernias

Two other congenital anomalies merit discussion as the cause of abdominal catastrophes in neonates or in slightly older children. The first is the most common cause of bowel obstruction in children, the hernia. Hernias in children are usually congenital defects that allow the bowel to protrude into a space where it doesn't belong. The bowel then gets caught, swells, and complications ensue. The most common site of hernia is the inguinal area (Fig. 4.31); however, internal hernias, particularly in areas where the bowel goes from retroperitoneum to an intraperitoneal location, are also possible (Fig. 4.32). Hernias can go on for a long time if the bowel does not become compromised, but they can become very symptomatic very fast in instances where the bowel is compromised (Fig. 4.33). Some

FIGURE 4.30 A contrast enema performed on the patient shown in Fig. 4.29 shows a very small (micro-) colon leading to a very dilated ileum distended with multiple filling defects. The filling defects are the impacted meconium, which gives meconium ileus its name. Remember that a microcolon means a distal obstruction.

A

B

FIGURE 4.31 **A:** Plain radiograph of the abdomen shows bowel lying below the inguinal ligament (*dotted line*). On a plain radiograph, the inguinal ligament is defined as the space between the symphysis pubis and the anterior superior iliac spine—in this case, the child had a large inguinal hernia filled with bowel. **B:** This baby, having a contrast study of the kidneys, had a protrusion of the lateral margin of his bladder into the right inguinal canal. A small protrusion can be normal; however, this large protrusion of bladder is associated with an inguinal hernia.

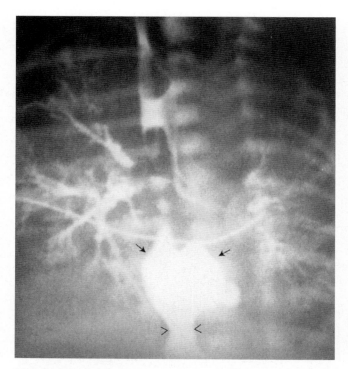

FIGURE 4.32 This neonate has a large hiatus hernia or protrusion of stomach above the diaphragm. The hernia pouch (*arrows*) is shown in the chest, whereas the narrowing of the esophageal hiatus (*arrowheads*) shows the area where the stomach herniates through the periesophageal hiatus. Note that there is contrast in the lungs. This hernia was so large that it caused the baby to reflux contrast from his stomach to his esophagus and then aspirate. Unlike this one, most hiatus hernias are relatively benign.

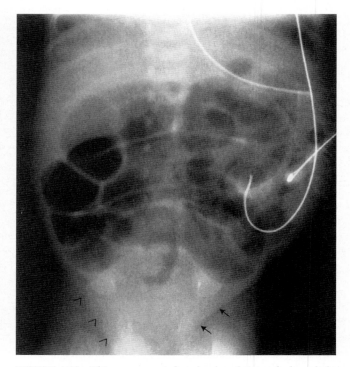

FIGURE 4.33 This premature infant developed signs of a bowel obstruction. Note the very dilated loops of small bowel on the film. The most important finding is the asymmetry of the inguinal folds, the right bulging in a concave fashion (*arrowheads*), whereas the left is straight (*arrows*). The bulge in the right groin is owing to an incarcerated inguinal hernia, a finding the clinicians missed until they took off the patient's diaper.

FIGURE 4.34 This baby with hydrocephalus had a ventricular peritoneal shunt. The radiopaque markers (*arrows*) show the course of the shunt. Notice that the shunt extends into an inguinal hernia. Because these babies have chronic ascites from the drainage of the cerebrospinal fluid into the abdomen, they are more prone to have inguinal hernias. Approximately one third of babies with ventricular peritoneal shunts develop inguinal hernias.

FIGURE 4.35 This 36-day-old infant began vomiting bilious material and became acutely ill. The plain abdominal radiograph is not diagnostic; however, note the gas-filled duodenal bulb (*arrowheads*). It is very unusual to see gas in a normal duodenal bulb. The subsequent upper GI proved that this patient had a midgut volvulus. The plain film findings in midgut volvulus range from normal to complete bowel obstruction. When in doubt with an infant with bilious vomiting, note that an upper GI is always indicated.

conditions of the neonate may enhance the possibility of a hernia, particularly conditions that involve chronic ascites, prematurity, or the presence of a ventricular peritoneal shunt for hydrocephalus (Fig. 4.34).

Malrotation

The other congenital abnormality worthy of special attention is that of malrotation. This condition occurs because of a congenital abnormality of fixation of the bowel. Remember that the bowel forms about the axis of the superior mesenteric artery (I bet you never thought you'd ever need that bit of embryology) and that the bowel herniates out of the body through the omphalus, then returns to the abdominal cavity. If, on return, the bowel does not rotate appropriately, it fixes in abnormal positions. This error in fixation of the bowel sets the scene for the bowel to twist and obstruct, causing the so-called midgut volvulus (Figs. 4.35 and 4.36). This is truly a surgical emergency and should be considered whenever you have an abnormal film suggesting obstruction as well as the presence of bilious vomiting in a child. Because the bowel twists about the superior mesenteric artery and vein, the major complication is vascular compromise of the bowel. If the bowel is not untwisted, the gut will die, leaving the child a nutritional cripple. Although malrotation is discussed with the neonatal diseases, be aware that it can present at any time in life. The majority of malrotation patients who get in trouble do so before 2 years of age; however, older children and adults can occasionally have malrotation-related problems.

FIGURE 4.36 Upper GI in a 27-day-old baby who suddenly developed bilious vomiting. Note that the duodenum descends in the midline, then passes off to the right at the duodenal–jejunal junction (*arrows*), never coming to the left of the spine and behind the stomach as is normal. This is characteristic of malrotation, an anomaly that occurs due to malfixation of the gut *in utero*. The greatest danger with these infants is midgut volvulus and infarction of the small bowel because of twisting about the vascular pedicle at the root of the mesentery.

A   B

FIGURE 4.37   A: This child's heart measures over 60% of the transverse diameter of the chest on the radiograph. In an adult, this would be a large heart; however, this is a normal child with a large thymus simulating cardiomegaly. **B:** Note that on lateral view, the heart does not protrude posterior to the airway (*arrows*).

CONGENITAL HEART DISEASE

Serious congenital heart disease has a prevalence of approximately 1 per 1000 live-born infants and, therefore, is a disease that you will likely encounter if you care for children. You could argue that this belongs in the neonatal section, but many children with serious heart disease present later, so I left it here—life is imperfect!

Although plain film is valuable for screening for congenital heart disease, it takes a tremendous amount of experience (and luck) before you can be specific as to the type of congenital heart disease. Several principles are very important. The first is that heart size in infants and children is more difficult to estimate than that in adults. The rule of thumb of 50% cardiothoracic ratio is not valid in children. When you're looking for cardiomegaly in a child, you need to be sure *that you are not looking at thymus, that the film has been taken on a good breath, and that lateral views are used extensively.* If the heart protrudes significantly beyond the visible airway on lateral view, the heart is usually enlarged. If on an anteroposterior view the heart appears large whereas on the lateral view it is normal, then you are usually dealing with a deceiving thymus (Fig. 4.37).

The second rule is that children can have very serious heart disease and a normal-sized heart. This is particularly true in conditions in which blood flow to the lungs is insufficient because of right-to-left shunting. As a good general rule, children's hearts, being resilient, tend to dilate owing to a volume rather than a pressure overload. Conditions that cause right-to-left shunting, like tetralogy of Fallot, do not give you an enlarged heart because the volume of blood traversing the heart is actually diminished (Fig. 4.38). A truly cyanotic neonate with a normal chest film (including heart size) usually has some variant of tetralogy of Fallot.

Rule number three is that if you think that the pulmonary vascularity is increased in a patient suspect for congenital heart disease, you are probably right; however, if you think it is decreased,

you are probably wrong. For some reason, it is much easier for humans to perceive an increase in vascularity than a decrease in vascularity in a chest film, probably because of the way our brains are wired. An enlarged heart and increased vascularity in an older child who is not cyanotic usually mean some form of left-to-right shunt such as a ventricular septal defect (Fig. 4.39).

Rule number four is applicable to neonates. We have already talked about the fact that being born is the ultimate time of transition. When you are *in utero*, very little blood goes through the pulmonary artery circuit. To understand this, think about physiology. *In utero*, the baby is not breathing air; therefore, there is no need for blood to bring oxygen to the

FIGURE 4.38   This cyanotic, extremely ill child has a relatively small but boot-shaped heart. The pulmonary vascularity is normal because of the presence of a patent ductus arteriosis. The findings are characteristic of a variant of tetralogy of Fallot.

FIGURE 4.39 The anteroposterior (**A**) and lateral (**B**) radiographs of a 2-month-old infant with respiratory distress when feeding, but no evidence of cyanosis, show a markedly increased pulmonary vascularity and a large heart. This combination in a child is characteristic of a congenital left-to-right shunt. The most common left-to-right shunt is a ventricular septal defect or a communication between the right and left ventricles.

baby from the lungs. Immediately following birth, the baby breathes air and the situation changes dramatically. It takes some time for the pulmonary arterial flow to reach adult levels of blood flow through the lungs. All neonates, therefore, have a relative state of pulmonary hypertension. Early on, lesions that should have increased vascularity, such as transposition of the great vessels, are not revealed by radiograph (Fig. 4.40).

FIGURE 4.40 This very cyanotic patient has a chest radiograph showing a large heart, narrow superior mediastinum, and pulmonary vascularity that is slightly, but not dramatically, increased. The patient is a 3-day-old infant with transposition of the great vessels; the vascularity is going through the transition between the very high vascular resistance *in utero* and the low vascular resistance of an air-breathing baby. Over the course of subsequent days, the vascular resistance will drop further and the lungs will become flooded.

The same logic explains why most left-to-right shunt lesions are not manifest until about 6 weeks of age (see rule three) when the pulmonary artery pressure has fallen significantly.

With those rules to consider, it is possible to set out a systematic approach to looking at the chest film of a newborn with congenital heart disease. First, see whether the heart is enlarged and whether you can determine which chamber is enlarged. Next, determine whether the vascularity is normal or increased, keeping in mind that the younger the baby, the less confident you can be to find increased vascularity. Finally, you need to talk to your clinical colleagues and find out whether the baby is truly cyanotic, as defined by arterial oxygen saturation of under 80% with a normal arterial CO_2 saturation. With those pieces of information you can look at Figs. 4.41 and 4.42 and make a rough estimate as to what type of congenital heart disease the baby may have (Figs. 4.43 to 4.45).

MEDIASTINAL MASSES

Other than the thymus and bronchi, the remainder of the structures in the pediatric mediastinum are relatively inconspicuous unless abnormal. Pediatric mediastinal abnormalities (masses) conform to a compartmental scheme. If you can accurately identify the compartment where a mass is located, you can provide an intelligent differential diagnosis. The anterior mediastinum is defined as part of the mediastinum visible in front of the airway on lateral view, and the posterior mediastinum is defined as that portion of the mediastinum just posterior to the anterior edge of the vertebral bodies on lateral view. Everything else is the middle mediastinal compartment (Fig. 4.46). The whole trick is telling these compartments apart, and there are a few rules:

1. *Clavicle cutoff sign*: The anterior chest is anatomically lower than the posterior chest, so if a mass stops at the inferior margin of the clavicle on the PA chest radiograph, it has to be in the anterior mediastinum (Fig. 4.47).

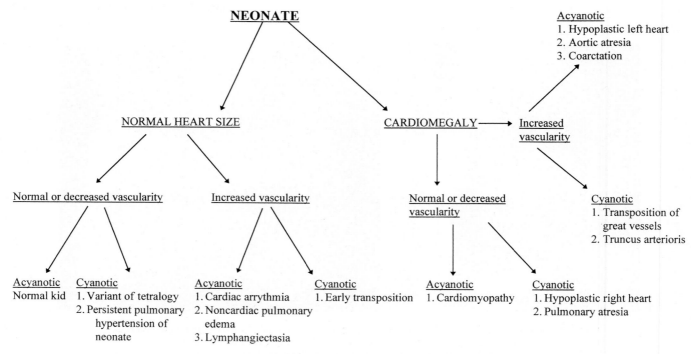

NEONATE

Acyanotic
1. Hypoplastic left heart
2. Aortic atresia
3. Coarctation

NORMAL HEART SIZE

CARDIOMEGALY → Increased vascularity

Normal or decreased vascularity

Increased vascularity

Normal or decreased vascularity

Cyanotic
1. Transposition of great vessels
2. Truncus arterioris

Acyanotic
Normal kid

Cyanotic
1. Variant of tetralogy
2. Persistent pulmonary hypertension of neonate

Acyanotic
1. Cardiac arrythmia
2. Noncardiac pulmonary edema
3. Lymphangiectasia

Cyanotic
1. Early transposition

Acyanotic
1. Cardiomyopathy

Cyanotic
1. Hypoplastic right heart
2. Pulmonary atresia

FIGURE 4.41 Flow diagram for neonates suspect for heart disease.

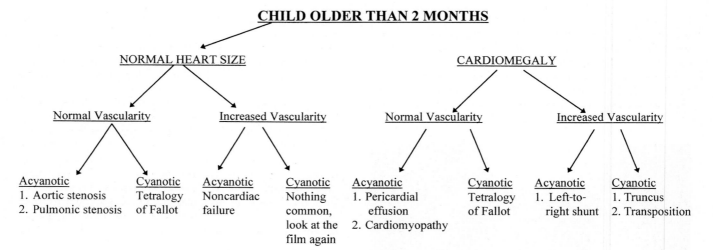

CHILD OLDER THAN 2 MONTHS

NORMAL HEART SIZE

CARDIOMEGALY

Normal Vascularity

Increased Vascularity

Normal Vascularity

Increased Vascularity

Acyanotic
1. Aortic stenosis
2. Pulmonic stenosis

Cyanotic
Tetralogy of Fallot

Acyanotic
Noncardiac failure

Cyanotic
Nothing common, look at the film again

Acyanotic
1. Pericardial effusion
2. Cardiomyopathy

Cyanotic
Tetralogy of Fallot

Acyanotic
1. Left-to-right shunt

Cyanotic
1. Truncus
2. Transposition

FIGURE 4.42 Flow diagram for older children suspect for heart disease.

FIGURE 4.43 This child has a huge heart. Note that the superior mediastinum has a large shadow to the right of the trachea, a right aortic arch. The vessels are large, flooding the lung. If we add the information that the child was cyanotic, then this becomes a characteristic truncus arteriosis. Approximately 40% of truncus patients have a right arch.

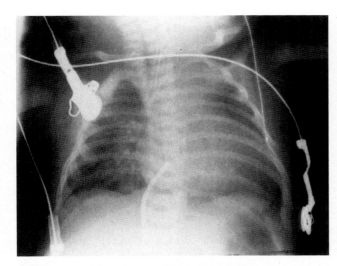

FIGURE 4.44 A large heart and increased vascularity; however, this time the child is not cyanotic. This usually means either a left heart obstructive lesion or a failure for some other reason. The child has a hypoplastic left heart.

FIGURE 4.46 A normal lateral view of the chest, with barium in the esophagus, delineates the boundaries of the anterior (A), middle (M), and posterior (P) mediastinum. When you consider mediastinal masses, it is important mentally to divide the mediastinum into these components as it helps you localize the likely diagnosis for the cause of the mass.

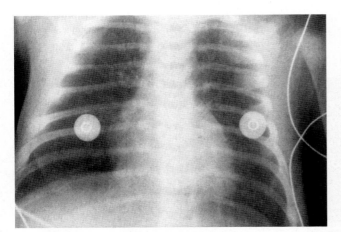

FIGURE 4.45 A large heart and increased vascularity in a 2-week-old baby—findings typical for transposition of the great vessels. Note the very thin mediastinum because the pulmonary artery is directly in front of the aorta as opposed to being slightly to the left of it. This is characteristic of the transposition of the great vessels.

FIGURE 4.47 This anterior mediastinal lymphoma stops right at the undersurface of the clavicles. Remember that the anterior portion of the chest is physically lower than the posterior portion of the chest; therefore, any mass that has the clavicle as its superior margin must be an anterior mediastinal mass.

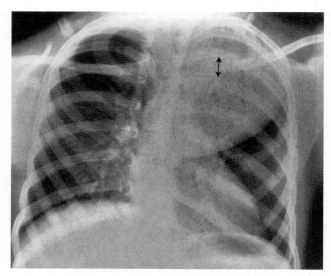

FIGURE 4.48 This teenager has an anterior mediastinal mass. Note that the descending branch of the right pulmonary artery (*arrows*) is visible through the mass, documenting that the tumor is not in the same plane as the vessel; otherwise, the silhouette sign would prevent the vessel from being visible. This is called the hilum overlay sign where masses out of plane of the hilum (usually anterior mediastinal masses) allow hilar structures to be visualized.

2. *Hilum overlay sign*: Structures in the far anterior mediastinum overlie the vessels at the lung hilum; therefore, the vessels are usually seen through these structures (Fig. 4.48).
3. *Posterior rib effacement*: Posterior mediastinal masses frequently spread the posterior ribs; therefore, distortion or asymmetry of the posterior ribs is a good sign that the mass is posterior (Fig. 4.49).

FIGURE 4.49 This child has a huge posterior mediastinal mass on the left. Note how the mass has spread the ribs posteriorly. Masses that distort the posterior ribs are almost always neural crest in origin, in this case a ganglioneuroblastoma.

4. *Airway distortion sign*: Masses that distort the esophagus or compress the airways are almost surely middle mediastinum (Fig. 4.50).

Once you have applied these rules and decided in which compartment to look, the pathologic processes tend to categorize themselves fairly easily. Anterior mediastinal masses are almost always lymphoma or thymus related with the occasional thyroid mass or teratoma. An Aunt Minnie applies here: If the anterior mediastinal mass contains calcium, always go for teratoma (Fig. 4.51). Middle mediastinal masses are generally

FIGURE 4.50   **A:** The large mass (*arrows*) near the mediastinum is displacing the upper lobe bronchus on the left. Note that the left lung is blacker than the right because the mass is causing partial obstruction of the left main stem bronchus, allowing air to get in but not to escape easily. The effect on the bronchus or blood vessels is characteristic of a middle mediastinum mass, in this case, a bronchogenic cyst. **B:** Lateral view shows the rounded mass (*arrows*) of the bronchogenic cyst in the same plane as the airway (*arrows*).

FIGURE 4.51 The mass lying anterior to the right hilum (*arrowheads*) contains a large glob of high-density calcium. Remember that anterior mediastinal mass plus calcium equals teratoma.

FIGURE 4.52 This 6-week-old infant had severe and pernicious vomiting that had become progressively worse over the course of a week. The impact on his nutrition was so severe that he had actually lost weight. Note the distended stomach (*arrowheads*). The presence of distal gas in his rectum shows that he was not completely obstructed, but the film is suggestive of a high-grade partial gastric outlet obstruction. About 90% of pyloric stenosis patients will have a plain film that looks like this.

either lymph nodes or anomalous vessels related to the aortic arch. Esophageal and bronchial duplications are less frequent but also occur in the middle mediastinum. Posterior mediastinum masses are neurogenic in origin, usually a neuroblastoma or ganglioneuroblastoma. When confronted with a suspected pediatric mediastinal mass, the first rule is to place it in the proper compartment; thereafter, it is a matter of pursuing the differential diagnosis.

PYLORIC STENOSIS

A common intra-abdominal condition worth discussion in babies (not brand new but 4 to 6 weeks old) is pyloric stenosis, which isn't a congenital anomaly. Pyloric stenosis is due to hypertrophy of the pyloric muscle induced by a heritable error in metabolism. Because of the heritable nature of the disease, it is somewhat a congenital defect, but it does not usually present right after birth because it takes some time for the abnormal chemistry to cause the pyloric muscle to hypertrophy to a sufficient degree to obstruct gastric outflow. The disease is male preponderant and classically presents with nonbilious vomiting and weight loss in a 6-week-old infant. The plain abdominal radiograph suggests a partial obstruction with a very dilated stomach. Upper GI will show elongation of the pyloric channel and the narrowing of that channel. Ultrasound is the current favored method for the definitive diagnosis, showing the very large pyloric muscle tumor in exquisite detail (Figs. 4.52 to 4.54).

CONDITIONS IN OLDER CHILDREN WITH CYSTIC FIBROSIS

When you are studying pediatric patients, it is always important to remember that the prevalence of congenital or heritable

FIGURE 4.53 The upper GI in this 6-week-old baby shows elongation and narrowing of the pyloric channel (*arrowheads*). On the stomach side, notice the rounded indentation (*arrows*) caused by the very hypertrophied pyloric muscle. This is called the shoulder sign. Together this combination of signs is diagnostic for pyloric stenosis.

FIGURE 4.54   **A:** A longitudinal ultrasound view of the pylorus in a 6-week-old boy with vomiting. The pyloric muscle appears black, whereas the mucosa of the central lumen appears white (*arrows*). During the entire period of observation, the configuration of the pyloric muscle did not change and measurement of the pyloric muscle revealed a thickness of 6 mm (normal is greater than 4 mm). This is diagnostic of pyloric stenosis. Note the intimate relationship of the pylorus to the right kidney (K). **B:** Transverse ultrasound view of the pylorus in the same infant as shown in A. Again the black or hypoechoic muscle surrounds the very echogenic mucosa. Arrows outline the transverse view of the pylorus. In pyloric stenosis, the muscle is thick and unchanging throughout the examination.

abnormalities is higher among the pediatric population than the adult population. Therefore, in looking at the radiographs of a child with recurrent pneumonias, you should think about heritable conditions that predispose the child to pneumonia, an example being cystic fibrosis. Cystic fibrosis, the most prevalent lethal genetic disease among the white population, begins with recurrent pneumonias but also has a number of features that allow a specific diagnosis from the films (Fig. 4.55). The lungs are usually hyperexpanded because of the blockage of

many of the smaller bronchi by mucous plugs. The presence of mucoid impactions, branch-shaped collections of intra-bronchial mucus, is very suggestive of cystic fibrosis. Generally, the children have very prominent hili due to the combination of the inflamed lymph nodes and pulmonary artery enlargement resulting from pulmonary hypertension caused by lung destruction. The last common finding of cystic fibrosis is that of peribronchial cuffing, or thickening of the walls of the bronchus, due to the intense inflammatory change induced by the disease (Fig. 4.56). None of these signs are

FIGURE 4.55   Typical chest film of a child with cystic fibrosis. Patchy infiltrates are present in both lung fields. The right hilus is very large and irregular owing to a combination of enlarged pulmonary artery and lymph nodes (*arrows*). Also note that the heart is very small because of markedly overly expanded lungs. The pulmonary arteries are large because of a pulmonary hypertension. This is a very typical appearance for cystic fibrosis.

FIGURE 4.56   A close-up of the lung showing peribronchiolar thickening. Note that the bronchus appears as a black dot amid a white cuff. This cuff is edema and inflammatory cage in the bronchial wall.

pathognomonic for cystic fibrosis; however, all of these signs taken in combination make the likelihood of this disease very high.

INTUSSUSCEPTION

Intussusception, a disease in which one segment of bowel telescopes into another, has its maximum prevalence between the ages of 6 months and 2 years. The bowel is constantly in motion because of normal peristaltic activity. Theoretically, an inflamed intramural lymph node or some other structure alters this peristaltic activity, such that one segment of bowel begins to be propelled at a differential rate, leading to prolapse of one segment (intussusceptum) into the next contiguous portion of bowel (intussuscipiens). The intussusceptum becomes edematous because the blood supply of the prolapsed bowel is compromised and the intussusceptum begins to swell. This compounds the problem and leads to further extension of the intussusception. The ultimate extension is protrusion of the intussusceptum from the rectum! In fact, in nineteenth century textbooks, the differential diagnosis of intussusception was rectal prolapse. The most common anatomic area involved in intussusception is the terminal ileum, and most intussusceptions are ileocecal.

Radiology plays a key role in the diagnosis as the child often presents with acute abdomen. Plain film shows evidence of partial bowel obstruction, and the intussusceptum is frequently visible on the plain film as a rounded density near the point of obstruction (Fig. 4.57). Diagnosis is confirmed either by ultrasound or by barium enema (Figs. 4.58 and 4.59). Radiology often plays both a diagnostic and a therapeutic role in intussusception. Between 50% and 80% of intussusceptions can be nonoperatively reduced using either an air enema or a contrast enema. These techniques are very specialized and should be performed only by trained personnel. They are, however, part of the standard armamentarium of any board-certified radiologist.

APPENDICITIS

Appendicitis is the most common abdominal surgical emergency of later childhood. Appendicitis is one of the great mimics in that the symptoms can be fairly protean and the diagnosis in many instances is obscure (Table 4.3). There is an old adage that the clinical certainty of appendicitis should be about 85%, meaning that 15% of the appendices that a surgeon removes should be normal or the surgeon is going to begin to miss some true-positive cases of appendicitis. Various radiology imaging techniques can narrow this false-positive rate somewhat, but really the value of imaging is in those cases in which the diagnosis is in serious doubt. Look at it in another way. If imaging tests can give you 95% sensitivity, whereas clinical tests are 85% sensitive, the imaging doesn't add much in a situation in which you are quite sure that

FIGURE 4.57 Notice the rounded density and a spiral gas pattern located in the right upper quadrant in this 2-year-old child with recurrent cramping, abdominal pain, and hematochezia (*arrows*). This plain film alone, if not diagnostic, is certainly very suspicious of intussusception. About 80% of the time you can make the diagnosis of intussusception on plain film by looking for a rounded mass and the spiral air pattern that is so characteristic.

appendicitis exists. On the other hand, in that case when you aren't sure or, let's say, you are only 30% sure, a 95% sensitivity test is crucial in deciding appropriate patient management. At current hospital prices, it is cheaper to do the test than to put the patient in the hospital overnight for observation. Appendicitis is discussed in detail in Chapter 3, so it will only be mentioned here.

TABLE 4.3

CLASSIC SIGNS OF APPENDICITIS[a]

1. Right lower quadrant pain
2. Leukocytosis
3. Anorexia/vomiting

[a]Only half of appendicitis patients younger than age 5 or older than age 50 exhibit these signs!

FIGURE 4.58   A: A longitudinal ultrasound view of an intussusception. Notice the intussusceptum (*arrowheads*) telescoping into the intussuscipiens. With a little imagination, you can almost see a coiled spring signal as the bowel wrinkles, with one loop of the bowel prolapsing into the other. **B:** A transverse view of an intussusception showing the target sign. The brightly echogenic material is the edematous mucosa, whereas the less echoic material is the wall of the intussusceptum.

FIGURE 4.59 **A:** The barium enema in this 2-year-old child shows a round defect in the area of the cecum. Notice how the barium infiltrates in a spiral pattern as it pushes its way between the intussusceptum and the intussuscipiens. This so-called coiled spring (*arrows*) is characteristic of intussusception. **B:** This is a CT scan of a child with known tumor affecting the bowel wall. The child presented with abdominal pain owing to an intussusception (*arrows*) caused by a metastasis to a lymph node near his ileocecal valve. Note on this CT how you can see the same signs: the blunt-headed intussusceptum and the stretched fat of the mesentery, as the intussusceptum is propelled forward into the intussuscipiens. Also note the multiple fluid-filled bowel loops (*arrowheads*) from dilated small bowel secondary to the partial small bowel obstruction from the intussusception.

SUMMARY

In this chapter, we have discussed the radiographs of children with particular emphasis on those conditions that are common and unique to pediatrics. As in any imaging, there will always be exceptions, but a few rules are key. Always remember the thymus as a deceiver in evaluating chest films in children, particularly younger children. Any anterior mediastinal mass is thymus, thymus, and thymus! Neonatal medical and surgical chest disease can be easily differentiated by remembering the rules of mediastinal shift and unilateral abnormality. If you apply carefully the rules of looking at congenital heart disease and mediastinal masses, you should be able to get into the ballpark about 80% of the time for making an accurate diagnosis of the correct lesion. That's a lot better than Babe Ruth did at batting, and look at how famous he is.

In summary, remember that it is normal for neonates to have considerable gas in their small bowel. As long as the walls are thin and the bowel loops are approximating each other, don't worry. Also remember that up to 6 months of age it is extremely difficult to tell large bowel from small bowel, and guesses as to whether a loop represents large or small bowel on plain film are exactly that—educated estimates. In babies with distended tummies, always look to the rectum to determine the presence of distal gas and thereby obstruction.

KEY POINTS—CHEST

■ In some babies, *in utero* lung fluid takes more than a few minutes to clear, resulting in TTN. This appears on radiographs as pleural effusions and streaky densities. TTN should resolve within the first 24 hours after birth.

■ TTN is indistinguishable on radiographs from early neonatal pneumonia.

■ The best clue to diagnosing congestive heart failure in babies is a radiograph displaying a streaky density pattern in the lungs and cardiomegaly. If the heart protrudes significantly beyond the visible airway on a lateral radiograph, the heart is generally enlarged.

- HMD displays four characteristic radiographic features: diffuse granularity, uniform disease, air bronchograms, and a relatively small lung volume.
- Generally, surgical conditions are unilateral and will displace the mediastinum away from the more abnormal side.
- Radiographic features of cystic fibrosis include hyperexpanded lungs, mucoid impactions, very prominent hili, and peribronchial cuffing.

KEY POINTS—ABDOMEN

- In summary, the rules for evaluating an infant's abdomen are different from those used for adults.
- The younger the child, the more discrepant the rules.
- Babies have a lot of air, and it is difficult to differentiate large from small bowel by plain film.
- Young children usually have congenital anomalies or atresias; slightly older children have manifestations of either congenital anomalies or heritable anomalies such as pyloric stenosis and malrotation.

- In children beyond 6 months, intussusception and appendicitis are the major clinical entities.
- In looking at abdominal films of children, remember that your odds are much better in diagnosing an unusual manifestation of a common disease (such as appendicitis) than in diagnosing a common manifestation of a rare disease.
- If you stick with the diagnosis and rules from this chapter, you will be right more often than you will be wrong.

References

1. Silverman FN, Kuhn JP. *Caffey's pediatric x-ray diagnosis: an integrated imaging approach,* 9th ed., vols. 1 and 2. St. Louis, MO: Mosby, 1993.
2. Franken EA Jr, Smith WL. *Gastrointestinal imaging in pediatrics,* 2nd ed. New York: Harper & Row, 1982.

Suggested Readings

Hedlund GL, Griscom NT, Cleveland RH, Kirks DR. Respiratory system. In: Kirks DR, Griscom NT, eds. *Practical pediatric imaging: diagnostic radiology of infants and children.* Philadelphia: Lippincott-Raven Publishers, 1998.
Strife JL, Bissett GS, Burrows PE. Cardiovascular system. In: Kirks DR, Griscom NT, eds. *Practical pediatric imaging: diagnostic radiology of infants and children.* Philadelphia: Lippincott-Raven Publishers, 1998.

CHAPTER 5 ■ MUSCULOSKELETAL SYSTEM

WILLIAM E. ERKONEN AND CAROL A. BOLES

NORMAL DEVELOPMENT

When you think about it, bones are visible on nearly all radiographs. Therefore, radiologic anatomy of the musculoskeletal system is extremely important, but it is time-consuming to learn. Entire textbooks are dedicated to isolated joints, and there are just no shortcuts to mastering this detailed material. As always, a solid knowledge of normal image anatomy is a prerequisite for intelligent image evaluation. Remember that the anatomic structures are all the same—we are merely viewing them differently. Let us begin with normal image anatomy of the hand and move systematically cephalad to the shoulder girdle. This will be followed by normal image anatomy of the lower extremity from the foot to the hip.

The bones develop in a rather systematic fashion. Bone formation is by either intramembranous (transformation of mesenchymal tissue) or endochondral (conversion of an intermediate cartilage form) formation, or by both methods.

Many flat bones, such as the skull and mandible, form by intramembranous bone formation. Both methods are found in the extremities, spine, and pelvis. With endochondral ossification, cartilage is replaced by bone initiated at specific sites called centers of ossification. These centers of ossification appear in such a predictable order that they may be used for estimation of age. (Table 5.1) Understanding this aids in evaluation of fractures in the pediatric population as a small bone adjacent to a joint may be assumed to be an ossification center when it is, in fact, a fracture. The area of cartilage between the centers of ossification is often called the growth plate, or physis. Eventually, the centers of ossification fuse across the physis.

Joints develop between the developing ends of bone. There are three types of joints: synchondrosis, symphysis, and synovial joints. A synchondrosis has hyaline cartilage between the ends of bone and not movable while symphysis joints have fibrocartilage and a small amount of motion. Synovial joints have mesenchymal tissue converted into synovium, which will eventually produce fluid to lubricate these movable joints.

NORMAL EXTREMITY IMAGES

Upper Extremity

People commonly injure their extremities because they actively encounter the environment with their arms and legs. Consequently, you will probably order many radiographs of the extremities in your clinical practice. Thus, we need a system to evaluate upper and lower extremity images (Table 5.2). Each bone in an image must be carefully evaluated for density, variations of normal, and fracture. Also, each joint must be evaluated for width, smoothness of the articular surfaces, dislocation, arthritis, fracture, and foreign body. The soft tissues should be evaluated for edema, hemorrhage, masses, calcifications, and foreign bodies.

The hand is so complex that it is a subspecialty in both orthopedics and plastic surgery, so don't expect to conquer the anatomy overnight. When you request radiographs of the hand, the standard study usually consists of posteroanterior (PA), oblique, and lateral views (Fig. 5.1). *Remember that one of the most difficult aspects of medicine is to learn the jargon*

TABLE 5.1

AVERAGE AGE OF APPEARANCE OF SOME MAJOR OSSIFICATION CENTERS

Ossification center	Average age (girls usually earlier than boys)
Head of humerus	2 weeks
Head of femur	4 mo
Distal radius	1 y
Patella	4 y
Elbow	
Capitellum	3 y
Radial head	5 y
Medial epicondyle	6 y
Trochlea	8 y
Lateral epicondyle	10 y
Olecranon	11 y
Acromion	13 y
Coracoid process of scapula	14 y
Ischial tuberosity	15 y
Inner margin clavicle	19 y

TABLE 5.2

OBSERVATION CHECKLIST FOR BONE RADIOGRAPHS

Each bone should be evaluated for
    Density
    Anomaly
    Fracture
    Tumor
    Foreign body
    Infection
Each joint should be evaluated for
    Articular surface smoothness
    Symmetry
    Fracture
    Dislocation
    Arthritis
    Foreign body
Soft tissues should be evaluated for
    Edema
    Hemorrhage
    Calcifications
    Masses
    Foreign bodies

and routines, so we need to get the hand terminology correct from the beginning. Each digit of the hand must be properly named to communicate and document information accurately. The proper terminology for each digit and the numbering system for the metacarpals are displayed in Fig. 5.1A. Simply numbering the digits does not suffice, especially in situations in which digits are missing. Would you refer to the index finger as the first or second finger when the thumb is missing? So, beginning on the radial side of the hand, the thumb is always

the thumb and not the first finger. Next is the index finger (not the second finger and not the first finger as some say there are four fingers and a thumb). Then the long finger (not the third or middle finger), the ring finger (not the fourth), and the small or little finger (not the fifth).

Metacarpals (Fig. 5.1A) are numbered logically with the thumb articulating with the first metacarpal, the index finger with the second metacarpal, and so on. As a general rule, each hand digit has three phalanges except the thumb, which has

Distal, middle, and proximal phalanges

Distal and proximal phalanges of thumb

Metatacarpal phalangeal joint (MCP)

Head shaft, base 1st metacarpal

Distal interphalangeal joint (DIP)

Proximal interphalangeal joint (PIP)

Thumb, index, long, ring, and short fingers

Sesamoid bone

1st, 2nd, 3rd, 4th, 5th metacarpals

Carpals

Ulna styloid

Radius styloid

Oblique   PA

FIGURE 5.1   A: Right-hand oblique and posteroanterior (PA) radiographs. Normal. (*continued*)

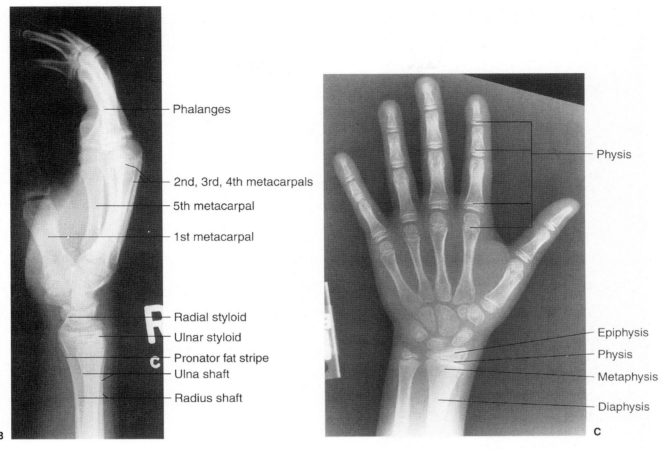

FIGURE 5.1 (*Continued*) **B:** Right-hand lateral radiograph. Normal. **C:** Left-hand PA radiograph. Normal physis, epiphysis, metaphysis, and diaphysis. The cartilaginous physis is a lucent area on a radiograph.

only two. The phalanges are named proximal, middle, and distal. The joint between the proximal phalanx and the metacarpal is called the metacarpophalangeal (MCP) joint (Fig. 5.1A). The joint between the proximal and middle phalanges is the proximal interphalangeal (PIP) joint. The joint between the distal and middle phalanges is called the distal interphalangeal (DIP) joint. The thumb, with only two phalanges, has an interphalangeal joint. The distal-most aspect of the metacarpals and phalanges is the head, whereas the proximal portions are the bases. The central aspects of these bones are the shafts.

Commonly used bone terms such as physis, epiphysis, metaphysis, and diaphysis can be confusing to the novice, but actually they are very simple. The locations of these entities are demonstrated in Fig. 5.1C. The physis (physeal or epiphyseal plate) is the growth plate as bone formation occurs on both sides (epiphysis and metaphysis) of the physis. The physis is the weakest part of a growing bone. The epiphysis is a secondary ossification center at the end of the bone, the metaphysis is just proximal to the physis, and the diaphysis (bone shaft) is between the proximal and distal metaphyses. Eventually, the epiphysis and the metaphysis fuse as the physis closes. The term apophysis is confusing and merely refers to an epiphysis that does not articulate with another bone and does not contribute to bone length growth but rather to bone contour. A typical example is the greater trochanter as seen in Fig. 5.23.

The wrist and forearm are common fracture sites, especially in children. If we are to intelligently understand and treat fractures in these areas, a thorough knowledge of wrist and forearm anatomy is very important. The appearance, location, and names of each carpal bone must be learned as well as their relationship to the distal radius and ulna. These relationships are well visualized on standard PA, lateral, and oblique radiographic views of the wrist (Fig. 5.2).

We generally obtain anteroposterior (AP) and lateral views of the forearm in children and adults (Fig. 5.3). Routine elbow radiographs consist of AP and lateral views (Fig. 5.4), but external rotation oblique views of the elbow may be requested on occasion (Fig. 5.5A). Radiographs of the humerus usually consist of AP (see Fig. 5.5A) and lateral views. Generally, an AP radiograph is obtained to evaluate the shoulder (Fig. 5.5B), and this is supplemented by either an axillary or lateral view of the shoulder depending on local practice. Musculoskeletal anatomy and disease can be nicely demonstrated by computed tomography (CT) and magnetic resonance imaging (MRI) (Table 5.3). CT imaging is especially good for bone detail, whereas MRI is good for soft tissue and bone marrow imaging, which can reveal edema caused by bone contusions or subtle fractures not seen on the radiographs. MRI is especially helpful in displaying the soft tissue structures around joints such as shoulder rotator cuff anatomy (Fig. 5.6).

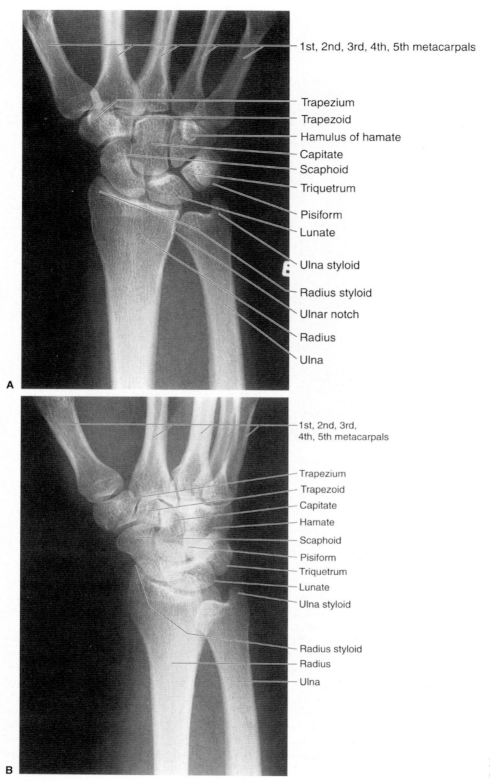

1st, 2nd, 3rd, 4th, 5th metacarpals

Trapezium
Trapezoid
Hamulus of hamate
Capitate
Scaphoid
Triquetrum

Pisiform
Lunate

Ulna styloid

Radius styloid
Ulnar notch
Radius
Ulna

A

1st, 2nd, 3rd, 4th, 5th metacarpals

Trapezium
Trapezoid
Capitate
Hamate
Scaphoid
Pisiform
Triquetrum
Lunate
Ulna styloid

Radius styloid
Radius
Ulna

B

FIGURE 5.2 Right wrist PA (**A**), oblique (**B**), and lateral (*continued*)

Sesamoid bone

1st metacarpal

Pisiform

Trapezium
Capitate
Scaphoid
Trapezoid
Lunate

Anterior fat pad

C

FIGURE 5.2 (*Continued*) (**C**) radiographs. Normal. Notice that the tip of the radial styloid is distal to the tip of the ulnar styloid and the radius articulates distally with the scaphoid and lunate carpals and laterally with the ulna (ulnar or sigmoid notch). The distal radial articular surface slopes toward the ulna and anteriorly (palmar). The distal ulna articulates with the radius laterally and wrist fibrocartilage distally. The ulna does not articulate directly with a carpal.

Scaphoid
Radial styloid
Lunate
Ulna styloid

R
S F

Radius shaft
Ulna shaft

Radial (biceps) tuberosity
Radial neck
Radial head

Lateral epicondyle

Ulna olecranon
Medial epicondyle

A

1st metacarpal

Scaphoid
Lunate

Ulnar styloid

Ulna shaft
Radius shaft

Radial (biceps) tuberosity
Radial neck
Radial head
Humerus trochlea
Ulna olecranon
Humerus shaft

B

FIGURE 5.3 Right forearm AP (**A**) and lateral (**B**) radiographs. Normal. Note that in the correct lateral of the forearm, both the elbow and the wrist are in the lateral position. The distal radius is large and the proximal radius is small, whereas the distal ulna is small and the proximal ulna is large. The radius is far more important than the ulna in the wrist joint, whereas the ulna is more important in the elbow joint than the radius.

FIGURE 5.4 Left elbow AP (**A**) and lateral (**B**) radiographs. Normal. The elbow is usually flexed 90 degrees to minimize the appearance of the anterior and posterior fat pads. The *dotted line* on **B** indicates the ulna coronoid process.

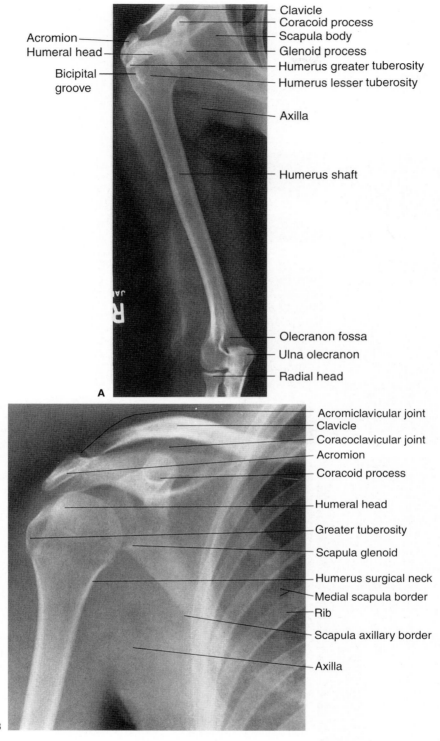

FIGURE 5.5   A: Right humerus AP radiograph with external rotation of the humerus. Normal. The right elbow is in an oblique position. **B:** Right shoulder AP radiograph with external rotation of the humerus. Normal. Note the prominence of the greater tuberosity.

TABLE 5.3

MUSCULOSKELETAL CT AND MRI INDICATIONS

Computed tomography
  Bone detail
  Fracture fragment evaluation
  Bone tumor workup

Magnetic resonance imaging
  Bone marrow imaging for occult fracture or metastasis
  Soft tissue evaluation: ligaments, tendons, cartilages, and
    vessels
  Bone tumor workup

— Fat

— Trapezius

— Acromion

— Supraspinatus m.

— Deltoid m.

— Humeral head
— Scapula glenoid
— Shoulder joint

FIGURE 5.6 Right shoulder coronal T1 MR image. Normal.

— Distal phalanx
— Distal interphalangeal joint (DIP)

— Middle phalanx

— Proximal interphalangeal joint (PIP)
— Proximal phalanx
— Sesamoid bones

— 1st, 2nd, 3rd, 4th, 5th metatarsals

— 1st (medial) cuneiform
— 2nd (intermediate) cuneiform
— 3rd (lateral) cuneiform

— Navicular

A

FIGURE 5.7 Right foot AP (**A**), oblique (*continued*)

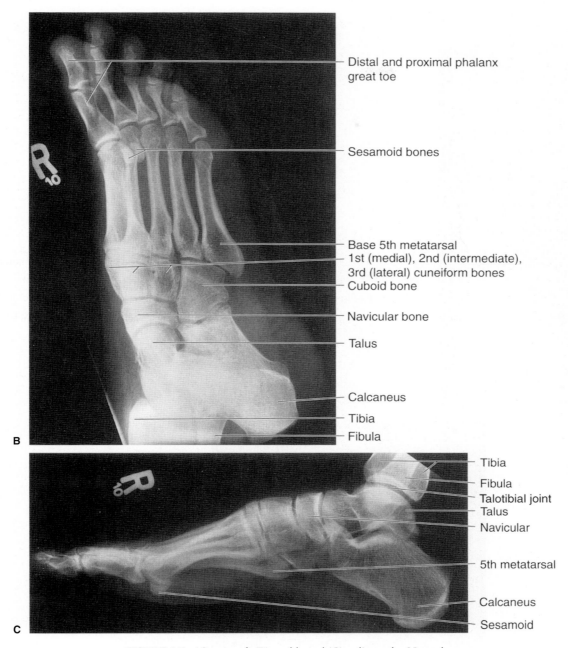

Distal and proximal phalanx great toe

Sesamoid bones

Base 5th metatarsal
1st (medial), 2nd (intermediate),
3rd (lateral) cuneiform bones
Cuboid bone

Navicular bone

Talus

Calcaneus

Tibia

Fibula

Tibia
Fibula
Talotibial joint
Talus
Navicular

5th metatarsal

Calcaneus

Sesamoid

FIGURE 5.7 *(Continued)* (B), and lateral (C) radiographs. Normal.

Lower Extremity

Now we approach lower extremity radiologic imaging by beginning with the foot and moving toward the hip. The standard views of the foot are AP, lateral, and oblique (Fig. 5.7). Naming of the toes is far easier than that of the fingers. The big toe or great toe may be referred to as the first toe, and the remaining toes are numbered sequentially ending with the little or fifth toe. Similarly, the metatarsals are numbered sequentially with the great toe articulating with the first metatarsal, the second toe articulating with the second metatarsal, and so forth. The ankle is usually imaged by AP, lateral, and either oblique or mortise-view (an internally rotated view) radiographs (Fig. 5.8). MRI may be used to image the ankle to de-

tect soft tissue injury (Fig. 5.9). Radiographs of the tibia and fibula usually consist of AP and lateral views (Fig. 5.10).

Routine knee radiographs consist of AP and lateral views, and they may be supplemented by AP standing radiographs (Fig. 5.11A–C) and/or oblique views. Axial, coronal, and sagittal magnetic resonance (MR) images of the knee (Fig. 5.12) are commonly requested to evaluate injuries of the knee, particularly the nonosseous structures, including the medial and lateral menisci, articular cartilage, ligaments, tendons, and muscles. *Remember that ligaments, tendons, and vessels have a low-intensity signal or appear black on MR images.*

The femur and the hip joint are radiographed in the AP and lateral views (Fig. 5.13). A cross-table lateral view of the hip is frequently obtained in a trauma setting as seen in Fig. 5.68B.

FIGURE 5.8 Left ankle AP (**A**), oblique/mortise (**B**), and lateral (**C**) radiographs. Normal. Note how the mortise view (**B**) allows improved visualization of the distal tibiofibular articulation.

Flexor hallucis longus
muscle
Tibia
Talotibial joint
Talus

Calcaneal (Achilles) tendon
Calcaneus
Tibialis anterior tendon

Navicular

Plantar fascia
Middle cuneiform

2nd metatarsal

FIGURE 5.9   Right ankle sagittal T1 MR image. Normal. Note that the calcaneal (Achilles) tendon has a homogeneous low-intensity (black) signal.

Intercondylar fossa
Tibia plateau
Fibula head
Fibula neck

Fibula shaft
Tibia shaft

Medial malleolus (tibia)
Talus
Lateral malleolus (fibula)

Femur
Tibia plateau

Tibia tuberosity

Calf muscles

Fibula shaft

Tibia shaft

Talus

FIGURE 5.10   Right tibiofibular AP (**A**) and lateral (**B**) radiographs. Normal.

A

- Patella
- Adductor tubercle
- Medial femur epicondyle
- Lateral femur epicondyle
- Lateral femoral condyle
- Medial femoral condyle
- Lateral and medial intercondylar eminences (spines)
- Tibia plateau
- Fibula

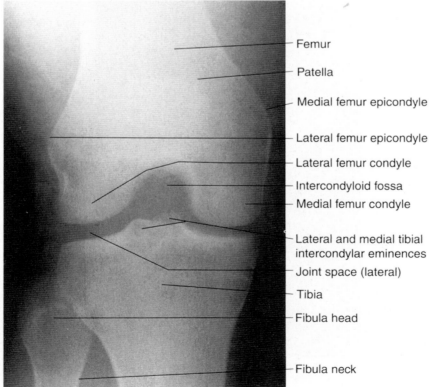

B

- Femur
- Patella
- Medial femur epicondyle
- Lateral femur epicondyle
- Lateral femur condyle
- Intercondyloid fossa
- Medial femur condyle
- Lateral and medial tibial intercondylar eminences
- Joint space (lateral)
- Tibia
- Fibula head
- Fibula neck

FIGURE 5.11   Right knee AP (**A**), AP standing (**B**), and lateral (*continued*)

- Patella
- Medial femur condyle
- Lateral femur condyle
- Lateral intercondylar eminence
- Medial intercondylar eminence
- Tibia plateau
- Fibula head
- Fibula neck
- Tibia tuberosity
- Fibula shaft

FIGURE 5.11 (*Continued*) (**C**) radiographs. Normal.

- Femur cortex
- Patella
- Anterior cruciate ligament
- Tibia cortex

FIGURE 5.12 A: Right knee proton-dense sagittal MR image. Normal anterior cruciate ligament in a 36-year-old man. (*continued*)

B

C

FIGURE 5.12 (*Continued*) **B:** Right knee proton-dense sagittal MR image in the same patient. Normal posterior cruciate ligament. The posterior cruciate ligament (*arrow*) is more homogeneous and has a lower intensity signal (blacker) than the anterior cruciate ligament. **C:** Right knee proton-dense medial-sagittal MR image in a 32-year-old man. Normal posterior horn (*straight arrow*) and anterior horn (*curved arrow*) of the medial meniscus.

— Acetabulum
— Hip joint
— Femoral head
— Greater trochanter

— Intertrochanteric crest
— Obturator foramen
— Lesser trochanter
— Ischial tuberosity

— Gluteal folds

— Femur shaft cortex

A

FIGURE 5.13 **A:** Right hip and proximal femur AP radiograph. Normal. Left hip AP (*continued*)

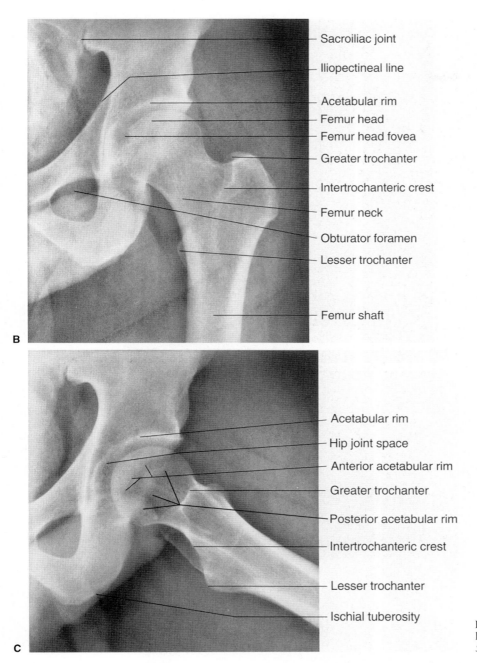

Sacroiliac joint
Iliopectineal line
Acetabular rim
Femur head
Femur head fovea
Greater trochanter
Intertrochanteric crest
Femur neck
Obturator foramen
Lesser trochanter
Femur shaft

B

Acetabular rim
Hip joint space
Anterior acetabular rim
Greater trochanter
Posterior acetabular rim
Intertrochanteric crest
Lesser trochanter
Ischial tuberosity

C

FIGURE 5.13 (*Continued*) (**B**) and frog-leg lateral (**C**) radiographs. Normal. See Fig. 5.68B for a true lateral of the hip.

VARIATIONS OF NORMAL

There are several osseous variations of normal that can cause confusion for the novice (Table 5.4). One such variation of normal is the *sesamoid bone*, which is merely a normal extra bone, usually within a tendon. Sesamoids occur at numerous sites and are commonly found in the plantar aspect of the foot near the head of the first metatarsal (see Fig. 5.7) and in the palmar aspect of the hand near the head of the first metacarpal (see Figs. 5.1A and 5.14A–C), where they are actually located in the volar plate rather than in a

TABLE 5.4
NORMAL OSSEOUS VARIATIONS
Sesamoid bones (located within a tendon like the patella) Ossicles (extra small bones) Supernumerary epiphyses Coalitions/fusions Bone islands

FIGURE 5.14   Left wrist PA (**A**), left-hand oblique (**B**), and lateral (**C**) radiographs. Multiple sesamoids (*arrows*). Bone islands (*curved arrows*) are present in the head of the fifth metacarpal and the capitate, and they have no clinical significance. **D:** Left foot AP radiograph. Os tibiale externum (*straight arrow*) and os peroneum (*curved arrow*). Right knee anterior radiograph (*continued*)

FIGURE 5.14 (*Continued*) (**E**), tangential radiograph of right patella (**F**), and axial fat-suppressed MR image (**G**). Bipartite patella. Note that the patella has two sections and the accessory bone (*curved arrows*) usually lies superior and lateral to the main body of the patella. The axial image (**G**) shows the continuous cartilage over the ossification center (*straight arrows*) differentiating it from a fracture, which is rare in this superolateral position. (*continued*)

FIGURE 5.14   (*Continued*) **H:** Right wrist PA radiograph. Normal distal right radial epiphysis spur. This 21-year-old woman fell and had a painful wrist. This spur (*arrow*) is a variant of normal and must not be confused with a fracture. **I:** Right ankle AP radiograph. Accessory epiphysis near the tip of the distal tibia epiphysis in the region of the medial malleolus (*arrow*). This is a variant of normal.

FIGURE 5.15 Left wrist PA and oblique radiographs. Congenital fusion. There is coalition of the lunate and triquetrum (*arrow*) and a prominent scaphoid tubercle (*curved arrow*). This tubercle should not be confused with a fracture. Compare with the normal carpals in Fig. 5.2.

tendon. When you think about it, the patella is actually a sesamoid bone or a bone within a tendon. Sesamoids function to decrease the moment arm and thus the work of a muscle. The quadriceps group of muscles becomes hypertrophied to compensate for increased work following removal of the patella.

Ossicles are another variant of normal. They are small supernumerary or extra bones found in a variety of places in juxtaposition to the skeletal system and usually named after the neighboring bone (Figs. 5.14D and 6.16). The bipartite or multipartite patella (Fig. 5.14E–G) is another example of an accessory bone that should not be mistaken for a fracture. The condition results when one or more of the patellar ossification centers fail to fuse with the main patellar body. The result is that the patella has two or more sections, and this variant occurs superolaterally approximately 75% of the time. There is a strong male predominance.

Epiphyses can vary in appearance and in their number of ossification centers and still be normal (Fig. 5.14H, I). A sometimes confusing variant is a prominent scaphoid tubercle. This prominence can be mistaken for a fracture by even experienced clinicians (Fig. 5.15).

CONGENITAL AND DEVELOPMENTAL ANOMALIES

Osseous congenital anomalies are not uncommon, and a few of the many variations are illustrated in Figs. 5.16 to 5.19 and listed in Table 5.5.

Coalition refers to the failure of segmentation of bones during development, resulting in a congenital fusion. This fusion may be bony or fibrous. Common locations involve the lunate and triquetrum in the wrist (Fig. 5.15) and the calcaneus and navicular or calcaneus and talus in the foot (Fig. 5.16).

Osteogenesis imperfecta is a congenital, non–sex-linked, hereditary abnormality with the primary defect in collagen synthesis with deficient bone matrix. These patients have abnormal bones (Fig. 5.20) that are fragile, fracture easily, and are often deformed. Achondroplasia is a hereditary, often sporadic, autosomal-dominant anomaly manifested by shortened long bones that results in this most common form of dwarfism (Fig. 5.21).

The hip joint is the most common site of congenital dislocation and has a strong female predominance. Developmental dysplasia of the hip (DDH) was formerly known as congenital dislocation of the hip or congenital hip dysplasia. This dysplasia, shown in Fig. 5.22, is usually diagnosed in infancy. DDH is an abnormal development of the hip joint resulting in an abnormal acetabulum and femoral head. There is displacement of the femoral head referable to the acetabular cartilage.

TABLE 5.5

SOME BONE ANOMALIES

Upper extremity
  Supernumerary digits or polydactylism
  Missing bones (fingers, radius)
  Coalition (carpals)
  Large digits or macrodactyly
  Supracondylar process

Lower extremity
  Polydactylism
  Coalition (calcaneus with talus or navicular)
  Developmental dysplasia hip
  Slipped capital femoral epiphysis
  Legg-Calvé-Perthes disease (avascular necrosis)
  Talipes equinovarus (club foot)
  Pes planus (flat foot)

Generalized
  Osteogenesis imperfecta
  Achondroplasia

FIGURE 5.16 Lateral radiograph of the left ankle (**A**) and coronal CT image of the same patient (**B**). There is a prominent C on the radiograph (*arrows*). Compare with the normal lateral in Fig. 5.8. The coronal CT clearly shows continuous bone bridging (*curved arrow*) between the talus (T) and calcaneus (C).

Two thumbs

1st metacarpal

Capitate

Hamate

Triquetrum

Distal radius epiphysis

Distal radius physis

FIGURE 5.17 Left-hand PA radiograph (child). Polydactylism. There are two thumbs and one first metacarpal. One thumb has three phalanges (*straight arrows*), and the other thumb has two phalanges (*curved arrows*).

FIGURE 5.18 Left forearm pronated, oblique radiograph. Absence of the radius, 1st metacarpal, and thumb. This 6-year-old had left hand and arm deformity at birth.

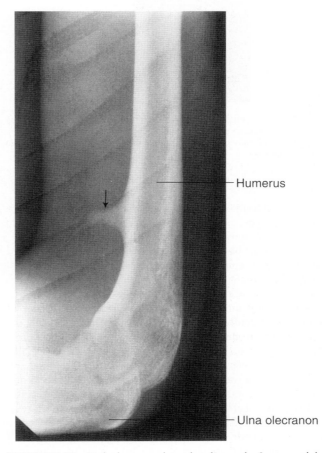

Humerus

Ulna olecranon

FIGURE 5.19 Right humerus lateral radiograph. Supracondylar process or spur (*arrow*). It is usually located in the anteromedial aspect of the distal humerus.

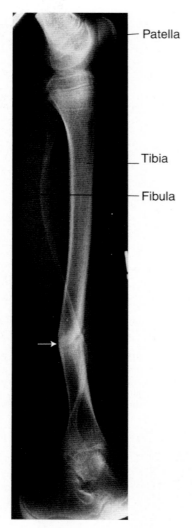

Patella

Tibia

Fibula

FIGURE 5.20 Left tibia and fibula lateral radiograph. Osteogenesis imperfecta. There is a healing, apex posterior, left tibia fracture (*arrow*). Note the thin serpentine appearance of the fibula and generalized osteoporosis.

The femoral head usually displaces superiorly but can displace posteriorly. The acetabulum becomes shallow and the angle between the femoral head and shaft is widened.

Two hip problems that can cause confusion are slipped capital femoral epiphysis (SCFE) and Legg-Calvé-Perthes disease (Table 5.6). SCFE (Fig. 5.23) is a hip problem that occurs during adolescence and is often associated with hip pain. The etiology is not understood, but there may be a history of trauma. Apparently, the physis becomes weakened during the rapid growth around puberty. The radiographic findings show the femoral head slipping or displacing posteriorly, medially, and inferiorly relative to the femoral neck. The proximal epiphysis becomes widened. Mild cases may go undetected and present with an earlier-than-expected onset of osteoarthritis.

Legg-Calvé-Perthes disease (Fig. 5.24A) is a form of avascular necrosis, and the etiology is unknown. It may be referred to as osteochondrosis or coxa plana. It typically occurs in a boy between 5 and 10 years of age who complains of hip pain

and walks with a limp. It occurs less frequently in females. The pain may be referred to the ipsilateral knee or the knee on the same side. Radiographic findings vary but may include increased density of the femoral capital epiphysis, femoral head flattening, rarefaction (bone demineralization) of the metaphysis, and medial joint space narrowing. In general, avascular necrosis or aseptic necrosis can occur in any joint (Fig. 5.24B, C) and can result from multiple other etiologies. Some of the other causes of avascular necrosis are listed in Table 5.7. The typical findings are sclerotic bone changes on one side of a joint that may go on to fragmentation and eventually to collapse or fracture. MRI (Fig. 5.24C) has proved particularly useful for the diagnosis of avascular necrosis prior to radiographic changes.

TRAUMA

Fractures and Dislocations

Extremity fractures are very common, so now is the time to discuss fractures in general. The initial imaging modality to evaluate for fracture should be a radiograph. *Because a fracture or other osseous abnormality may be visible on only one of the radiographs, we obtain at least two views of a bone or joint that are 90 degrees to each other.* Give yourself every opportunity to detect a fracture or other abnormality by obtaining as many views of an area as is practical. *Never accept just one radiographic*

FIGURE 5.21 Pelvis and lower extremities AP radiograph. Achondroplasia. The proximal long bones are shorter and wider than normal, especially the proximal tibias (*straight arrows*). The iliac bones are rounded (*double arrows*), and the acetabula are flat (*curved arrow*).

TABLE 5.6

COMPARISON OF SLIPPED CAPITAL FEMORAL EPIPHYSIS (SCFE) AND LEGG-CALVÉ-PERTHES DISEASE (LCP)

Feature	SCFE	LCP
Age	Adolescence	4–10 y
Gender	Boys more than girls (usually overweight)	Boys more than girls
Etiology	Unknown (usually during growth spurt)	Unknown
Symptoms	Hip and/or knee pain	Hip or knee pain and limping
Radiographic capital	Capital epiphysis slips posterior, medial, and inferior to the femoral neck	Flat and sclerotic epiphysis

Spina bifida occulta (sacrum)

Gonadal shield

FIGURE 5.22 Pelvis AP radiograph. Developmental dysplasia (DDH) of the right hip in a 14-year-old. The right hip is abnormal with a flattened femoral head (*single arrow*) and a poorly formed acetabulum (*curved arrow*). Compare the right hip to the normal left hip and note how the femoral heads remodel to conform to the shape of their corresponding acetabulum.

FIGURE 5.23 Pelvis AP radiograph. Bilateral slipped capital femoral epiphyses (SCFE) in a 15-year-old with chronic renal failure and on dialysis. The capital (proximal) femoral epiphyses (*straight arrows*) are displaced from their normal anatomic position. Usually, they are displaced inferiorly and posteromedially. There are monitoring electrodes projecting over the pelvis (*curved arrows*).

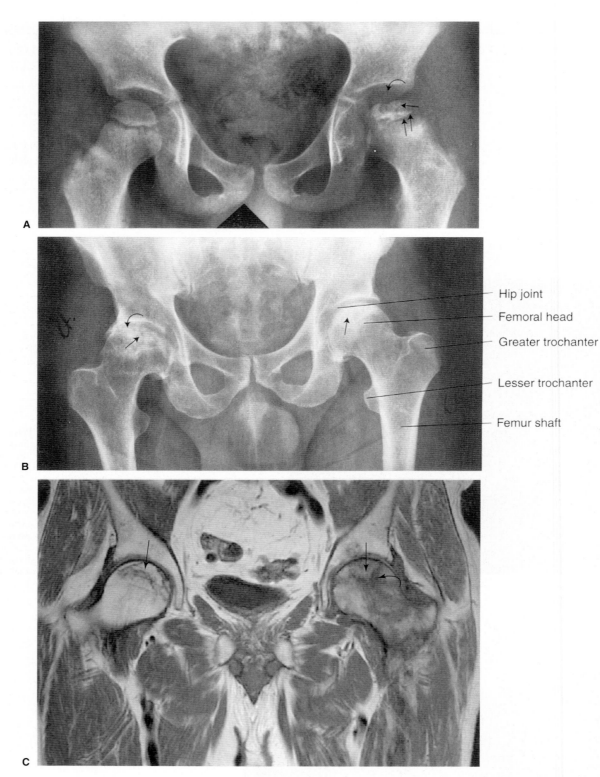

FIGURE 5.24   A: Pelvis AP radiograph. Legg-Calvé-Perthes disease. The right femoral head is normal. Note the irregular contour, flattened articular surface, and increased density of the left femoral head (*straight arrow*). The left hip joint space is widened (*curved arrow*). The left proximal femoral epiphysis is widened (*double arrows*), and the metaphysis is irregular. Note that the acetabulum is normal. **B:** Pelvis AP radiograph. Bilateral femoral head avascular necrosis of unknown etiology in a 42-year-old man. Both femoral heads (*straight arrows*) are sclerotic in appearance, and the right femoral head is deformed because of mild collapse or fracture. The right hip joint is narrowed laterally (*curved arrow*). **C:** Coronal T1-weighted MRI. Femoral head osteonecrosis in a patient on chronic steroids. The crescentic area formed by low-signal lines (*straight arrows*) represents the infracted regions. The left hip has a large amount of low-signal edema (*curved arrows*), suggesting a more acute infarction.

TABLE 5.7

A PARTIAL LIST OF AVASCULAR NECROSIS ETIOLOGIES

Steroids and anti-inflammatory drugs
Trauma including fractures and dislocations
Sickle cell anemia
Hemophilia
Alcohol
Systemic lupus erythematosus
Renal transplant
Infection
Diabetes

view of a bone or joint. When there is persistent concern for a fracture and the radiographs are normal, a clinical assessment is then needed. In many circumstances, the area of concern can be immobilized for a week and repeat radiographs obtained to see whether an occult fracture has now become visible. Other fractures are of such clinical importance that it is important to find out right away. The classic example is a hip fracture in an elderly patient for which an MRI should be obtained if the initial radiographs do not demonstrate a fracture. CT scans are the screening method of choice for cervical spine fractures are often used to better define a fracture prior to treatment.

In general, fractures can be conveniently divided into two major clinical categories:

1. Simple or closed fracture means that there are bone fragments and the skin is intact.
2. Compound or open fracture means the skin is not intact near the fracture. The skin has been penetrated by one or more of the bone fragments or by a penetrating foreign body.

Many terms applied to fractures are very descriptive and quite specific (Fig. 5.25A, B). Examples of straightforward common terms for describing fractures include the following:

1. Spiral, transverse, oblique
2. Nondisplaced
3. Overriding
4. Distracted
5. Angulated
6. Offset, or displacement, usually described by the percentage of the fracture fragments abutting or touching each other

Some fracture terms (Fig. 5.25C) that are not quite so obvious include the following:

1. Torus fracture of the distal radius looks like the bump at the base of a Greek column and has nothing to do with a bull. This is an incomplete fracture that occurs in children. The bump is created by a buckling of the cortex without an obvious fracture line.
2. Greenstick fracture describes a bone that fractures by bending like a green twig and is also incomplete.
3. Comminuted or complex fracture indicates more than two bone fragments.

4. Pathologic fracture is one that passes through abnormal bone such as a metastasis, a primary bone tumor, or a bone cyst.
5. Stress fractures are secondary to unusual or excess stress, for example, tibial fractures in runners who overdo it.
6. Insufficiency fractures describe fractures in bone with decreased strength, for example, caused by osteoporosis. Such a fracture may result from a normal stress such as merely walking across a room.
7. An avulsion fracture is usually a fracture that occurs at the site of a tendon attachment. This fracture results when the tendon and muscle remain intact while the bone gives way (avulses) at the site of the tendon attachment to the bone.

The Salter-Harris classification of fractures (Fig. 5.25D) is helpful in describing and understanding fractures around a physis. *Remember that the physis represents the weakest point in a bone.*

Type I: The fracture involves only the physis.
Type II: The fracture involves the physis and metaphysis.
Type III: The fracture involves the physis and epiphysis.
Type IV: The fracture involves the physis, metaphysis, and epiphysis.
Type V: The fracture involves only the physis, but there is compression of the physis. This type is more serious than Type 1 because there is a high risk of the physis fusing as the fracture heals. As a result, the bone stops growing and is shorter than the opposite side.

When describing the position of displaced fracture fragments, we use another set of terms. Unfortunately, much confusion can be created by the nomenclature. Traditionally, the distal fragment is described relative to the proximal fragment. An alternative nomenclature uses the apex of the angle created by the fracture fragments as the key. If the apex of the fracture fragments points lateral, the fracture is described as apex lateral. (This same fracture is described as medially angulated by the other nomenclature. You can see where confusion may arise.) I prefer using the word apex in the description so that everyone understands which system is used. If the apex of the fracture fragments points medial, then it is apex medial angulation (Fig. 5.25E). One may substitute medial with volar, dorsal, radial, ulnar, or any other appropriate direction of angulation. Varus and valgus angulation are other common terms to describe angulation and are also illustrated in Fig. 5.25E. Another useful rule for describing fracture alignment describes the direction in which the distal fracture fragment is displaced (Fig. 5.25F).

Fracture Healing

The rate at which a fracture heals depends on the fracture site, type of fracture, patient age, adequacy of immobilization, nutrition, and presence or absence of infection. When a fracture occurs, there usually is an associated hemorrhage into the fracture site with subsequent hematoma formation around and between the fracture fragments. The fibrin in a hematoma serves as a framework for fibroblasts, osteoblasts, and a general

A **Oblique**   **Transverse**   **Spiral**

B **Overriding**   **Distraction**

C **Torus**   **Greenstick**   **Comminuted**

FIGURE 5.25 A, B: Some common fractures (*arrows*) and the terms used to describe them and their alignment. **C:** Other common terms used to describe fractures (*arrows*). (*continued*)

I
Fracture through
the physis

II
Fracture through
physis and metaphysis

III
Fracture through
physis and epiphysis

IV
Fracture through
physis, metaphysis,
and epiphysis

V
Fracture through
physis with
compression

D

**Apex medial
angulation
or
valgus deformity**

**Lateral apex
angulation
or
varus definity**

E

**Medial
displacement**

**Lateral
displacement**

F

FIGURE 5.25 (*Continued*) **D:** The Salter-Harris classification of physis fractures. The solid black line indicates the fracture (*arrows*), whereas the physis is indicated by the vertical black and white lines. **E:** Illustrations of the nomenclature used to describe fracture angulation. **F:** Nomenclature used to describe the direction of displacement of the distal fracture fragments.

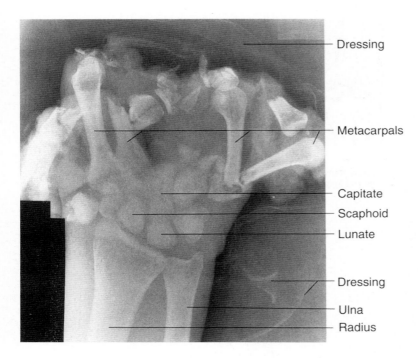

Dressing

Metacarpals

Capitate
Scaphoid
Lunate

Dressing
Ulna
Radius

FIGURE 5.26 Left-hand AP radiograph. Obvious severe hand injuries secondary to a corn-picking accident. The phalanges are essentially missing, and there are fractures of the metacarpals and carpals.

inflammatory reaction. Bone matrix or osteoid appears in the repair process after a few days, and this is called soft callus or provisional callus. The soft callus is not visible on a radiograph. As calcium salts precipitate in the soft callus and new bone grows, this is called callus. As the callus gradually becomes more dense, it becomes visible on a radiograph. Eventually the callus becomes solid, and bone union is established between the fracture fragments.

In a few days following a fracture, some absorption or removal of bone occurs as a part of the repair process near the ends of the fracture fragments. Because of this bone absorption, the fracture line becomes more visible on subsequent radiographs. This explains why some subtle fractures may not be visible on radiographs obtained immediately following injury but become visible approximately 7 to 10 days postinjury.

Self-explanatory terms used to describe problems in the fracture healing process include the following:

1. Nonunion or nonhealing
2. Delayed union
3. Malunion

Upper Extremity

Fractures of the hands result from a wide variety of activities (Table 5.7). Some fractures and injuries are so obvious that the average citizen could spot them on a radiograph (Fig. 5.26). Subtle fractures can involve any bone and are common in the phalanges of the hand (Figs. 5.27 and 5.28). Joint dislocations occur in almost all joints, and the hand phalangeal joints are common dislocation sites, notably related to sports (Fig. 5.29). Metacarpal fractures are also common, and fractures of the fifth metacarpal often result from punching a solid object. These fractures are appropriately called boxer fractures although they clearly demonstrate an amateur status because professionals would strike using the second and third metacarpals (Fig. 5.30).

The most commonly fractured carpal is the scaphoid (Fig. 5.31). The carpal scaphoid is occasionally referred to as the navicular (an archaic term) by clinicians, but anatomists correctly call it the scaphoid. To add to the confusion, there is a tarsal navicular. Scaphoid fractures result from the injury lines of force being transmitted along the long axis of the thumb, and the majority of these fractures are located in the scaphoid waist. Because of the location of their blood supply and variable arterial branches, scaphoid fractures may develop complications

A   B

FIGURE 5.27 Left thumb PA (**A**) and lateral (**B**) radiographs. Comminuted fracture (*straight arrows*) that extends to the articular surface of the interphalangeal joint (*curved arrow*). There is mild apex palmar angulation at the fracture site (*double arrows*).

FIGURE 5.28 Right index finger lateral radiograph. Mallet finger. The distal phalanx demonstrates a slightly flexed attitude due to fracture (*arrow*) at site of the insertion of the extensor digitorum mechanism. The loss of the extensor mechanism continuity with the distal phalanx allows the distal phalanx to assume a flexed position or a mallet finger.

FIGURE 5.30 Right-hand PA oblique radiograph. Boxer or Saturday night fracture. The apex dorsal angulated fracture (*arrow*) is through the neck of the right fifth metacarpal.

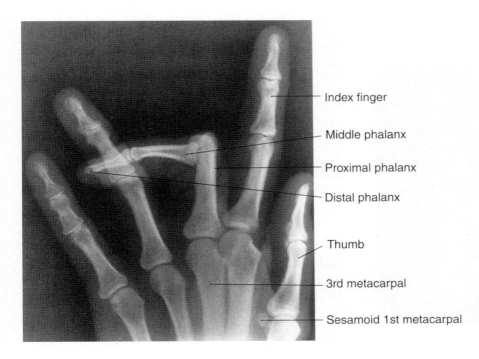

— Index finger

— Middle phalanx

— Proximal phalanx

— Distal phalanx

— Thumb

— 3rd metacarpal

— Sesamoid 1st metacarpal

FIGURE 5.29 Left-hand PA radiograph. Dislocation at the proximal interphalangeal (PIP) joint of the left long finger. The middle and distal phalanges are completely dislocated relative to the proximal phalanx. There are no fractures.

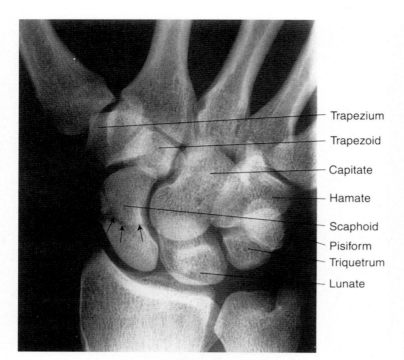

Trapezium
Trapezoid
Capitate
Hamate
Scaphoid
Pisiform
Triquetrum
Lunate

FIGURE 5.31   Right wrist PA radiograph. Essentially nondisplaced fracture (*arrows*) of the scaphoid waist.

such as nonunion and avascular necrosis, which may result in secondary development of arthritis. These complications are more apt to occur when there is delayed diagnosis and delayed or inadequate treatment. If a scaphoid fracture is suspected but the initial radiographs are negative, additional radiography, CT, or MR is indicated (Fig. 5.32).

FIGURE 5.32   STIR (short tau inversion recovery) MR image of the right wrist. The initial radiograph was normal, but suspicion for fracture led to the MR scan. In this sequence fat is suppressed, so the bone marrow appears dark. Cartilage is gray and fluid is white. There is fluid signal within the scaphoid centered at the scaphoid waist (*arrow*) with adjacent cortical disruption confirming the suspected scaphoid fracture.

Using arms and outstretched hands to cushion falls often results in fractures about the wrist. Whereas young adults typically fracture the scaphoid, children and older adults are more likely to fracture the distal radius and ulna. One such common fracture is called the Colles fracture (Fig. 5.33). It is imperative to reduce these fractured bones as close to their normal anatomic alignment as possible. Anything less than anatomic realignment may result in a painful and/or poorly functioning wrist. Therefore, it is important to know that the radial styloid tip is 1 to 1.5 cm distal to the ulnar styloid tip, and the distal radial articular surface slopes 15 to 25 degrees toward the ulna and 10 to 25 degrees volar or anteriorly. These important relationships are summarized in Table 5.8. Children, however, have a remarkable ability to remodel and anatomic realignment is not usually needed, depending on the age of the child. In fact, to avoid future limb length discrepancy, anatomic realignment may be purposely avoided.

TABLE 5.8

COMMON CAUSES OF UPPER EXTREMITY FRACTURES

Work injuries
Home falls
Recreational activities
Sports
Motor vehicle accidents
Fisticuffs

PA   Oblique   Lateral

FIGURE 5.33 Right wrist PA, oblique, and lateral radiographs. Colles fracture. There are fractures of the distal radius (*straight arrows*) and the ulna styloid (*curved arrows*) with dorsal tilting of the distal radius fracture fragment. The pronator fat stripe is obliterated when compared with Fig. 5.1B. The ulna styloid is minimally displaced radially. Note that the radial length is maintained and the distal radius articular surface slopes toward the ulna on the PA view. However, the distal radius articular surface now slopes posteriorly on the lateral view; reduction will try to bring this to neutral or restore the volar (anterior) tilt.

A subtle fracture in the distal forearm of children is the torus fracture (Fig. 5.34). Torus does not refer to a bull but rather the convex molding/projection (torus) located at the base of a classical column. The torus fracture on a radiograph usually appears as a minimal bump on the bone without a visible fracture line. It represents a buckling of the bone cortex. However, most fractures of the radius and ulna that are encountered in practice are much more obvious (Fig. 5.35).

Elbow fractures (Figs. 5.36 to 5.38) and dislocations (Fig. 5.39A–D) can occur when children and adults fall directly on their elbow or on an extended arm or hand. In children, supracondylar fractures of the distal humerus are more common, but in adults, radial head or neck fracture predominates. In general, children are more likely to have a supracondylar fracture of the distal humerus and adults a radial head fracture. Dislocations of the elbow are named for the direction the radius and ulna dislocate relative to the humerus. When the radius and ulna dislocate anterior to the humerus, it is an anterior dislocation.

The radiographic anatomy of the elbow is complicated. This is especially true in children because of the presence or absence of multiple ossification centers. *When in doubt about an elbow fracture or dislocation, the noninvolved elbow may be useful for comparative purposes as seen in* Fig. 5.38A and B. This principle of comparative views applies to all areas of difficult anatomy. However, knowledge of the

anatomy and ordered development of the ossification and fusion of the physes is fundamentally more important. Note that fractures and dislocations of the elbow can be a threat to the brachial artery because of its proximity to the distal humerus (Fig. 5.39E).

A very common injury to the shoulder occurs when a senior citizen trips on the rug or stairs. If they land on their extended hand and do not fracture their wrist, they may sustain a fracture of the surgical neck of the humerus (Fig. 5.40). Generally, this is very easily treated with a sling or a light hanging cast but may require an extended time for healing due to the patient's age and the fewer stresses compared to a weight-bearing bone. A similar fracture can occur through the physis of the proximal humerus in children (Fig. 5.41).

Dislocation of the shoulder is another common injury that can occur in all age groups. In anterior dislocation of the shoulder, the humeral head becomes caudad or inferior to the glenoid cavity on an AP radiograph and an impaction fracture of the greater tuberosity, a Hillsach's deformity, may result (Fig. 5.42A–C). Alternatively, the greater tuberosity may fracture during dislocation (Fig. 5.42D). In a posterior dislocation, the humeral head is often slightly cephalad to the glenoid cavity. However, a dislocation is often very difficult to diagnose on a single anterior view, and an axillary or scapular Y view should be obtained (Fig 5.42E). Anterior dislocation of the shoulder is much more common than a posterior dislocation.

FIGURE 5.34   A: Left wrist PA, oblique, and lateral radiographs. Torus fracture (*arrows*) or a nondisplaced fracture of the distal left radius. Left wrist PA (**B**) and lateral (**C**) radiographs. Healing left radius torus fracture 6 weeks following the radiograph shown in A. The dense white zone (*arrows*) is the typical appearance of a healing fracture.

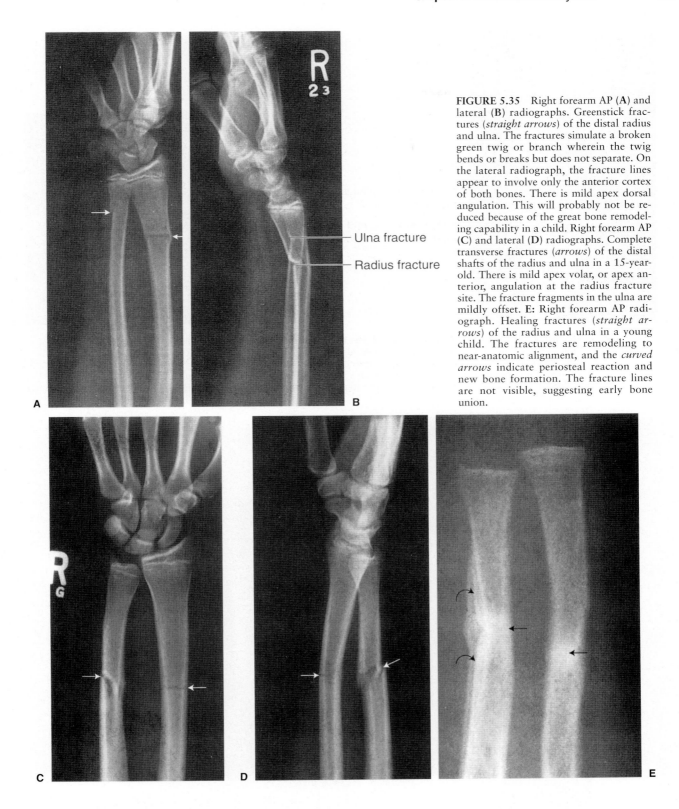

FIGURE 5.35 Right forearm AP (**A**) and lateral (**B**) radiographs. Greenstick fractures (*straight arrows*) of the distal radius and ulna. The fractures simulate a broken green twig or branch wherein the twig bends or breaks but does not separate. On the lateral radiograph, the fracture lines appear to involve only the anterior cortex of both bones. There is mild apex dorsal angulation. This will probably not be reduced because of the great bone remodeling capability in a child. Right forearm AP (**C**) and lateral (**D**) radiographs. Complete transverse fractures (*arrows*) of the distal shafts of the radius and ulna in a 15-year-old. There is mild apex volar, or apex anterior, angulation at the radius fracture site. The fracture fragments in the ulna are mildly offset. **E:** Right forearm AP radiograph. Healing fractures (*straight arrows*) of the radius and ulna in a young child. The fractures are remodeling to near-anatomic alignment, and the *curved arrows* indicate periosteal reaction and new bone formation. The fracture lines are not visible, suggesting early bone union.

Ulna fracture

Radius fracture

Trochlea and capitulum
epiphyses

Radius epiphysis and
physis

FIGURE 5.36 Left elbow AP (**A**) and lateral (**B**) radiographs. Radial neck fracture. The *straight arrows* indicate the site of the fracture, and the radial head is tilted laterally on the AP view. The fracture is very difficult to see on the lateral view (*straight arrows*). A positive fat pad sign is faintly visible posterior to the distal humerus (*curved arrow*) on the lateral view, and this always means that one should carefully evaluate for a fracture. A visible fat pad anterior to the distal humerus is normal so long as it is not overly prominent (see Fig. 5.4).

FIGURE 5.37 Left elbow AP (**A**), lateral (**B**), and oblique (**C**) radiographs. Fracture of the radius neck. The patient fell from a bicycle and complained of a painful elbow. A fracture is not definitely visible on the AP and lateral radiographs; however, it should be strongly suspected because the anterior fat pad (*single arrows*) is more prominent than normal and a posterior fat pad (*curved arrow*) is present. The fracture (*straight arrow*) can be clearly visualized on the oblique radiograph. This demonstrates the importance of obtaining multiple views of a suspected fracture site and reiterates the significance of a positive posterior fat pad sign and a prominent anterior fat pad. (*continued*)

FIGURE 5.37 *(Continued)*

Associated fractures of the humerus or scapula and rotator cuff tears may occur. Neural and vascular injuries are much less frequent.

Occasionally, a severe fracture or other disease process of the proximal humerus necessitates a shoulder prosthesis (Fig. 5.43). Fractures of the scapula are not common and usually result from a high-force injury as in motor vehicle accidents (MVAs; Fig. 5.44). These are frequently evaluated by CT to determine whether the fracture involves the glenoid or the suprascapular notch where the nerve to the supraspinatus and infraspinatus muscle travels (Fig. 5.45). Fractures of the clavicle are very common, especially in children who fall (Fig. 5.46). The most common site for clavicle fractures is at the junction of the middle and distal thirds.

MRI is a powerful tool for evaluating shoulder rotator cuff integrity, and a complete interruption of the rotator cuff is shown in Fig. 5.47. An arthrogram is performed by distending a joint, usually with fluid that will provide contrast to the structures of interest. MR arthrograms are especially helpful for evaluating tears of the glenoid labrum (Fig. 5.48). Remember that MRI is excellent for demonstrating the bone marrow and soft tissue detail, whereas CT imaging is better for trabecular and cortical detail.

Sudeck's atrophy, or reflex sympathetic dystrophy or chronic regional pain syndrome (Fig. 5.49), is a poorly understood phenomenon that can be the result of a fracture or almost any type of mild or severe injury. It is frequently associated with pain, swelling, and stiffness.

FIGURE 5.38 **A:** Left elbow AP radiograph. Avulsion fracture of the medial epicondyle epiphysis (*straight arrow*) in a 13-year-old. There is considerable soft tissue prominence (*curved arrows*), probably due to edema and hemorrhage secondary to the avulsion fracture. Remember that the pronators and flexors of the forearm attach to the medial epicondyle and the extensors and supinators to the lateral epicondyle. **B:** Right elbow AP radiograph for comparison. Normal. The medial epicondyle epiphysis (*straight arrows*) is normal. *(continued)*

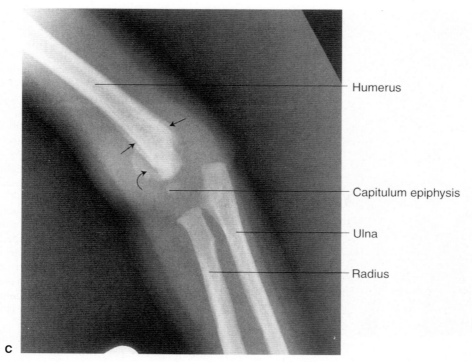

Humerus

Capitulum epiphysis

Ulna

Radius

C

FIGURE 5.38 (*Continued*) **C:** Right elbow oblique radiograph. Bucket-handle fracture of the distal humerus (*curved arrow*) in a 14-month-old child. Bucket-handle-type fractures can be found in child abuse situations. The *straight arrows* indicate periosteal reaction that occurs as a part of the healing process.

A

B

FIGURE 5.39 Left elbow (**A**) and right elbow (**B**) lateral radiographs. Anterior dislocation of the left (*arrow*). The right elbow lateral radiograph is normal and was obtained for comparative purposes as elbow anatomy may be especially difficult in children. Note the significant difference in position of the proximal left radius relative to the left humerus compared to the normal right proximal radius relative to the right humerus. Right elbow AP (**C**) and lateral (**D**) radiographs. Posterior dislocation of the elbow in a 23-year-old. The proximal ulna and the radial head are posterior to their normal articulations with the distal humerus, and this is best appreciated on the lateral view. There are no fractures. (*continued*)

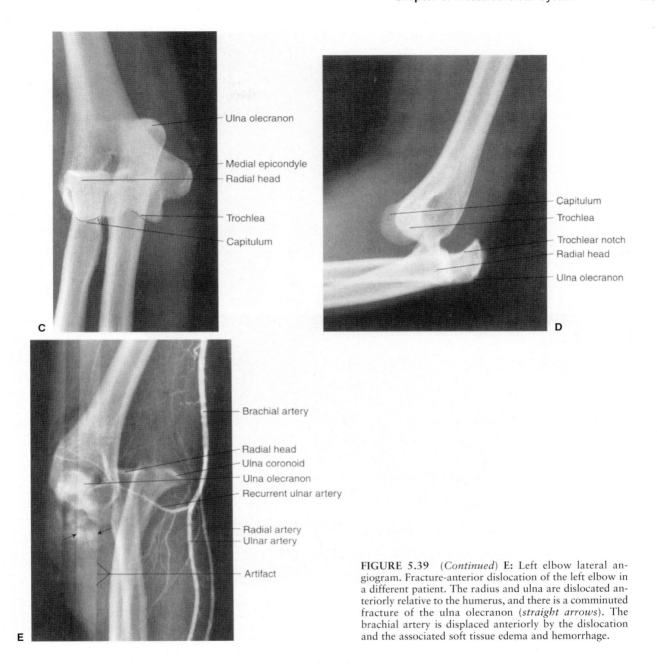

FIGURE 5.39 (*Continued*) E: Left elbow lateral angiogram. Fracture-anterior dislocation of the left elbow in a different patient. The radius and ulna are dislocated anteriorly relative to the humerus, and there is a comminuted fracture of the ulna olecranon (*straight arrows*). The brachial artery is displaced anteriorly by the dislocation and the associated soft tissue edema and hemorrhage.

Lower Extremity

The etiologies of lower extremity injuries are similar to those in upper extremity injuries (see Table 5.9). Injuries to the feet are very common, as this is where our body meets the ground (see Figs. 5.50 to 5.55 for a gallery of common foot injuries). CT is often used to evaluate complex ankle and calcaneal fractures (Fig. 5.55). Remember that a lateral radiolucent line near the base of the fifth metatarsal that runs parallel to the long axis of the metatarsal in a growing person represents a normal apophysis (Fig. 5.51C), whereas *a transverse lucent line at the base of the fifth metatarsal always represents a fracture* (Fig. 5.51D). An apophysis is a growth center (like the epiphysis) that does not contribute to bone length. It alters bone contour and usually is not located in a joint but typically has tendons attached to it.

TABLE 5.9

IMPORTANT DISTAL RADIUS ANATOMIC RELATIONSHIPS

Radius styloid tip lies 1–1.5 cm distal to the ulnar styloid tip
Distal radius articular surface slopes 15–25 degrees toward ulna (inclination)
Distal radius articular surface slopes 10–25 degrees anteriorly (volar tilt)

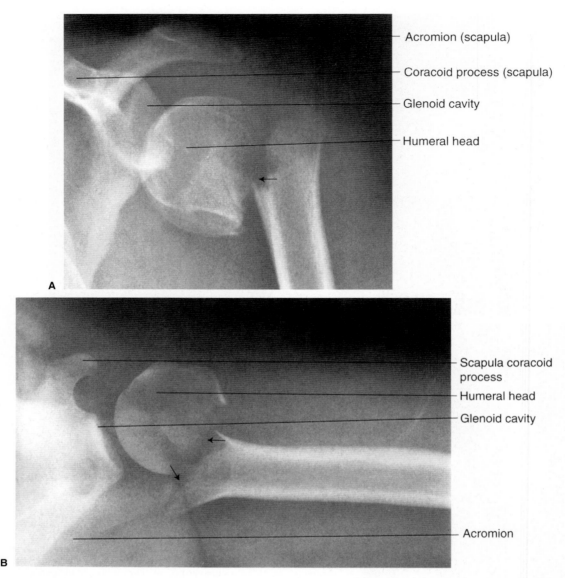

Acromion (scapula)

Coracoid process (scapula)

Glenoid cavity

Humeral head

Scapula coracoid
process

Humeral head

Glenoid cavity

Acromion

FIGURE 5.40   A: Left shoulder AP radiograph. Fracture (*straight arrow*) of the humerus surgical neck with offset of the fracture fragments in a 19-year-old patient. The humeral head is rotated and subluxed medially on the AP view resulting in an abnormal relationship between the humerus head and the scapula glenoid cavity. **B:** Left shoulder axillary radiograph of the same patient as in A. The central x-ray beam travels through the axilla to demonstrate nicely the offset fracture fragments (*arrows*). Note that the humeral head now is in a normal relationship with the scapula. The scapula coracoid process projects anteriorly, and the base of the scapula acromion projects posterior to the glenoid cavity on this view. Surgical internal fixation was required.

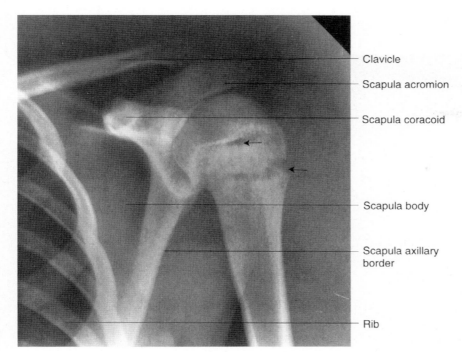

Clavicle

Scapula acromion

Scapula coracoid

Scapula body

Scapula axillary border

Rib

FIGURE 5.41 Left shoulder AP radiograph. Salter I fracture (*straight arrows*) through the proximal physis of the left humerus in a 15-year-old patient. The patient fell on an outstretched arm. The major clue to the presence of a fracture is that the physis width is greater than normal. Be careful not to overcall the normal physis a fracture—see Figs. 5.42 and 5.45.

Clavicle

Acromion

Scapula coracoid

Glenoid cavity

Greater tubercle

Intertubercular groove

Humeral head

Scapula inferior angle

A

H

G

B

FIGURE 5.42 A: Left shoulder AP radiograph. Anterior dislocation of the shoulder without fracture. The humeral head is inferior to the glenoid cavity, and this is the classic position of the humeral head in an anterior dislocation. The intertubercular (bicipital) groove is well visualized and within it rests the tendon of the long head of the biceps brachii. **B:** Left shoulder axial CT of an anterior dislocation. Note how the humeral head (H) may impact the glenoid (G). (*continued*)

FIGURE 5.42 (*Continued*) **C:** Right shoulder AP radiograph. Postreduction study demonstrates a Hill-sach's deformity (*arrow*) from impaction fracture. **D:** AP radiograph of left shoulder. Anterior disloca-tion with fracture of the greater tuberosity (*straight arrow*). Note a fat–fluid level (*curved arrow*) on this upright study. Fat from the marrow floats in blood. **E:** Scapular Y-view. Anterior dislocation. The cora-coid, acromion, and scapular body form the limbs Y. The glenoid (*dotted circle*) is located at the inter-section. The humeral head should contact this intersection.

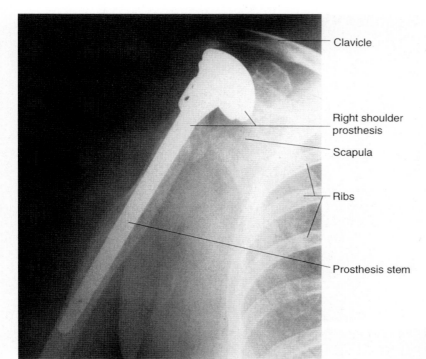

Clavicle

Right shoulder prosthesis

Scapula

Ribs

Prosthesis stem

FIGURE 5.43 Right shoulder AP radiograph. Right shoulder prosthesis. The prosthesis was necessitated by a severe old fracture deformity of the proximal humerus.

The ankle is frequently injured, and the injuries vary from minor sprains to severe trimalleolar fracture dislocations (Figs. 5.56 to 5.59). Fractures of the shafts of the tibia and fibula are common in sports, especially contact sports and skiing. A fracture that fails to heal and has persistent motion about it is called a nonunion fracture. Nonunion fractures have a variety of causes, some of which are listed in Table 5.10. Nonunions are frequently found in the mid- and distal tibia where the blood supply can be a problem (Fig. 5.60). Severe fractures of the tibia may require internal fixation to facilitate immobilization and healing (Fig. 5.61). The tibia is also the site of stress fractures in all age groups, especially in runners (Fig. 5.62).

A wide variety of fractures occur in and around the knee, and examples are demonstrated in Figs. 5.63 to 5.65. These figures demonstrate that not all fractures are visible on the initial radiographs around the time of injury. Whenever symptoms persist following an injury and the original radiographs were negative, you must consider follow-up imaging that might include radiographs, MRI, CT, or radionuclide scans. CT scans are often used for obvious tibial plateau fractures (Fig. 5.64) to better demonstrate the number and position of fragments and depth of depression of articular surface.

The patella is a large, superficial sesamoid bone. It is not uncommonly fractured in falls and MVAs (Fig. 5.66). Osteochondritis dissecans (Fig. 5.67A, B) is a common abnormality

FIGURE 5.44 Right shoulder AP radiograph. Acute fracture (*straight arrow*) of the scapula body and an old healed fracture (*curved arrow*) of the right midclavicle with deformity (malunion). The radiolucent line, or pseudofracture (*double arrows*), in the proximal right humerus is secondary to overlying soft tissues.

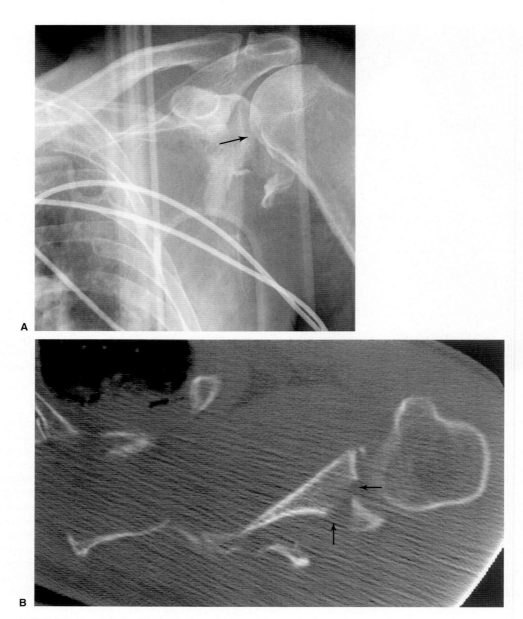

FIGURE 5.45   Left shoulder AP radiograph (**A**) and axial CT (**B**). Scapular fracture. The most important finding is involvement of the glenoid (*arrows*), which can lead to arthritis.

Clavicle
Scapula acromion
Scapula coracoid
Scapula body

FIGURE 5.46   A: Right and left clavicles AP radiograph. Subtle greenstick fracture of the middle third of the right clavicle (*arrow*) in a 3-year-old child. There is minimal apex cephalad angulation at the fracture site. The fracture is more apparent when compared to the normal left clavicle. **B:** Right clavicle AP radiograph in the same patient 4 weeks later. Healing fracture. The white material surrounding the fracture site in the middle third of the right clavicle (*arrows*) is callus. The bone has remodeled the angulation, and the clavicle alignment is normal.

Acromion
Trapezius
Supraspinatus muscle
Deltoid
Glenoid
Humeral head

**FIGURE 5.47   **Right shoulder fat-suppressed T2 coronal MR image. Rotator cuff complete tear in a 55-year-old man. The area of high intensity or white signal (*straight arrow*) represents blood, edema, and joint fluid in the laceration of the supraspinatus tendon. The free margin of the torn supraspinatus tendon is indicated by the *curved arrow*. Note that the bone cortex is black on the MR image. Note the edema (brighter signal) in the supraspinatus muscle.

FIGURE 5.48   Axial fat-suppressed T1 MR shoulder arthrogram. Labral tear. MR contrast is bright on the T1-weighted sequence (normal joint fluid is dark on the same sequence). The anterior labrum (*arrow*) is detached from the glenoid (G).

FIGURE 5.49   Right- and left-hand PA radiographs. Sudeck's atrophy of the left hand compared to the normal right hand. This patient's left upper extremity had been immobilized in a cast for 3 weeks. Sudeck's atrophy typically has patchy osteoporosis (*single arrows*) accompanied by soft tissue swelling (*double arrows*), and the latter is minimal in this 58-year-old patient. Disuse from immobilization may also lead to osteoporosis, and clinical information is necessary in this case.

FIGURE 5.50   Left great toe lateral, oblique, and AP radiographs. Nondisplaced fracture (*arrows*) of the distal phalanx. As is commonly the case, this patient dropped a heavy object on the great, or big, toe.

Medial and lateral sesamoids

FIGURE 5.51   Left foot oblique (**A**) and lateral (**B**) radiographs. Nondisplaced transverse fracture of the proximal left fifth metatarsal shaft (*arrows*). **C:** Right foot AP radiograph. Normal in a 14-year-old boy. The normal apophysis (*arrow*) at the base of the fifth metatarsal appears as a longitudinal radiolucent or black line and should not be confused with a fracture. **D:** Right foot oblique radiograph. Transverse nondisplaced fracture (*straight arrow*) involving the fifth metatarsal base. This injury usually results from an inversion stress on the peroneus brevis that attaches to the base of the fifth metatarsal.

Tibia

Lateral malleolus
(fibula)

Cuboid

5th metatarsal
base

Calcaneus

FIGURE 5.52 Right ankle lateral radiograph. Midtalus distracted fracture (*curved arrow*). The fracture fragments (*straight arrows*) are markedly distracted, and the soft tissue edema and/or blood is indicated by the *double arrows*. The fracture resulted from a dorsiflexion injury.

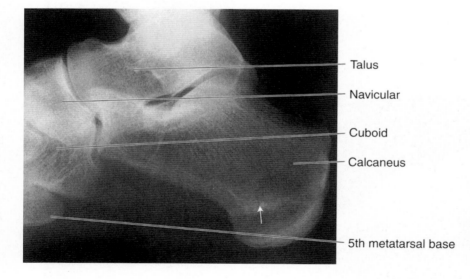

Talus

Navicular

Cuboid

Calcaneus

5th metatarsal base

FIGURE 5.53 Right calcaneus lateral radiograph. Calcaneus insufficiency fracture in a 53-year-old woman. The white line (*arrow*) indicates a healing mildly impacted fracture that was not visible on radiographs 2 months prior to this study. The shape and height of the calcaneus are fairly well maintained. She had been on steroids for inflammatory bowel disease, and the steroids caused osteoporosis. As a consequence of the osteoporosis, the bone was not strong enough to prevent fracture.

First metatarsal

Medial cuneiform

Navicular

Talus

FIGURE 5.54 Long axis fat-suppressed T2-weighted MR of the right foot in a runner. Stress fracture. Second metatarsal stress fracture has some callus, which is black (*straight arrow*), and a large amount of edema in the bone and soft tissues, which is white (*curved arrows*).

A

FIGURE 5.55 A: Right calcaneus lateral radiograph. Calcaneus fracture (*arrow*) with impaction and collapse of the vertical height of the calcaneus. Compare the shape of the calcaneus in this patient to the calcaneus in Fig. 5.52. Axial (**B**) and coronal reformatted (**C**) CT images better demonstrate the extent and comminution of the fracture. (*continued*)

Navicular

Calcaneus

B

Tibia

Medial malleolus
of tibia

Talus

Sustentaculum talus
of calcaneus

C

FIGURE 5.55   (*Continued*)

FIGURE 5.56 Right ankle oblique radiograph. Mildly distracted fracture (*straight arrows*) through the base of the medial malleolus in an adult. The fracture extends onto the articular surface of the distal tibia. The white lines (*curved arrows*) represent previous physis location and arrested growth lines.

FIGURE 5.57 Right ankle AP (**A**) and lateral (**B**) radiographs. Displaced trimalleolar fractures and talotibial dislocation. The medial and posterior tibial malleoli fracture fragments and the fibula lateral malleolus fracture fragments are all displaced. The talus is severely displaced laterally and posteriorly relative to the tibia. This is an eversion injury.

— Tibia physis

— Fibula physis

— Distal tibia epiphysis
— Distal fibula epiphysis

FIGURE 5.58 Left ankle AP radiograph. Salter III fracture of the left distal tibia in a 12-year-old. The fracture line (*arrow*) extends from the physis through the distal tibial epiphysis to the articular surface.

— Tibia physis

FIGURE 5.59 Right ankle AP radiograph. Salter IV fracture of the distal tibia. The fracture line (*straight arrow*) extends from the distal tibial physis through the epiphysis to the tibial articular surface. The fracture also involves the medial tibia metaphysis (*curved arrow*). There is an associated fracture of the distal fibula (*double arrows*).

A   **B**

FIGURE 5.60 Left tibia and fibula AP (**A**) and lateral (**B**) radiographs. Osteomyelitis and nonunion of a tibia fracture. The fracture line (*arrows*) is clearly visible 3 months following the injury, and this indicates a nonunion or nonhealing fracture. Infection at the fracture site caused the nonunion.

TABLE 5.10

CAUSES OF FRACTURE NONUNION

Infection and osteomyelitis
Inadequate immobilization
Poor blood supply
Interposition of muscle or other structure between the fracture fragments
Combinations of the above

— Knee joint space

— Tibia osteochondroma

— Intramedullary rod

— Cast

— Metallic screw

— Ankle joint space

FIGURE 5.61 Left tibia and fibula AP radiograph. Intramedullary rod internally fixating a transverse fracture in the distal one third of the left tibia (*straight arrow*). There is an offset overriding transverse fracture in the distal one third of the fibula (*curved arrows*). The fibula is non–weight-bearing, so the displacement is not important to a good functional outcome.

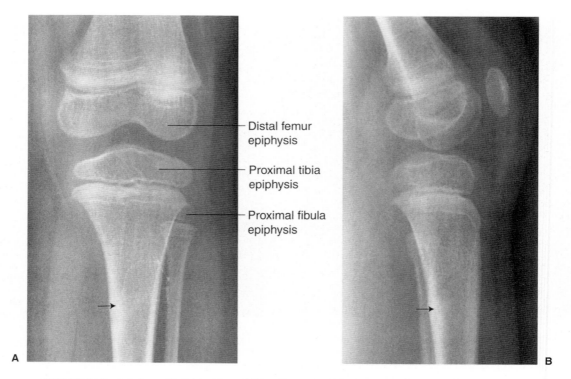

FIGURE 5.62   Left knee AP (**A**) and lateral (**B**) radiographs. A healing stress fracture in this 5-year-old is indicated by the zone of increased density in the posteromedial proximal tibia (*arrows*). The fracture resulted from excessive usage or stress.

FIGURE 5.63   **A:** Right knee AP radiograph. This AP radiograph and a lateral (*not shown*) radiograph were interpreted as normal. The radiographs were obtained because of right knee pain immediately following knee trauma in a 31-year-old man. **B:** Right knee coronal T1 MR image. Lateral tibial plateau fracture. This study was obtained 2 weeks following the initial radiograph in A because of persistent knee pain and a clinical suspicion of an anterior cruciate ligament injury. The *arrows* indicate an area of low-intensity signal (dark) caused by blood and edema replacing the bone marrow fat (white) in the tibial plateau fracture site. The anterior cruciate ligament was intact. The fracture eventually became apparent on subsequent radiographs.

FIGURE 5.64 Coronal CT of the knee reformatted from axial images. Lateral tibial plateau fracture. CT is often used to better evaluate the amount of depression of the articular surface (*straight arrow*) and number and location of fragments. The irregular bone formation along the medial femur (*curved arrow*) is the result of a prior medial collateral ligament injury.

FIGURE 5.66 Right knee lateral radiograph. Midpatella fracture secondary to a motor vehicle accident. There are two distracted fracture fragments (*straight arrows*) secondary to the fracture through the midpatella. The *curved arrows* indicate blood and increased synovial fluid in the supra-, pre-, and retropatellar spaces of the knee.

FIGURE 5.65 Coronal inversion recovery MRI of the right knee. Insufficiency fracture of the medial tibia in an elderly patient with pain. The fracture line (*arrow*) is white on this sequence from blood and edema.

involving the knee in adolescents and young adults. It occurs most frequently along the lateral aspect of the medial femoral condyle, but it can be found elsewhere in the knee and in other joints including the hip, shoulder, ankle, and elbow. It is thought to be a localized ischemic or avascular necrosis that often occurs after injury and results in a button of necrotic bone that may or may not detach from the donor site. When it becomes detached, it is a joint loose body. In middle-aged to older adults, the abnormality is typically the weight-bearing aspect of the medial femoral condyle and the term spontaneous osteonecrosis is often used (Fig. 5.67C, D). In the older age group, these lesions may be due to subchondral insufficiency fractures. Avascular necrosis is bone ischemia and localized bone death. The clinical presentations of bone ischemia (Table 5.11) vary with the bone site and size as well as bone age (Fig. 5.24). Osteonecrosis has a variety of causes.

TABLE 5.11

SOME CLINICAL PRESENTATIONS OF BONE ISCHEMIA

Osteochondritis dissecans
Legg-Calvé-Perthes disease
Avascular necrosis
Aseptic necrosis
Bone infarcts

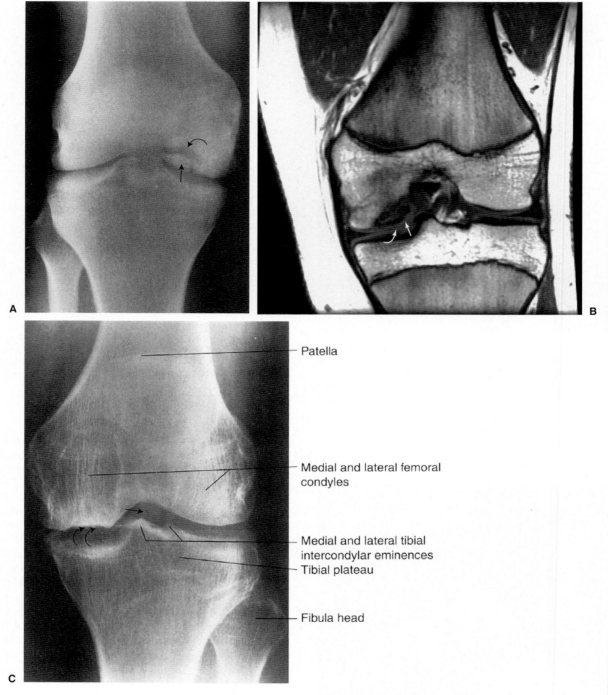

FIGURE 5.67 **A:** Right knee AP radiograph. Osteochondritis dissecans. The bone fragment (*straight arrow*) is not displaced from the donor site (*curved arrow*) on the lateral aspect of the medial femoral condyle. **B:** Coronal T1-weighted MR right knee in a different patient. The fragment (*straight arrow*) is clearly seen and cartilage covers it (*curved arrow*). **C:** Left knee AP radiograph in a different patient. Spontaneous osteonecrosis. There is a displaced bone fragment or loose body (*straight arrow*) in the joint space. The radiolucent defect surrounded by the sclerotic zone (*curved arrow*) in the weight-bearing portion of the medial femoral condyle is the donor site of the loose body.

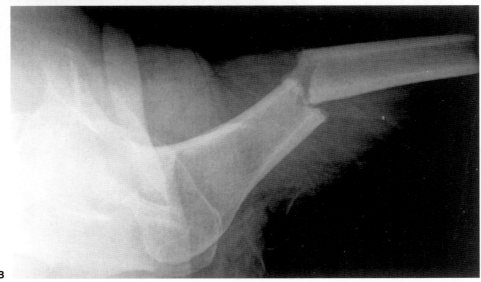

FIGURE 5.68   Left femur frog-leg (**A**) and true (**B**) lateral radiographs. Transverse fracture of the femur in a 26-year-old automobile accident victim. There is apex anterior angulation. Note how the fracture fragments can change when the patient is moved. Displacement is posterior in the frog-leg lateral but was anterior on the true lateral. The patient is supine and the x-ray beam horizontal on the true lateral.

The term infarct is used when the dead bone is not near a joint (Fig. 5.102C).

As a general rule, femoral shaft fractures are easy to detect both clinically and radiographically, as the patient experiences severe pain at the fracture site and is usually unable to bear weight (Fig. 5.68). This is an uncommon area for stress fractures, but they may occur here in young athletes.

The hip is another area commonly injured in MVAs and falls, especially in the elderly (Fig. 5.69). MRI has become the standard in evaluating for hip fracture with seemingly normal radiographs (Fig. 5.70). Dislocations of the hip are not common and require violent trauma as in MVAs (Fig. 5.71). As opposed to the shoulder, posterior dislocations of the hip are much more frequent than anterior. CT is quite useful in the assessment of complex pelvic and acetabular fractures (see figures in Chapter 6). However, patients with a hip prosthesis may on occasion dislocate the prosthetic head with a minimal amount of stress (Fig. 5.72).

There are estimates that over 900,000 children are abused each year and 4 children die per day as a result of abuse in the United States alone. Boys and girls are affected equally. It is thought that radiographic abnormalities can be detected in up to 70% of cases. Although 90% of child abuse deaths are secondary to head injuries, nonaccidental trauma can involve

FIGURE 5.69 **A:** Right hip AP radiograph. Femoral neck fracture. There is a mildly impacted fracture (*arrow*) through the midfemoral neck. The *curved arrow* denotes a small fracture fragment. The patient complained of right hip pain and inability to bear weight on the right leg following a minor fall. **B:** Coronal T1-weighted MR in a different patient. A left subcapital fracture is easily seen (*arrow*).

all parts of the skeletal system. An appropriate workup for suspected abuse includes a radiographic survey of the long bones, pelvis, spine, ribs, and skull. Bone scanning may also be useful.

The metaphyseal fractures demonstrated in Fig. 5.73A are typical of the findings in some child abuse cases, and these metaphyseal fractures are probably due to a twisting mechanism. Subperiosteal hemorrhage on a radiograph is another twisting type of injury that should make you highly suspicious of nonaccidental trauma (Fig. 5.73B). Bucket-handle fractures (see Fig. 5.37C) are also associated with abuse. Skeletal injuries and fractures that should make the observer highly suspicious for nonaccidental trauma are summarized in Table 5.12, and the common child abuse fracture sites out-

side the skull are shown in Table 5.13. Suspicious findings must be differentiated from normal periostitis found in infancy, osteogenesis imperfecta, congenital insensitivity to pain, and metabolic and vitamin deficiency disorders such as scurvy (vitamin C deficiency).

Soft Tissue Injury

One of the commonest injuries of the lower extremity is the sprained ankle. A sprain is simply an injury to a ligament around the ankle (or any other joint), and it varies in severity from a strain or stretching of the ligament to a complete

FIGURE 5.70 AP radiograph (**A**) of the left hip was interpreted as normal. This avid runner complained of persistent pain and an MR was obtained. Coronal fat-suppressed T2-weighted image (**B**) demonstrates edema (white) around the developing stress fracture (*arrow*). Left untreated, this might well progress to a complete fracture.

FIGURE 5.71 Pelvis AP radiograph. Posterior dislocation of the left hip without fracture secondary to a motor vehicle accident. The left femoral head is displaced cephalad and lateral relative to the acetabulum (*straight arrows*). The right hip is normal and makes an excellent comparison.

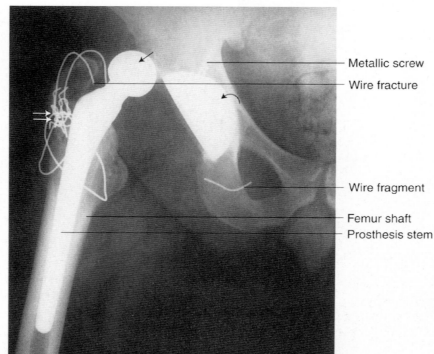

Metallic screw
Wire fracture

Wire fragment

Femur shaft
Prosthesis stem

A

FIGURE 5.72 **A:** AP radiographs of the right hip. There is posterior dislocation of the right hip prosthesis head (*straight arrow*) in relation to the acetabular component (*curved arrow*). The dislocation occurred while bending over to pick up a grandchild. Wires (*double arrows*) anchor the greater trochanter to the femur, and at least one of the wires is fractured. A fragment of loose wire lies inferior to the prosthesis acetabular component. (*continued*)

(*continued*)

TABLE 5.12

OSSEOUS INJURIES SUSPICIOUS FOR CHILD ABUSE

Corner fractures
Periosteal hemorrhage
Bucket-handle fractures

TABLE 5.13

COMMON FRACTURE SITES IN ABUSED CHILDREN

Lower extremity: femur (commonest), tibia
Elbow
Shoulder
Ribs

FIGURE 5.72 (*Continued*) **B:** Following closed reduction (no surgery) under general anesthesia, the prosthetic head has been returned to its proper position relative to the acetabular prosthetic component.

FIGURE 5.73 **A:** Left knee AP radiograph. Metaphyseal corner fractures (*arrows*). This battered child complained of knee pain and had an obvious limp. **B:** Right and left lower extremities radiograph. Subperiosteal hemorrhage. The *straight arrows* indicate the appearance of blood beneath the periosteum secondary to severe squeezing and twisting of the extremities. This appearance is highly suspicious for child abuse and should be investigated further.

FIGURE 5.74 Left ankle inversion stress AP radiograph. Ankle sprain. The talus is tilted laterally (*arrow*) secondary to disruption of the lateral collateral ligament in an inversion or adduction injury. There are no fractures.

disruption. Sprains usually result from a turning or twisting of the ankle joint while walking or running. When the foot turns outward, there is an eversion or abduction injury. When the foot turns inward, there is an inversion or adduction injury. Sprains occur with and without associated fractures.

A dramatic example of a severe sprain is demonstrated in Fig. 5.74.

Because ankle sprains are usually treated by casting in the United States, MRI is not commonly used to image ankle sprains, and the imaging usually is limited to radiographs; one exception is high-performance athletes. However, MRI of the ankle is used for specific problems such as Achilles tendon tears. The Achilles tendon or calcaneal tendon is a common injury site (Fig. 5.75). This injury can result from violent sport activities or simply stepping in a hole, and the diagnosis usually is made by the history of pain in the Achilles tendon. When there is a complete tear or disruption of the Achilles tendon, physical examination often shows pinpoint tenderness at the site of injury and inability to plantarflex the foot. An MRI is usually requested to confirm a clinical diagnosis or suspicion and evaluate the degree of separation. This will aid in the decision for casting versus surgical intervention. Alternatively, ultrasound has also been used to evaluate the Achilles tendon (Fig. 5.76).

Injuries to muscles are often diagnosed clinically. Some muscular injuries may require further evaluation—frequently using MRI. Muscle avulsions or tears of the hamstrings (Fig. 5.77A, B) or pectoralis muscle. A muscle may also tear in its substance. The extent of this intramuscular tear and hematoma is particularly important to the elite athlete since length of rehabilitation and long-term prognosis are affected by the severity of the muscular injury. Following injury to muscles there may be subsequent calcification and/or ossification at the injury site called *myositis ossificans*. Common locations include the quadriceps and brachialis muscles.

— Flexor hallucis longus tendon
— Tibialis anterior tendon

— Flexor digitorum brevis muscle

FIGURE 5.75 Right ankle midsagittal T1 MR image. Calcaneal (Achilles) tendon tear. The tear site is manifest by a high-intensity signal due to blood and edema within the tear (*arrow*).

FIGURE 5.76 Transverse ultrasound image of an Achilles tendon. Partial tear. The normal portion of the tendon is echogenic (*curved arrow*). The anterior portion, which is normally flat or concave, is rounded (*arrows*) and has low echogenicity (*double arrow*) due to edema and blood.

FIGURE 5.77 A: AP radiograph of the pelvis shows a partial avulsion at the hamstring origin on the right ischium (*arrow*). Note the asymmetry from the other side. **B:** Coronal plane fat-suppressed T2-weighted MR image at the plane of the ischial tuberosities. The bright signal in the left posterior thigh is edema and blood surrounding the tear of the biceps femoris muscle of the hamstrings (*arrow*).

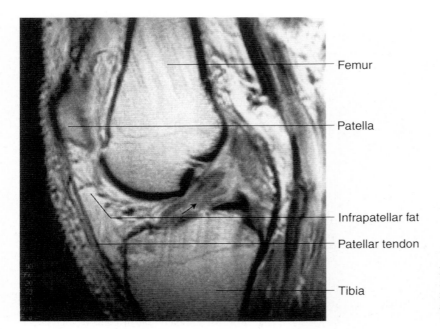

Femur

Patella

Infrapatellar fat

Patellar tendon

Tibia

FIGURE 5.78   Right knee sagittal proton-density MR image. Anterior cruciate ligament tear in a 41-year-old man. The arrow indicates the site of the anterior cruciate ligament tear manifested by a wavy high-intensity (white) signal.

FIGURE 5.79   Sagittal fat-suppressed proton-density MR image through medial meniscus. Tear of the posterior horn in a 45-year-old woman. The high-intensity signal (*arrow*) likely represents edema and synovial fluid within the tear. The anterior horn of the meniscus (*curved arrow*) is normal.

FIGURE 5.80   Axial fat-suppressed T2 MR right knee. Post patellar dislocation. The patella (P) is laterally subluxed: It should closely articulate with the trochlea of the femur. There is edema of the lateral femur (*arrow*) where the patella impacted. A cartilage defect (*curved arrow*) was created in the patella during the dislocation or relocation.

FIGURE 5.81 Sagittal proton-density MR right knee. Patellar tendon tear. There is disruption of the patellar tendon (ligament) at its patellar attachment (*arrow*).

FIGURE 5.83 Coronal fat-suppressed proton-density MRI of left wrist. Triangular fibrocartilage tear. There is disruption and slight retraction of the triangular fibrocartilage from its radial attachment (*straight arrow*). Wrist MRIs are also useful in evaluating the scapholunate ligament (*curved arrow*), which is normal in this patient.

MRI is a wonderful imaging tool for evaluating cartilage, menisci, tendons, and ligaments in and around the knee. Usually the radiographs are negative in such injuries, but based on the physical findings and the patient's symptoms, an MR image is requested for a more definitive evaluation of these soft tissue structures (Figs. 5.78 to 5.83).

Many foreign bodies in soft tissue and bone are radiopaque and readily identified on radiographs (Fig. 5.84A, B). Occasionally, a nonopaque foreign body in an extremity is suspected. If a foreign body is not visible on a radiograph, an ultrasound, CT, or MR study can be requested to assist in the detection and location of the foreign body (Fig. 5.84C).

FIGURE 5.82 Sagittal inversion recovery MRI of left foot. Plantar fasciitis. The plantar fascia is thickened (*arrow*) and has surrounding edema (white). Mild edema is also seen in the adjacent calcaneus (C).

— Eyelets for boot laces

A

FIGURE 5.84 Left foot AP (**A**) and lateral (**B**) radiographs taken through the boot. Metallic nail (*arrows*) piercing the boot and lodged in the calcaneus. The nail was driven into its present location by a power tool. **C:** Left foot axial T2 MR image. Foreign body (*straight arrow*) in a different patient. The site of the foreign body entry wound (*curved arrow*) is marked by the white pill containing fat. The foreign body tract (*double arrows*) is white, probably because it is filled with edema, blood, granulation tissue, or inflammatory cells.

— Eyelet for boot laces

— Calcaneus

— Boot sole

B

—1st metatarsal

—2nd, 3rd, 4th metatarsals

—5th metatarsal

C

ARTHRITIDES

Osteoarthritis

Osteoarthritis (degenerative arthritis) is the most common form of arthritis. You can categorize osteoarthritis into two types. Secondary osteoarthritis, or degenerative joint disease, can occur at all ages but tends to appear with increasing age as a result of wearing-out processes. It may involve almost all of the joints of the extremities and spine (Figs. 5.85 to 5.87) but favors the DIP joints and thumb carpometacarpal joint in the hand, hips, and knees. In younger individuals, secondary arthritis may result from trauma, infection, or any other process that may disrupt the normal joint. Primary osteoarthritis is probably familial and involves the DIP joints of the hands, hips, and the first metacarpal–carpal joint. Another frequent location of arthritis is the great toe (metatarsophalangeal [MTP]) joint. A bunion may develop from a familial predisposition or related to shoeware, particularly high heels. The apex at the MTP joint is medial and becomes more prominent. Overlying soft tissue irritation may develop or osteoarthritis may result from the now incongruent joint (Fig. 5.88).

The radiograph is the primary tool for evaluating osteoarthritis as well as all other arthritides. Some important facts and radiographic findings of osteoarthritis are listed in Table 5.14 and include asymmetric, irregular joint narrowing because of articular cartilage destruction, osteosclerosis, and osteophyte formation. When advanced osteoarthritis involves the medial knee compartment, a genu varus deformity or bowed leg usually results. When advanced osteoarthritis involves the lateral knee compartment, a genu valgus deformity or knock-knee often results. When advanced osteoarthritis involves the hip, the femoral head migrates cephalad because of asymmetric cartilage destruction, whereas in rheumatoid arthritis the femoral head tends to drift centrally from uniform

FIGURE 5.85 A: Right- and left-hand PA radiograph. Osteoarthritis or erosive osteoarthritis. This 63-year-old woman worked as a typist for 20 years. Note the advanced osteoarthritic changes (*straight arrows*) involving the distal interphalangeal (DIP) joints of both hands. The DIP joints are markedly narrowed and osteophytes (*curved arrows*) are present. Erosions are also present (*double arrows*). **B:** Left index and long finger lateral radiograph. Osteoarthritis DIP joints. For many years this 60-year-old woman operated an adding machine with her left hand. There is narrowing of the DIP joint spaces due to articular cartilage destruction. There are soft tissue prominences (*curved arrows*) overlying bone excrescences near the DIP joints. These bone excrescences or protuberances are called Heberden nodes (*straight arrows*)

FIGURE 5.86 Right knee AP radiograph. Osteoarthritis. The medial joint space or medial knee compartment is markedly narrowed, the articular surfaces are irregular (*straight arrow*), osteophyte formation (*curved arrow*) is present, and there is varus deformity. Note that the medial joint space has all but disappeared compared to the lateral joint space.

A

B

Cement

Cement

FIGURE 5.87 A: Pelvis AP radiograph. Bilateral hip osteoarthritis in a 61-year-old. The hip joint spaces are irregularly narrowed, and the femoral heads are typically migrating in a cephalad direction (*straight arrows*). The femoral heads are cystic and sclerotic in appearance. Osteophyte formation is present along the periphery of the joints (*curved arrows*). Osteophyte formation is also present in the lower lumbar spine (*double curved arrows*). **B:** Pelvis AP radiograph. Osteoarthritis of the right hip, left hip prosthesis, and bilateral inguinal hernias. There is irregular narrowing of the right hip joint and cephalad migration of the femoral head (*straight arrow*). A left hip prosthesis is in place. The *curved arrows* indicate the prosthetic femoral head and acetabular components. Large bilateral inguinal hernias contain air-filled loops of bowel (*double arrows*).

FIGURE 5.88 Anterior (**A**) and lateral (**B**) radiographs of the right foot in a 64-year old woman. Hallux valgus. The head of the first metatarsal is uncovered as the great toe is directed laterally (*curved arrow*). The great toe is also pronated and the sesamoids of the first metatarsal are subluxed laterally. This person also has a flat foot deformity (pes planus). The head of the talus is directed medially and plantar (*arrows*).

A

B

TABLE 5.14

TYPICAL SYMPTOMS AND RADIOGRAPHIC FINDINGS IN OSTEOARTHRITIS AND RHEUMATOID ARTHRITIS

Osteoarthritis
  Pain, deformity, and limitation of joint motion
  Involves all joints of the extremities and spine
  Typically involves the hand distal interphalangeal (DIP)
    joints and the first metacarpophalangeal (MCP) joint
  Irregular joint narrowing
  Sclerotic bone changes
  Cysts or pseudocysts
  Osteophyte formation
  Usually absence of osteoporosis
  Genu valgus and varus deformities
  Cephalad and sometimes lateral migration of the femoral
    head
Rheumatoid arthritis
  Pain, stiffness, limitation of motion, especially in the hands
    and feet
  Involves all joints of the extremities and spine and all
    synovial joints
  Typically involves the hand MCP joints
  Symmetric joint narrowing
  Periarticular osteoporosis (prominent feature)
  Periarticular soft tissue thickening and swelling
  Marginal and central osseous erosions
  MCP subluxation and ulnar deviation
  Medial migration of the femoral head and acetabular
    protrusio
  Pencil appearance of the distal clavicle

cartilage loss. Acetabular protrusion may result from softening of the bones due to osteoporosis.

Rheumatoid Arthritis

Rheumatoid is another type of arthritis that is frequently encountered in the everyday practice of medicine (Figs. 5.89 to 5.92). It is an inflammatory arthritis of unknown etiology that involves synovial joints and is characterized by symmetric joint narrowing secondary to articular cartilage destruction by pannus, which is granulation tissue derived from the synovium. Some important facts and radiographic findings are listed in Table 5.14. As in osteoarthritis, any or all of the joints in the extremities and spine can be involved. The most commonly affected joints, in decreasing frequency, are the MCP, wrist, PIP, knee, MTP, shoulder, ankle, cervical spine, hip, elbow, and temporomandibular joints. Often the initial symptoms of rheumatoid arthritis are stiffness, pain, limitation of movement, and swelling in the hands and/or feet. Usually, the first joints involved are the MP joints, and this tends to be symmetric. Potentially, the earliest abnormality detectable on a radiograph is periarticular soft tissue thickening. Additional radiographic findings include periarticular osteoporosis due to hyperemia, symmetric joint narrowing, and marginal central erosions. As the disease progresses, joint deformity may develop due to subluxation and ulnar deviation of the fingers at the MCP joints. This later finding is quite characteristic of rheumatoid arthritis. When joint cartilage destruction becomes far advanced, bony ankylosis of the joint

TABLE 5.15

THE DIFFERENTIAL DIAGNOSIS OF RHEUMATOID ARTHRITIS

Gouty arthritis
Infectious arthritis
Sudeck's atrophy
Sarcoid
Osteoarthritis
Ankylosing spondylitis
Scleroderma
Systemic lupus erythematosus

FIGURE 5.90 Right shoulder AP radiograph. Rheumatoid arthritis. There is characteristic osteoporosis, a pointed distal clavicle, and mild cephalad drift of the humeral head. The cephalad drift of the humeral head suggests rotator cuff damage that is common in this disease. There are articular bone erosions (*straight arrows*) and sclerosis (*curved arrows*).

may result. The differential diagnosis of rheumatoid arthritis is shown in Table 5.15.

In gout, osteoporosis is usually absent, and articular and juxta-articular erosions are more sharply defined. In osteomyelitis and infectious arthritis, the osteoporosis is greatest near the infection site. In Sudeck's atrophy, the osteoporosis is severe but the articular margins remain sharp. In osteoarthritis, osteoporosis is usually absent and osteophytes are often present.

Psoriatic Arthritis

Psoriatic arthritis is found in 2% to 6% of patients with skin manifestations of psoriasis although the vast majority of those with psoriatic arthritis have had a long history of psoriatic skin disease and particularly associated with psoriatic nail changes. There are five clinical spectra of the arthritis: (1) polyarthritis with DIP joint involvement, (2) a markedly deforming condition (arthritis mutilans) with widespread ankylosis

(fusion across joints) and destruction, (3) symmetric arthritis resembling rheumatoid arthritis, (4) single or asymmetric, few joint involvement, and (5) sacroiliitis and spondylitis, which may resemble ankylosing spondylitis. The arthritis is characterized by involvement of small joints with asymmetric distribution. There are bone erosions, but, unlike rheumatoid arthritis, there is more frequent ankylosis. Bony proliferation adjacent to joints and at muscle and tendon attachment sites is characteristic (Fig. 5.93).

— Narrowed PIP joints

— Fusiform soft tissue changes

— Narrowed carpal joints

— Ulnar soft tissue prominence

FIGURE 5.89 Right- and left-hand PA radiograph. Rheumatoid arthritis. The radiographic findings include periarticular osteoporosis (*curved arrows*), swan neck deformities of the little fingers, narrowing of the proximal interphalangeal (PIP) joints with associated fusiform soft tissue swelling, narrowing of the carpal and PIP joints, and soft tissue thickening or prominence around the distal ulna. Also, there are erosions involving the carpals, ulnar styloids, and metacarpal heads (*straight arrows*). The fusiform soft tissue swelling surrounding the joints represents edema and effusion. The soft tissue prominence around the distal ulna is secondary to edema and thickening around the external carpi ulnaris.

FIGURE 5.91 Right and left knees AP radiograph. Rheumatoid arthritis in a 27-year-old. There are symmetric narrowing of the knee joints (*straight arrows*), periarticular cysts (*curved arrows*), erosions (*double arrows*), and osteoporosis.

Gout, Pseudogout, and Hemophilic Arthritis

Some arthritides that are associated with metabolic diseases and blood dyscrasias are listed in Table 5.16. Gout arthritis (Fig. 5.94) is secondary to hyperuricemia or elevated serum uric acid levels, and it is characterized by exacerbations and remissions. The patients classically present with podagra or pain and inflammatory changes near the medial aspect of the first MTP joint. The disease usually is present for a number of years before it is detectable on a radiograph; the radiographic findings of gout are listed in Table 5.17.

Chondrocalcinosis means calcification of cartilage, and it is most often noted in the knee. It can be associated with a number of conditions that are listed in Table 5.18. The arthritis of calcium pyrophosphate deposition (CPPD), or the clinical exacerbation termed pseudogout, is found in middle-aged or older people and is caused by the deposition of calcium pyrophosphate dihydrate crystals in the soft tissues of a joint, including menisci, ligaments, articular cartilage, and the joint capsule (Fig. 5.95).

FIGURE 5.92 Pelvis AP radiograph. Rheumatoid arthritis in a 27-year-old. There is generalized osteoporosis. The entire left hip joint space is symmetrically narrowed (*straight arrow*). There is characteristic medial drift of the right femoral head and acetabular protrusio (*curved arrow*). Note that the sacroiliac joints are not involved.

FIGURE 5.93 Anterior radiograph of the left hand second metacarpal-phalangeal joint. There are joint space narrowing and small erosions with a fluffy proliferation of new bone at the joint margins typical of psoriatic arthritis.

TABLE 5.16

ARTHRITIDES ASSOCIATED WITH METABOLIC DISEASES AND BLOOD DYSCRASIAS

Gout
Calcium pyrophosphate deposition (CPPD) disease
Hemophilia

TABLE 5.17

RADIOGRAPHIC FEATURES OF GOUT

Sharply marginated and sometimes sclerotic bordered erosions with overhanging edges near a joint
Tophus formation or soft tissue nodules
Usually osteoporosis is absent
Occasionally joint deformity

TABLE 5.18

CAUSES OF CHONDROCALCINOSIS

Calcium pyrophosphate deposition (CPPD)
Gout
Aging
Hyperparathyroidism

FIGURE 5.94   Right-hand PA radiograph. Gout arthritis. The proximal interphalangeal (PIP) joint spaces are at least partially preserved, and the lucent areas (*double arrows*) are typical of the sharply marginated periarticular erosions. Erosions that extend into the joint often have an overhanging edge (*single straight arrow*). Note the classic appearance of a tophus (*curved arrow*). A tophus is an asymmetric swelling about the joint that may or may not be calcified.

FIGURE 5.95   Left knee AP radiograph. Calcium pyrophosphate deposition (CPPD) disease or pseudogout. There are calcifications in the lateral meniscus (*single straight arrow*) and the medial meniscus (*double straight arrows*). There is also calcification of the articular cartilage (*curved arrow*).

FIGURE 5.96 A: Right shoulder AP radiograph. Hemophilia in a 15-year-old boy. There are cystic changes (*straight arrows*) in the humeral head secondary to repeated bleeds, and there is widening of the shoulder joint (*curved arrow*) due to hemarthrosis. **B:** Knee AP radiograph. Hemophilia in the same patient as in A. He has a widened intercondylar notch (*arrows*) secondary to repeated episodes of hemarthrosis. There is osteoporosis.

The joints in patients with hemophilia are gradually injured by repeated bleeding into the joints. Cystic changes develop in the bones neighboring the injured joints, and osteoporosis is a common feature (Fig. 5.96). In general, osteoporosis is a common feature in rheumatoid arthritis, blood dyscrasias, and osteomyelitis but not in osteoarthritis and gout.

Neuropathic Joints

Chronic trauma to a joint that has lost pain sensation can result in a neuropathic or Charcot's joint (Fig. 5.97). Some common causes are shown in Table 5.19. Diabetic neuropathic joints are most common in the lower extremity, whereas syringomyelia-related neuropathic joints are usually found in the shoulders and upper extremities. The radiographic findings include joint space narrowing, fragmentation of sclerotic subchondral bone, articular bone cortex destruction, joint loose bodies, and bone mass formation at the articular margins. Some of the neuropathic joint findings are similar to those found in osteoarthritis. It is generally not true that patients do not feel pain in their neuropathic joints; rather, the degree of pain is disproportionate to the amount of damage.

Other

Periarticular calcifications can result from acute and chronic trauma (Fig. 5.98). Although they do not involve joints, bone spurs are sometimes considered a form of arthritis. Bone spurs cause pain and may be clinically difficult to differentiate from arthritis. Also, bursitis may cause periarticular pain and can sometimes be demonstrated radiographically. Scleroderma is a connective tissue disorder that potentially involves the musculoskeletal system. Multiple soft tissue calcifications are commonly seen in these patients (Fig. 5.99). Other radiographic changes in scleroderma include atrophy of the finger tips and loss of bone at the tips of the distal phalanges. If joint changes are present, they may simulate rheumatoid arthritis.

TUMORS

Benign

There are a number of benign bone lesions, and it is important to recognize them as such (Table 5.20). A bone island, or enostosis, is the most common bone lesion. It is essentially cortical bone that is found in the medullary cavity and appears as a small sclerotic focus. It blends with the surrounding trabeculae and has no aggressive features (Figs. 5.14 and 5.107D). Fibrous cortical defects or nonossifying fibroma may appear similarly in adults but are closely related to the cortex.

TABLE 5.19

CAUSES OF NEUROPATHIC OR CHARCOT'S JOINTS

Diabetes mellitus
Syringomyelia
Congenital indifference to pain
Meningomyelocele
Peripheral nerve injury

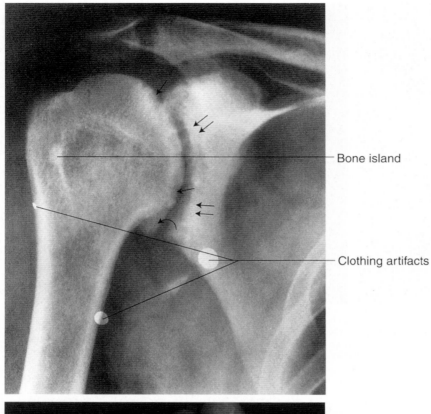

Bone island

Clothing artifacts

A

B

FIGURE 5.97 **A:** Right shoulder AP radiograph. Neuropathic joint or Charcot's joint in a patient with syringomyelia. There is characteristic irregularity of the articular surfaces secondary to destruction of bone and joint cartilage (*single arrows*). There are sclerotic changes or increased density (*double arrows*) of the bone surrounding the joint and an osteophyte (*curved arrow*). **B:** Oblique radiograph of the left foot in a diabetic person. Neuropathic joints. There are healed fracture deformities of the metatarsal heads (*arrows*). The great toe has been amputated because of infection. Note the destruction of the fifth metatarsal head (*curved arrow*) and adjacent ulcer (*double arrow*) from current osteomyelitis.

FIGURE 5.98 Left shoulder AP radiograph with the humerus in external rotation. Calcific tendinitis. There is posttraumatic calcification (*arrow*) in the region of the supraspinatus mechanism.

These are fibroosseous lesions that are lucent and may expand the cortex in children and adolescents. They are typically small and found incidentally but are occasionally large and may focally weaken the cortex where fractures may occur. They heal or involute as the child matures (Fig. 5.100). An osteochondroma or osteocartilaginous exostosis is a common benign bone lesion and can occur in nearly all bones. They are bony projections from the external surface of a bone with a cartilage cap and are most commonly found in the metaphysis

TABLE 5.20
SOME BENIGN BONE LESIONS
Bone island
Nonossifying fibroma/fibrous cortical defect
Osteochondroma
Osteoma
Osteoid osteoma
Enchondroma
Bone cyst
Fibrous dysplasia
Chondroblastoma
Osteoblastoma
Hemangioma

of long bones, especially around the knee and shoulder. These lesions can result in bone deformities and/or cause pressure on surrounding structures. The cartilaginous cap of osteochondromas undergoes malignant transformation to chondrosarcoma in less than 1% of the cases. Multiple osteochondromas or multiple or familial multiple exostoses are a hereditary autosomal-dominant disorder (Fig. 5.101). Growth abnormalities and malignant transformation (5% to 15%) are more common in multiple osteochondromas than in a single osteochondroma.

Another benign bone lesion is the enchondroma (Fig. 5.102A, B). It is a slow-growing cartilaginous tumor usually found in the hand phalanges and in the distal metacarpals. Small calcifications may be present within the lesions, and they may be difficult to differentiate from bone infarcts. Bone

FIGURE 5.99 Right- and left-hand PA radiograph. Scleroderma. Scleroderma is a connective tissue disease that may involve the musculoskeletal system. There are soft tissue calcifications (*straight arrows*), and the soft tissues at the tip of the fingers are atrophic (*curved arrows*). The joints are normal.

FIGURE 5.100 Anterior (**A**) and lateral (**B**) left ankle radiographs in a 12-year-old girl. Nonossifying fibroma. The bony lesion has a sclerotic margin (*arrows*), is slightly lobulated, and arises form the cortex. This benign fibroosseous lesion will eventually become sclerotic and appear as a focal area of cortical thickening when she is an adult.

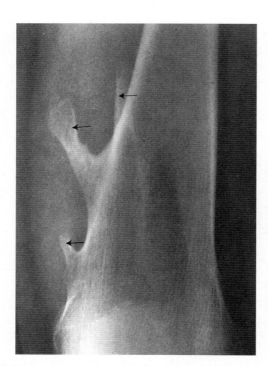

FIGURE 5.101 Left femur AP radiograph. Multiple osteochondromas or familial multiple exostoses. The osteochondromas (*arrows*) point away from the knee joint, simulating a coat hook.

infarcts (Fig. 5.102C) are most commonly present in long bones, and they may or may not be symptomatic. Bone infarcts usually have a well-defined and sclerotic border, whereas enchondromas do not. On occasion, infarcts may have a more permeative appearance, mimicking a malignant primary bone tumor that necessitates a bone biopsy. Some etiologies of bone infarcts include steroid use, sickle cell anemia, systemic lupus erythematosus, Caisson's disease, and pancreatitis.

A simple benign bone cyst (Fig. 5.103) is commonly found in the metaphysis of the proximal humerus and femur, but it can occur in almost any bone. Usually this lesion occurs in patients before the age of 25, and a common complication is a pathologic fracture.

Fibrous dysplasia is a benign fibrous–osseous lesion that arises centrally in the bone, and it can affect one bone (monostotic) or multiple bones (polyostotic). The exact etiology is unknown, and these lesions may or may not be symptomatic. The radiographic features include expansive bone lesions, bone cortex thinning, radiolucent lesions of variable density, and pathologic fractures. The differential diagnosis includes Paget's disease, hyperparathyroidism, and simple bone cyst.

Osteoid osteoma (Fig. 5.104) is a benign bone lesion of unknown etiology, and the typical symptom is night pain relieved by aspirin. It can occur in almost every bone but is most often found in the femoral neck and the tibia. Approximately 75% to 80% of these lesions are intracortical and have multiple radiographic appearances, but the classical appearance is

FIGURE 5.102   A: Right-hand PA radiograph. Enchondroma of the distal fourth metacarpal (*straight arrow*). This slow-growing tumor typically causes thinning and scalloping (*curved arrows*) of the inner bone cortex. **B:** Right knee radiograph. Enchondroma. In a large bone, scalloping of the cortex is less common. The calcification of cartilage often appears as small balls (*straight arrows*) or as arcs (*curved arrows*) and rings. Note osteoarthritis predominantly in the medial compartment of the knee. **C:** Right and left knees AP radiograph. Multiple bone infarcts. The multiple infarcts are manifested by thin zones of sclerosis surrounding lucencies (*straight arrows*) and marrow calcifications (*curved arrows*). The etiology in this patient is unknown.

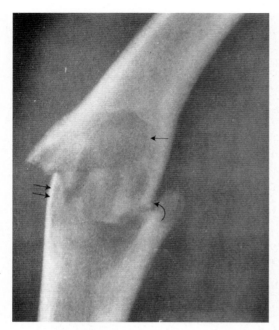

FIGURE 5.103   Right femur AP radiograph. Benign cyst (*straight arrow*) with pathologic fracture (*curved arrow*) in a 10-year-old child. There is apex lateral angulation and mild offset of the fracture fragments. Note the thinning of the bone cortex (*double straight arrows*) caused by the expanding benign cyst.

sclerosis surrounding a radiolucent center or nidus. In some instances, there may be calcifications within this lucent zone mimicking a sequestra of osteomyelitis. The differential diagnosis would also include stress fracture, bone island, infection, and metastatic disease.

Osteoid osteoma has intense activity on a radionuclide bone scan (Fig. 104B), whereas bone islands have none or very little activity (Table 5.21). CT is usually diagnostic, demonstrating the classic nidus (Fig. 5.104C). MRI may also show the nidus but may be confusing because of the large amount of bone edema surrounding it (Fig. 5.104D).

A chondroblastoma (Fig. 5.105) is an uncommon benign bone lesion found in the epiphysis, usually before skeletal maturity. These radiolucent lesions generally have sclerotic borders and sometimes contain scattered calcifications. The

---

TABLE 5.21

USING THE RADIONUCLIDE BONE SCAN TO DIFFERENTIATE BONE LESIONS

Positive bone scans
  Osteoid osteoma
  Primary bone tumors
  Metastases
  Paget's disease

Negative bone scans
  Multiple myeloma
  Bone island
  Enchondroma

---

differential diagnosis should include infection, giant cell tumor, osteoid osteoma, and metastatic disease.

Giant cell tumors occur in young adults following skeletal maturity (Fig. 5.106). These lesions are eccentrically located in the end of long bones such as the tibia, femur, radius, and humerus. They usually have sharp nonsclerotic borders without periosteal reaction and usually abut the articular surface. Based on their radiographic appearance, it is difficult to determine whether they are benign or malignant. Approximately 15% will recur following simple curettage and packing of the defect. They are rarely malignant if metastases are considered a malignant indicator.

Malignant

Metastatic lesions (Fig. 5.107 A–C) are the most common malignant bone tumors and represent spread from a wide variety of primary neoplasms. Bone metastases may be single, multiple, osteolytic (radiolucent or black), osteoblastic (white), or mixed. The majority of metastases are osteolytic radiolucent, but osteoblastic metastases frequently result from cancers of the prostate and breast (Table 5.22). A bone island (Fig. 5.107D) should not be confused with an osteoblastic metastatic lesion. Bone islands are benign, asymptomatic, and distributed widely and usually sparingly in the skeletal system.

Multiple myeloma originates in the bone marrow and is the most common primary malignant bone tumor (Table 5.23). The patient usually complains of pain in the involved area. Although any bone can be involved, the most commonly affected sites include the skull, spine, ribs, and pelvis. Unlike Ewing's sarcoma, this disease occurs in the over-40 age group. The typical radiographic appearance (Fig. 5.108) consists of multiple osteolytic areas with a punched-out appearance. At times it is difficult to differentiate multiple myeloma from osteolytic metastatic disease. *Urine and serum protein electrophoresis is important in the diagnosis of multiple myeloma.*

Osteosarcoma is a primary malignant bone tumor that commonly occurs during the second decade of life. It can occur in many locations but is usually found in the metaphysis of a long bone. It has a wide variety of radiographic appearances but classically produces an abundance of new, irregular bone (Fig. 5.109). In some primary bone tumors a Codman's triangle may be identified, and the triangle represents periosteal new bone formation reacting to the growing tumor. Osteosarcomas may have a Codman's triangle as well as a sunburst or ray appearance that is secondary to bone formation in the tumor (Fig. 5.109). On occasion, it can be difficult to differentiate osteosarcomas from metastatic disease and other primary bone tumors, especially Ewing's sarcoma.

Ewing's sarcoma usually occurs in children and young adults (Fig. 5.110). The classic appearance is a permeative or moth-eaten pattern, but it may have a variety of other associated bone changes such as sclerosis. Occasionally, Ewing's sarcoma has a layered periosteal reaction secondary to the tumor's presence that looks like onion skin. Other lesions in children with periosteal reaction include osteomyelitis, fracture, eosinophilic granuloma, neuroblastoma, and osteosarcoma. The soft tissue extension of Ewing's sarcoma usually will not contain bone or cartilage calcification, whereas the soft tissue extensions of osteosarcomas tend to produce bone.

A

B

Lumbar
spine

Iliac crest

Urinary
bladder

Obturator
foramen

C

D

M 20

FIGURE 5.104 **A:** Left hip AP radiograph. Osteoid osteoma in a 20-year-old patient. The patient experienced left hip night pain that was typically relieved by aspirin. The lucent zone (*arrow*) in the inferior aspect of the left femur subcapital region is the osteoid osteoma. **B:** Anterior pelvis radionuclide scan on the same patient. The single area of increased radionuclide uptake (*arrow*) in the left femoral neck corresponds to the radiolucent abnormality visualized in A. The bone scan is otherwise normal. **C:** Axial CT distal tibia. Osteoid osteoma. The cortical lucent nidus (*arrow*) is nicely demonstrated by CT. Rarely, there is a central dot of calcification in the lucency. **D:** Coronal T1 MR in the same patient does not show the nidus as well as CT (*curved arrow*), but the large amount of edema (gray) is easy to see (*straight arrows*).

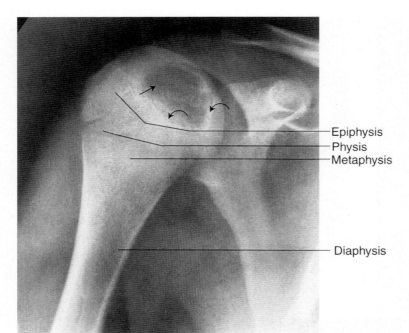

Epiphysis
Physis
Metaphysis

Diaphysis

FIGURE 5.105 Right shoulder AP radiograph. Benign chondroblastoma (*straight arrow*) of the proximal humerus epiphysis in a 14-year-old patient. The typical sclerotic border is present (*curved arrows*).

FIGURE 5.106 Left wrist PA radiograph. Giant cell tumor (*arrow*) of the distal radius. This is the classic appearance and common location of this tumor.

TABLE 5.22

RADIOGRAPHIC APPEARANCE OF BONE METASTASES

Osteoblastic or sclerotic
Prostate
Breast
Carcinoid
Neuroblastoma
Mixed (lytic and blastic)
Breast
Cervix
Bladder
Osteolytic
Nearly all neoplasms

TABLE 5.23

SOME MALIGNANT BONE LESIONS

Primary
Multiple myeloma
Osteosarcoma
Ewing's sarcoma
Chondrosarcoma
Secondary
Metastases

FIGURE 5.107 **A:** Left hip AP radiograph. Metastatic carcinoma of the lung. The radiolucent area in the left iliac bone (*arrow*) represents a suspected osteolytic metastasis. **B:** Pelvis axial CT image in the same patient. Two osteolytic metastases (*arrows*) in the left iliac bone. The CT image confirmed the presence and extent of two bone lesions. **C:** Pelvis AP radiograph. Osteoblastic metastases from carcinoma of the prostate. The *arrows* indicate multiple bilateral osteoblastic (white) metastatic lesions (*arrows*). **D:** Pelvis AP radiograph. Bone island (*straight arrow*). Bone islands are usually ovoid or oblong with a spiculated contour. They are benign and generally asymptomatic.

FIGURE 5.108   Left humerus AP radiograph (**A**) and lateral skull radiograph (**B**). Multiple myeloma. The lucent or black areas indicated by the *arrows* represent the classic appearance of multiple myeloma in bone.

FIGURE 5.109   Left humerus AP radiograph in a 6-year-old. Large osteosarcoma of the humerus metaphysis and diaphysis. The tumor (*single straight arrows*) has not crossed the physis (*arrow head*). Codman's triangle (*double straight arrows*) represents periosteal new bone formation reacting to the tumor growth, and the sunburst or ray appearance (*curved arrow*) represents tumor bone.

Humeral head
Deltoid muscle
Subcutaneous fat
Humeral shaft

FIGURE 5.110   A: Left humerus AP radiograph. Ewing's sarcoma. This 27-year-old presented with left arm and shoulder pain, and the radiographic appearance is typical: a permeative or moth-eaten appearance (*straight arrows*), ill-defined borders, and periosteal reaction (*curved arrows*). **B:** Left humerus coronal T1 MR image on the same patient. Ewing's sarcoma. The tumor replaces nearly all the proximal humerus bone marrow (*straight arrows*). Note how much of the tumor extends into the soft tissue surrounding the proximal humerus (*curved arrow*). This latter finding cannot be fully appreciated on the radiograph. An osteosarcoma could have this same appearance.

METABOLIC DISEASES

Some metabolic diseases have the potential to affect bones significantly. A few examples are listed in Table 5.24.

Paget's Disease

Paget's disease is a common, chronic, and progressive metabolic bone disease of unknown etiology that occurs in adults over the age of 40. This disease can involve all bones (Figs. 5.111 and 6.53). The radiographic features of Paget's disease are listed in Table 5.25. On radiographs, the bone cortices are thick and sclerotic in appearance and the trabecular pattern is thickened and prominent. Rarefaction and bone destruction may occur. Occurring secondary to bone softening are bone deformities such as bowing of long bones and protrusio acetabula. The two most significant complications are pathologic fractures and sarcomatous degeneration. The differential diagnosis should include osteoblastic metastatic disease, fibrous dysplasia, lymphoma, and osteosclerosis.

Osteoporosis and Osteomalacia

Osteoporosis (Figs. 5.20, 5.48, 5.87 to 5.90, 5.93B) is secondary to a reduced amount of bone matrix (osteoid) with normal mineralization, whereas osteomalacia is a normal bone matrix (osteoid) with a reduced amount of mineralization. Osteoporosis has become a major public health problem with 1.5 million related fractures per year and probably costing an estimated 14 billion dollars per year. Osteoporosis accounts for 70% of all fractures in patients over the age of 45 in the United States. Of these, 700,000 are vertebral fractures

TABLE 5.24

SOME METABOLIC DISEASES THAT MAY AFFECT BONES

Paget's disease
Hypothyroidism
Scurvy
Acromegaly
Rickets
Diabetes mellitus
Hyperparathyroidism

TABLE 5.25

RADIOGRAPHIC FEATURES OF PAGET'S DISEASE

Thick and sclerotic bone cortices
Thick and prominent trabecular pattern
Long bone bowing
Acetabular protrusio
Pathologic fractures

FIGURE 5.111 Right tibia and fibula AP (**A**) and lateral (**B**) radiographs. Paget's disease. The tibia cortices are sclerotic in appearance (*straight arrows*) because of widening and thickening of the cortices and a prominent trabecular pattern. The tibia is bowed anterolaterally. The fibula is spared. The typical transverse pathologic fractures are best visualized on the lateral radiograph (*curved arrows*), and they are the most common complication of this disease. There is osteoporosis.

and 300,000 are hip fractures. Ten million Americans have osteoporosis, 80% of these are women. It is estimated that 18 million more are undiagnosed. There is a long list of osteoporosis etiologies, and a partial list of etiologies is shown in Table 5.26. Radiographs are insensitive for evaluation of osteoporosis. Dual x-ray absorptiometry is currently the standard screening method (Fig. 5.112A,B).

TABLE 5.26

SOME ETIOLOGIES OF OSTEOPOROSIS

Immobilization
Sudek's atrophy
Estrogen deficiency or postmenopausal
Steroid therapy
Cushing's disease
Hyperparathyroidism
Diabetes mellitus
Anemia
Paget's disease
Malnutrition
Osteogenesis imperfecta

Rickets

Rickets is a good example of osteomalacia and osteopenia in children. It is found in the growing portions of infant bones and is caused by poor calcification of the osteoid matrix that may result from vitamin D deficiency, renal disease, or intestinal malabsorption diseases. The radiographic findings include widened and irregular physes, cupping of the metaphyses, bowing of the legs, and osteopenia (Fig. 5.113). When this disease occurs in adults, it does not affect the growth plates and is termed osteomalacia.

INFECTION

Osteomyelitis (Fig. 5.114) can occur in all age groups, and the classic clinical presentation is bone or joint pain and fever. There are multiple etiologies including trauma and hematogenous spread of infection (Fig. 5.115). In adults, particularly diabetics, the bone destruction is usually adjacent to a soft tissue ulcer and known infection (see Fig. 5.97B). However, the radiographic appearance of osteomyelitis can be similar to a bone tumor with bone and joint destruction, periosteal reaction, and a soft tissue component. It can be especially confusing when found in the center of bone, such as at a site of prior fracture. Unlike tumors, infections may occasionally have gas in the soft tissues secondary to gas-forming organisms. MRI is

Dual Femur Bone Density

Image not for diagnosis

Reference: Total

BMD (g/cm²)   YA *T*-Score

	BMD[1,6]	Young-Adult[2,7]		Age-Matched[3]	
Region	(g/cm²)	(%)	T-Score	(%)	Z-Score
Neck					
Left	0.685	64	−3.0	79	−1.4
Right	0.667	62	−3.1	77	−1.5
Mean	0.676	63	−3.0	78	−1.4
Difference	0.018	2	0.1	2	0.1
Total					
Left	0.705	64	−2.7	77	−1.5
Right	0.654	59	−3.1	71	−1.9
Mean	0.679	62	−2.9	74	−1.7
Difference	0.052	5	0.4	6	0.4

A

B

FIGURE 5.112 A: Dual x-ray absorptiometry evaluation of bone mineral density in the hips in an 83-year-old man. A *T*-score value of 2.5 or less indicates osteoporosis. This gentleman's is −3.0 on the left and −3.1 on the right. **B:** Coronal T1-weighted MR image of the hips obtained after a minor fall on the same gentleman demonstrates an incomplete intertrochanteric hip fracture (*arrow*).

FIGURE 5.113   Right and left knees AP radiographs. Rickets. The physes are widened (*straight arrows*), and the metaphases are cupped (*curved arrows*).

A

FIGURE 5.114 **A:** Left foot AP radiograph. Osteomyelitis in a patient with diabetes mellitus. There are destructive changes (*straight arrows*) involving the base of the proximal phalanx of the fourth toe as well as the fourth metatarsal head. Also, there are destructive changes in the fourth metatarsophalangeal joint manifested by narrowing of the joint space. The infection has characteristically caused destructive joint changes as well as bone destruction on both sides of the joint. Loose bone fragments have resulted from the osteomyelitis (*curved arrows*). **B:** Left foot axial T1 MR image in the same patient. When compared to the other metatarsal heads, the fourth metatarsal head is not visible because the infection (*arrow*) has destroyed and replaced the bone marrow.

Skin marker

1st, 2nd, 3rd metatarsal heads

5th metatarsal head

B

A

B

FIGURE 5.115 **A:** AP radiograph of the left knee in a child. Osteomyelitis. Focal lucency is noted in the epiphysis (*arrows*). **B:** Coronal fat-suppressed T2 MR in the same patient shows the abscess crosses the physis and involves the metaphysic as well (*arrows*).

a very useful tool for the demonstration of bone and soft tissue involvement by infection. However, it can be a confusing picture in a diabetic foot, which may also have abnormalities and fractures due to neuropathic changes (Fig. 5.97B). Osteomyelitis in children is more likely from hematologic seeding and is most often found in the metaphyseal regions of bones where it is thought that the normal loop in the bone's feeding blood vessels creates a slow flow of blood and increased chance for bacteria to deposit.

APPROACH TO COMMON CLINICAL PROBLEMS

When evaluating the musculoskeletal system, a thorough physical examination should dictate the next appropriate steps in imaging. Radiographs are typically the initial screening tool but should be used appropriately. For example, if a patient presents with pain after falling on an outstretched arm, one would not order a radiograph of the upper arm. Nor should one order radiographs of the humerus and forearm in an attempt to screen for injuries to the shoulder, humerus, elbow, forearm, and wrist. A bone is best imaged when the x-ray beam is centered at that bone or joint. Elbow joint effusions are typically not seen on films of the humerus and forearm. Similarly, radial head fractures or scaphoid fractures may be seen only on specialized dedicated views. If our hypothetical patient has focal tenderness over the radial head or has pain with pronation and supination, a dedicated elbow radiographic series is the appropriate choice. If a shoulder dislocation is suspect, a shoulder series to include an axillary or transcapular Y-view is the appropriate study of choice.

When the radiographs are normal, the clinical setting and degree of suspicion of injury will dictate how to proceed. Often, immobilization with repeat radiographs in 1 week is sufficient to evaluate for an occult fracture. This is not appropriate, however, for a potential hip fracture in an elderly person as immobilization could have devastating effects. An emergent MRI has been shown to be the imaging procedure of choice in this circumstance.

KEY POINTS

- It is important to recognize sesamoid bones and ossicles as normal variants. Sesamoids are bones within a tendon. Ossicles are extra or supernumerary bones next to the skeleton and usually named after the neighboring bone.
- MRI is useful for injuries to the shoulder rotator cuff, knee ligaments and menisci, ankle ligaments, and Achilles

tendon. CT imaging is good for bone detail, fracture diagnosis, locating fracture fragments, and evaluating matrix formation in bone tumors.

- The Salter-Harris classification describes fractures around the physis, which is considered the weakest point in a growing bone.
- Because fractures and other abnormalities may not be visualized on all radiographic views, always insist on at least two views of an injured or diseased area that are 90 degrees to each other.
- Fractures may not be visible on the first radiographs but may become visible after time (7 days) because of bone resorption at the ends of the fracture fragments.
- A transverse lucent line at the base of the fifth metatarsal always represents a fracture, whereas the normal apophysis in this area is lateral and parallel to the long axis of the metatarsal.
- Osteoarthritis is the most common form of arthritis and often results from asymmetric cartilage wear.
- The radiographic features of osteoarthritis include irregular joint narrowing, sclerosis, absence of osteoporosis, and osteophyte formation.
- The radiographic features of rheumatoid arthritis include periarticular thickening, symmetric joint narrowing, marginal erosions, periarticular osteoporosis, and joint deformity.
- Metastatic cancer is the most common malignant bone tumor. The majority of metastatic lesions are osteolytic or radiolucent. Osteoblastic metastatic lesions most commonly are secondary to prostate and breast neoplasms.
- Multiple myeloma is the most common primary malignant bone tumor, and it originates in the bone marrow.
- Ewing's sarcoma usually occurs in children and young adults. They may have a permeative type of lesion and an onion-skin–like periosteal reaction.
- Osteomyelitis and septic joints typically present with localized pain and fever. The radiographic features include bone and joint destruction, periosteal reaction, and occasionally, a soft tissue component.

Further Readings

Chew FS, Kline MJ, Bui-Mansfield LT. *Core curriculum: musculoskeletal imaging,* Philadelphia: Lippincott Williams & Wilkins, 2003.

El-Khoury GY. *Essentials of musculoskeletal imaging.* New York: Churchill Livingstone, 2003.

El-Khoury GY, Bergman RA, Montgomery WJ. *Sectional anatomy by MRI,* 2nd ed. New York: Churchill Livingstone, 1995.

CHAPTER 6 ■ SPINE AND PELVIS

CAROL A. BOLES

The axial skeleton is the next focus for our consideration. It consists of the skull (which is covered separately), the spine, and the pelvis. It is the main structural support for the body and, as a result, is subjected to many stresses. The spine consists of cervical, thoracic, lumbar, and sacral divisions composed of bones, joints, ligaments, muscular attachments, and nerves. The pelvis articulates with the sacrum on each side, supports many soft tissue structures, articulates with the femurs, and is the proximal attachment for many muscles involved in locomotion.

Back pain is a problem for the majority of our patients at some time in their lives. Most people recover from their back pain with little or no medical care. Occupation-related back injuries are common, and other common etiologies of back pain are listed in Table 6.1. When patients do seek medical care for back pain, radiologic imaging often becomes an important diagnostic tool. Following a thorough history and physical examination, routine anteroposterior (AP) and lateral radiographs often are the first radiologic consultation to be requested to evaluate the symptomatic region of the spine. These images may be supplemented with oblique and coned-down views to better visualize an area, and occasionally lateral flexion and extension views are requested to document spine motion and stability.

Computed tomography (CT) and magnetic resonance imaging (MRI) are extremely useful noninvasive diagnostic tools in visualizing the spine, and their use is increasing while use of the invasive myelogram is decreasing. CT delineates anatomy and pathology more clearly than does myelography. One significant shortcoming of myelography is its inability to demonstrate lateral disc herniations and lateral stenosis. For this reason, CT is obtained following myelography to better delineate the contrast distribution in the dural sac and visualize the in-

tervertebral discs. CT is excellent for bone detail and is useful for diagnosing fractures not visible on plain radiographs as well as better defining the extent of injury. CT is helpful for localizing the exact position of vertebral fracture fragments, particularly important when the fracture fragments are displaced into the spinal canal. Lateral radiographs are used to assess for instability with flexion–extension views. Full series are useful during follow-up of cervical spine injuries, so a thorough understanding of the radiographs remains important. CT is also useful in screening for disc disease and degenerative disease but has largely been replaced by MRI for this purpose. MRI is very good for imaging soft tissues and the bone marrow and allows a wonderful view of the spinal cord and the intervertebral discs. MRI is also used when a spine fracture is present and an associated cord injury is suspected. However, MRI costs approximately twice as much as CT imaging (Table 6.2). In addition, some patients may not be able to have an MRI because the strong magnetic field may disrupt a pacemaker or displace an aneurysm clip, or the patient may not tolerate the relatively confined space.

NORMAL IMAGES

Cervical Spine

As previously emphasized in other anatomic regions, a systematic approach for evaluating the spine is needed. You will eventually develop your own system, but the following one will work until you do (Table 6.3). Start with the lateral radiograph (Fig. 6.1A) as it is the most important cervical spine radiograph. Glance at the entire image to see whether something obvious jumps out at you. If it does, put that aside

TABLE 6.1

BACK PAIN ETIOLOGIES

Congenital
  Meningocele and myelomeningocele
  Scoliosis
  Transitional vertebra with pseudarthrosis
Acquired
  Arthritis—degenerative, rheumatoid, ankylosing
    spondylitis
  Infection—staphylococcus, tuberculosis
  Metabolic—osteoporosis, osteomalacia, Paget's disease,
    sickle cell anemia
  Neoplasm—benign and malignant primary bone tumors,
    metastases
  Trauma—fracture, muscle and ligament injury,
    spondylolysis, and spondylolisthesis
Extraspinal
  Cardiovascular system—referred myocardial pain, aortic
    aneurysm
  Gastrointestinal disease
  Genitourinary system—renal and ureteral pain
  Muscle strain
  Psychosomatic or functional

and force yourself to look at the entire study. It is not uncommon to stop looking once one abnormality is found. This can lead to serious consequences! On the lateral radiograph, the normal cervical curve should be mildly convex anteriorly (lordotic). When the patient has pain, straightening of the spine may occur secondary to muscle spasm. A

TABLE 6.2

INDICATIONS FOR THE USE OF IMAGING MODALITIES IN THE SPINE AND PELVIS

Radiographs

Routine
  Cervical spine—AP and lateral
  Thoracic spine—AP and lateral
  Lumbar spine—AP and lateral
  Pelvis—AP
Optional when indicated
  Cervical spine—AP open-mouth view and/or swimmer's
    view in trauma, flexion, and extension views for
    mobility and stability, oblique views for the neural
    foramina
  Lumbar spine—flexion and extension views for stability
    and mobility, oblique views for spondylolysis
  Sacroiliac joints—oblique views, modified outlet view
CT
  Fractures and disc disease
MRI
  Soft tissues and bone marrow
  Spinal cord and disc disease
  Fractures with suspected cord injury
Myelogram
  Disc disease, spinal stenosis, cord, and extradural tumors

TABLE 6.3

CHECKLIST FOR SPINAL RADIOGRAPH OBSERVATIONS

Lateral radiograph
  Alignment (three lines in cervical spine)
  Must visualize seven cervical vertebrae
  Vertebral body heights
  Disc space heights
  Osseous density
AP radiograph
  Alignment
  Vertebral body heights
  Disc space heights
  Bone density
  Pedicles (lower cervical)

patient in a hard cervical collar also has a straightened curvature. Make note of the normal lines that should be intact on this view (Fig. 6.1B). Now simply count the cervical vertebrae. Things you must see include all seven cervical vertebrae, the entire C7 and T1 intervertebral disc space, and, ideally, the T1 vertebral body. This is especially important in trauma situations as a fracture could be lurking in nonvisualized areas of the spine, and the result could be catastrophic. For example, if the C7 vertebra is not included on the lateral cervical spine radiograph, a fracture of C7 might go unrecognized. An unrecognized and displaced fracture has the potential to cause a serious cord injury. *Always* gauge the vertical heights of the vertebral bodies and the intervertebral disc spaces. The vertical heights of each vertebral body and intervertebral disc space should be approximately equal to those immediately above and below. Note the osseous densities in general. Some common causes for decreased (osteopenia)

TABLE 6.4

SOME COMMON CAUSES FOR INCREASED AND DECREASED BONE DENSITY

Decreased
  Osteolytic metastases
  Osteomalacia
  Osteomyelitis
  Osteoporosis
  Primary bone tumor, especially multiple myeloma
  Rheumatoid arthritis, ankylosing spondylitis
Increased
  Bone infarcts
  Bone island
  Callus formation—fractures
  Endplate sclerosis—disc degeneration
  Fibrous dysplasia
  Lymphoma
  Osteoblastic metastases (prostate and breast)
  Osteopetrosis
  Paget's disease
  Primary bone tumors (<5% of multiple myeloma)

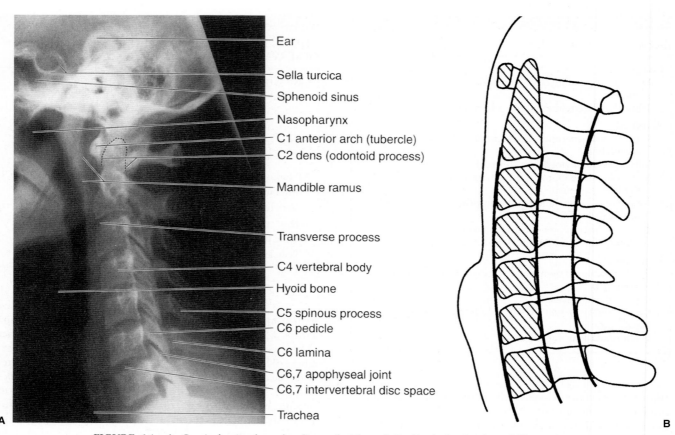

FIGURE 6.1 **A:** Cervical spine lateral radiograph. Normal. **B:** Cervical spine lateral illustration. Normal lines found on the normal lateral radiograph.

Labels on figure: Ear; Sella turcica; Sphenoid sinus; Nasopharynx; C1 anterior arch (tubercle); C2 dens (odontoid process); Mandible ramus; Transverse process; C4 vertebral body; Hyoid bone; C5 spinous process; C6 pedicle; C6 lamina; C6,7 apophyseal joint; C6,7 intervertebral disc space; Trachea

and increased bone density are shown in Table 6.4. Metastatic bone disease from prostate, breast, and other malignancies can result in an increased bone density or osteosclerotic appearance.

Next, look at the AP radiograph (Fig. 6.2A) and again check the alignment of the cervical spine. The spine should be straight on this view. Again note the heights of the vertebral bodies and intervertebral disc spaces. When disease or injury is suspected at the C1 and C2 levels, an AP radiograph of the upper cervical spine is obtained by directing the central x-ray beam through the patient's open mouth. This is called the *open-mouth view* (Fig. 6.2B), and it allows visualization of the dens, or odontoid process, of the C2 vertebra and the C1 and C2 alignments and joints. An extremely important observation to make is the presence or absence of the vertebral pedicles. Pedicles look like the headlights of the vertebrae in the low cervical, thoracic, and lumbar regions but are obliquely oriented in the upper and mid cervical spine and best seen on cervical oblique views. They are often involved by metastatic disease because of their abundant blood supply. *If one or more pedicles are absent, metastatic involvement or some other destructive process must be strongly suspected.* There are benign causes such as a meningocele or congenital absence of the pedicle, but these need to be proven rather than assumed.

Occasionally, oblique views (Fig. 6.3) are obtained and the same observations are made as on the other views. The intervertebral foramina, through which the spinal nerves pass, are well seen on these views. Any disease process that narrows the foramina could potentially cause pressure on the nerve exiting through that neural foramen, resulting in radiculopathy, or pain along the distribution of the involved nerve. Some processes that can impinge on the intervertebral foramina include intervertebral disc disease, arthritis, and primary and secondary neoplasms. In the trauma setting, these oblique views allow for evaluation of the facet joints to look for fractures or dislocations.

Lateral flexion and extension views may be necessary to evaluate stability of the spine and assess for ligamentous injury. They should not routinely be obtained when a fracture is present. The majority of motion occurs in the upper cervical spine. When the lower cervical vertebrae cannot be visualized on the lateral view, a swimmer's view is indicated (Fig. 6.4). CT is often used to diagnose occult cervical spine fractures, determine the extent of fractures, and localize fracture fragments. At many medical centers, severe trauma patients are routinely screened with a CT of the entire cervical spine. The CT data can then be reformatted into coronal and sagittal plane images (see Fig. 6.29B). As already mentioned, MRI is especially useful for evaluating the spinal

- Mandible angle
- Transverse process
- Intervertebral disc space
- C5 vertebral body
- Spinous process
- C7 pedicles
- Trachea
- T1 transverse process
- 1st rib
- Lung

A

- Tooth
- Odontoid
- C1 inferior articular facet
- C2 superior articular facet
- C2 vertebral body
- Bifid spinous process
- Mandible teeth
- Mandible body

B

FIGURE 6.2 A: Cervical spine AP radiograph. Normal. **B:** Cervical spine AP open-mouth radiograph of the upper cervical spine. Normal.

cord and the intervertebral discs and for assessing ligamentous injury (Fig. 6.5).

Thoracic (Dorsal) Spine

Routine radiographic study of the thoracic spine consists of AP and lateral radiographs (Fig. 6.6). When viewing the thoracic spine, it is easiest to begin with the lateral view and follow the same method of evaluation as used for the lateral cervical spine radiograph. The normal dorsal curve should be mildly convex posterior (kyphotic). Again, assess the vertical heights of the dorsal vertebral bodies and intervertebral disc spaces. As always, check the overall densities of the bones. The lamina and spinous processes are not well seen because the ribs project over them (Fig. 6.6B). It is difficult to number the vertebral bodies without using the anterior view to determine the size of the twelfth ribs.

Next, evaluate the AP thoracic spine radiograph; the spinal alignment should be straight. Assess the vertical height of each dorsal vertebral body and each dorsal intervertebral disc space. The paraspinal line along the left side of the

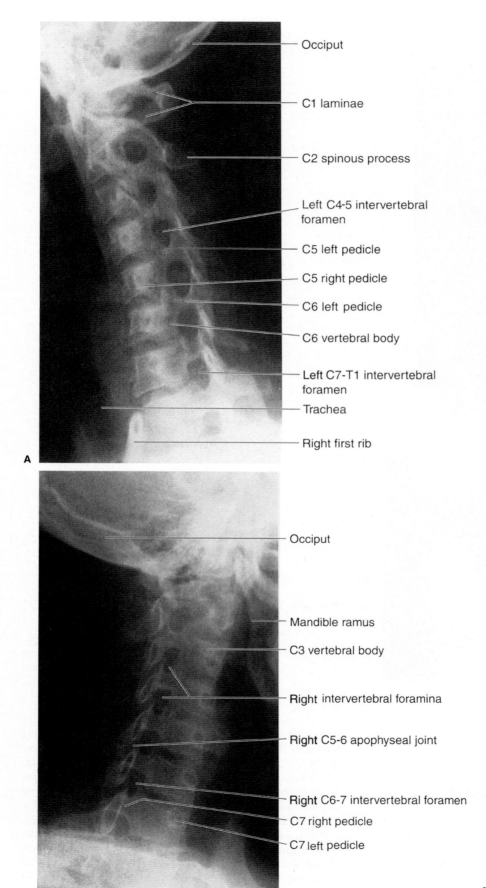

Occiput

C1 laminae

C2 spinous process

Left C4-5 intervertebral foramen

C5 left pedicle

C5 right pedicle

C6 left pedicle

C6 vertebral body

Left C7-T1 intervertebral foramen

Trachea

Right first rib

A

Occiput

Mandible ramus

C3 vertebral body

Right intervertebral foramina

Right C5-6 apophyseal joint

Right C6-7 intervertebral foramen

C7 right pedicle

C7 left pedicle

B

FIGURE 6.3 Cervical spine right (**A**) and left (**B**) oblique radiographs. Normal.

C1 anterior arch

C2 spinous process

Apophyseal joint

C4 vertebral body

C7 vertebral body

T1 vertebral body

FIGURE 6.4 Cervical spine lateral swimmer's view. Normal. The patient is almost always radiographed supine with one arm, usually the left, abducted upward alongside the head, whereas the other arm is lowered. This position makes patients appear as if they are swimming the backstroke. The central x-ray beam is directed to the C7-T1 level from the patient's side on which the arm is lowered, usually the right. The *straight arrows* indicate the raised arm humerus projecting over the spine. The *curved arrows* outline the humeral head. Note how well the C7 vertebra is visualized as well as a portion of the T1 vertebra and the apophyseal joints. In this view, it is considered a good technique when you can see the entire C7 vertebra and at least the upper one third of the T1 vertebral body.

vertebra should be narrow and straight. A focal bulge may be your first indication of a fracture. The pedicles look like headlights on the vertebral bodies, and every attempt should be made to visualize all of them. On AP radiographs, the spinous processes project over the midvertebral bodies at all levels in the spine. Assess the number of rib-bearing vertebra. T12 typically has two short ribs, but transverse processes may instead be present. Similarly, L1 may have rudimentary ribs, so it is important to count from the top down. Occasionally, C7 will have short ribs, but these do not have the typical curved appearance of the true first rib and are usually not a cause of mislabeling. MRI and CT (Fig. 6.7) imaging are useful in the dorsal spine for the same indications as in the cervical spine.

Lumbar Spine

Pain in the lumbar spine region is a major cause of disability, lost work time, and health dollar expenditure. The etiology of back pain is complicated, varied, and poorly understood. Following a careful history and physical examination of the lower back, the next step in the evalua-

tion process usually includes radiographs. Routine lumbar radiographs generally consist of AP and lateral views (Fig. 6.8). As previously noted, look first at the lateral view using the same system as described for the lateral cervical and dorsal spine radiographs. In general, note the lumbar spine alignment, which is normally convex anterior (lordotic). When muscle spasm or disease processes are present, this normal curvature may be lost and the spine may appear straight. In addition, observe the overall osseous densities. Next, carefully evaluate the vertical heights of the lumbar vertebral bodies and the intervertebral disc spaces; they should be approximately equal to those immediately above and below but gradually become taller as you progress distally. As a general rule, the L4-5 intervertebral disc space height is greater than the other lumbar disc spaces. If the L4-5 disc space is the same height as those above or below, you should suspect L4-5 disc disease. This also means that the L5-S1 disc level is typically narrower than that at L4-5 and should not be considered abnormal because of decreased height alone. Approximately 15% of the population will have variability in the appearance at the lumbosacral junction. There may be partial or complete lumbarization of S1 or sacralization of L5. Numbering of the lumbar spine

Cerebellum

C2 dens (odontoid)

C2 vertebral body

Cervical spinal cord

C3 vertebral body

Intervertebral disc

Nuchal ligament

Cerebral spinal fluid

Spinous process

A

Cerebellum

C2 dens (odontoid)

C2 vertebral body

Cervical spinal cord

C3 vertebral body

Intervertebral disc

Nuchal ligament

Cerebral spinal fluid

Spinous process

B

FIGURE 6.5   A: Cervical spine sagittal T1 MR image. Normal. The cerebral spinal fluid is black on a T1 image and white on a T2 image. The bone marrow fat appears whiter (high-intensity signal) on a T1 image than on a T2 image. **B:** Cervical spine sagittal T2 MR image. Normal.

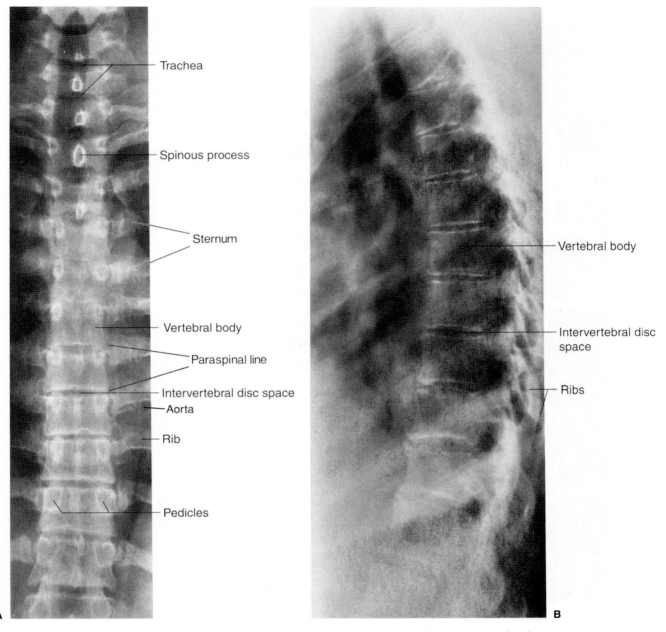

FIGURE 6.6   A: Thoracic spine AP radiograph. Normal. The pedicles on each vertebra have an appearance similar to automobile headlights. **B:** Thoracic spine lateral radiograph. Normal.

A: — Aorta
— Dorsal vertebral body
— Diaphragm crus
— Spinal canal
— Costovertebral articulation
— 12th rib
— Transverse process
— Spinous process
Pedicle —
Lamina —
A

B: — Aorta
— Left kidney
— Diaphragm crura
— Vertebral body
— Basivertebral vein
— Costovertebral joint
— Pedicle
— 12th rib
— Lamina
— Mamillary process
— Spinous process
B

FIGURE 6.7   A: Thoracic spine axial CT image at the T12 level. Normal. **B:** Thoracic spine axial CT image at the T12 level. Normal. The spinal cord (*straight arrow*), nerve roots (*curved arrows*), and the contrast-filled subarachnoid space (*double arrows*) are well visualized. The contrast media was introduced into the subarachnoid space as part of a myelogram while the CT imaging followed the myelogram. Note how well the osseous structures of the spine are demonstrated.

can be very difficult, and every attempt should be made to number correctly using chest radiographs if needed to count the number of ribs. It is incorrect to assume that the first non–rib-bearing vertebra on the anterior view is L1 and the vertebra above the sacrum on lateral view is L5. I have seen the same vertebral body numbered differently on the AP and lateral views!

Always observe the pars interarticularis region of each vertebra for a possible defect; an interruption of bone continuity in the pars interarticularis is abnormal and called *spondylolysis*. The pars can be seen on lateral view but is difficult on the anterior projection. It is easiest to see on the oblique view. Similar observations are made on the AP radiograph regarding alignment, density, vertical heights of the lumbar vertebral bodies, and the lumbar intervertebral disc spaces. Again, be certain that all of the pedicles are present. Depending on the angulation at L5-S1, it may be difficult to see the L5 pedicles. Occasionally, an angled anterior view is obtained to better evaluate L5 (Fig. 6.9). This view also nicely displays the sacroiliac (SI) joints. Also note that

— 12th left rib

— Transverse process L1

— L1 spinous process

— L2 pedicles

— L3 vertebral body

— L3-4 intervertebral joint space

— Sacrum

A

— 12th ribs

— L1-L2 intervertebral disc space

— L2 vertebral body

— Transverse process

— Pars interarticularis

— L4 pedicle

— L5 spinous process

— Sacrum first segment

B

FIGURE 6.8 Lumbar spine AP (**A**) and lateral (**B**) radiographs. Normal. The *arrows* on the AP radiograph indicate the pars interarticularis region.

— Left pedicle L5

— L5-S1 disc space

— SI joint

FIGURE 6.9 Lumbar spine angled view of lumbosacral junction. Note how the L5-S1 disc is now easily seen when compared to Fig. 6.8. The facets are prominent because of arthritis. The *small straight arrows* show the arcuate line of the right S1 anterior sacral foramen.

oblique radiographs (Fig. 6.10) are sometimes necessary to better assess the pars interarticularis when spondylolysis is suspected. Once again, the observation checklist for spine radiographs is outlined in Table 6.3.

MRI of the lumbar spine is often requested to evaluate the vertebrae, intervertebral disc spaces, and the spinal cord (Fig. 6.11), which usually ends at the level of L1. As elsewhere in the spine, CT imaging may be requested to determine the presence and extent of fractures and the presence of intervertebral disc disease (Fig. 6.12).

In the past, the myelogram was the gold standard for the diagnosis of disease in and around the neural canal. The myelogram is an invasive procedure that is accompanied by discomfort. It is accomplished by injecting contrast material into the subarachnoid space via a lumbar or cervical puncture, and typical images are shown in Fig. 6.13. Fortunately, water-soluble myelographic contrast agents do not require physical removal as oil-based contrast once did. CT rou-

tinely follows the injection to better define the disc and nerve pathology. Understandably, CT and magnetic resonance (MR) examinations are more acceptable to the patient than the invasive spinal puncture associated with myelography.

The sacrum should be evaluated with both the spine and the pelvis, playing a role in both. Unfortunately, it may be difficult to evaluate, especially in an older patient with osteoporosis. The normal sacrum has an anterior concavity and is tilted posteriorly at the L5-S1 junction. The arcuate lines of the neural foramina should be evaluated closely on the AP view. They should be smoothly curved and symmetric (Fig. 6.14). Asymmetry may be the result of fracture or tumor involvement. The SI joints should be evaluated as they are important in the evaluation of several arthritides and may be widened as a result of trauma. Both CT and MRI can be useful in the evaluation of the sacrum and SI joints.

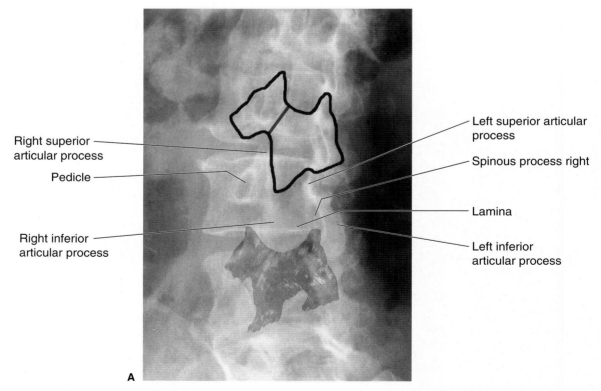

FIGURE 6.10   **A:** Visible "Scotty dog" and the anatomy that it represents on oblique lumbar spine radiographs. The neck of the Scotty dog represents the pars interarticularis. When the Scotty dog neck is absent, the condition is called spondylolysis. (*continued*)

- Transverse process
- Pedicle
- Transverse process
- Sacroiliac joint

- L1 vertebral body
- L2 superior articular process
- L2 pedicle
- L2 inferior articular process
- Sacroiliac joint

FIGURE 6.10 (*Continued*) **B, C:** Lumbar spine right (**B**) and left (**C**) oblique radiographs. Normal. Note on these oblique views how well you visualize the normal pars interarticularis or the neck of the Scotty dog (*straight arrows*) and the normal apophyseal (facet) joints between the superior and inferior articular processes (*curved arrows*).

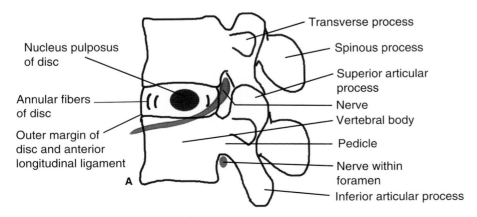

- Nucleus pulposus of disc
- Annular fibers of disc
- Outer margin of disc and anterior longitudinal ligament
- Transverse process
- Spinous process
- Superior articular process
- Nerve
- Vertebral body
- Pedicle
- Nerve within foramen
- Inferior articular process

FIGURE 6.11 **A:** Lumbar spine lateral illustration. Normal. (*continued*)

FIGURE 6.11 (*Continued*) **B, C:** Lumbar spine T1 (**A**) and T2 (**B**) sagittal MR images. Normal. Notice again that the cerebral spinal fluid is black on a T1 image and white on a T2 image. Also, the bone marrow fat is whiter (high-intensity signal) on the T1 image. The intervertebral disc is whiter on the T2 image. **D:** Lumbar spine T1 axial image. Normal. Note that the nerve roots (*curved arrows*) are well visualized. **E:** Lumbar spine T1 coronal MR image. Normal. The coronal plane passes through the upper lumbar vertebral bodies and the lower lumbar neural sac.

A

— Lumbar intervertebral disc

— Right kidney

— Psoas muscle

— Apophyseal joint

— Ligamentum flavum

B

— Aorta

— Inferior vena cava

— Lumbar vertebral body

— Pedicle

— Lamina

— Transverse process

— Inferior articular process

— Spinous process

C

— Intervertebral disc

— Psoas muscle

— Ligamentum flavum

— Apophyseal joint

FIGURE 6.12 **A:** Lumbar spine axial CT image through the L1-2 intervertebral disc level. Normal. The *straight arrows* indicate the cauda equina surrounded by contrast media in the subarachnoid space cerebral spinal fluid (*curved arrow*). **B:** Lumbar spine axial CT image through a lumbar vertebra. Normal. The *straight arrows* indicate multiple nerve roots. Notice how the inferior articular processes of the vertebra articulate with the superior articular processes (*curved arrows*) from the vertebra below to form the apophyseal joints (*double arrows*). **C:** Lumbar spine axial CT image through a lumbar intertebral disc. Normal. The *straight arrow* indicates nerve roots in the posterior aspect of the subarachnoid space, whereas the *curved arrows* indicate nerve roots about to exit through the neural foramina. (*continued*)

12th rib

Spinal cord

L1 pedicle

Nerves

D

FIGURE 6.12 (*Continued*) **D:** Lumbar spine coronal reformatted CT. The image was obtained following a myelogram and reformatted through the thecal space. This has a similar appearance to the conventional myelogram radiographs and shows the conus quite well.

Pelvis

An AP pelvis radiograph is the standard view (Fig. 6.15). A lateral view is not obtained, but on occasion up- and down-tilt AP (outlet and inlet) views are indicated to assess fracture displacement. A modified outlet view is also useful for assessing the SI joints. As elsewhere, you must know the anatomy and have a system for looking at the pelvis radiograph. First, look at the sacrum and coccyx followed by the iliac bones bilaterally. Compare the SI joints as they may be narrowed or even absent in diseases like ankylosing spondylitis (see Fig. 6.47C). Then check out the ischial bones bilaterally as well as the pubic rami and the symphysis pubis. *Remember that the hamstring muscles arise from the ischial tuberosity*; this explains why someone with a hamstring injury runs off the athletic field clutching his or her buttock. As you know, all of the pelvic bones must be evaluated for fractures, density, anomalies, and metastatic lesions.

ANOMALIES

Anomalies of the spine and pelvis (Table 6.5) vary in severity from mild to severe. *As a general rule, most mild spinal anomalies are asymptomatic.* Small extra bones or supernumerary

TABLE 6.5

A PARTIAL LIST OF SPINE AND PELVIS ANOMALIES

Mild
  Accessory ossicles
  Cervical ribs
  Hemivertebra
  Osteitis condensans ilii
  Scoliosis
  Spina bifida
  Transitional vertebrae
Severe
  Absence of the sacrum
  Meningocele and myelomeningocele
  Scoliosis
  Symphysis diastasis

bones called *accessory ossicles* are usually asymptomatic, and they may be located near many different bones including the spine. Examples of accessory ossicles are shown in Fig. 6.16A and B. Accessory ossicles are simply normal variants and should not be confused with a fracture. The smoothly corticated, usually rounded margins help differentiate them from fractures.

Occasionally, extra ribs arise from the cervical spine, and they are called *cervical ribs* (Fig. 6.16C). Cervical ribs are generally asymptomatic but have the potential to cause symptoms secondary to extrinsic pressure on the brachial plexus and the vessels of the upper extremities. A common anomaly at the lumbosacral junction is a *transitional vertebra* in which the L5 vertebra begins to have the appearance of the sacrum or the sacrum begins to look like a lumbar vertebra. *Partial sacralization* of L5 is the term used when fusion exists between a portion of the L5 vertebra and the sacrum (Fig. 6.17A). Usually one of the L5 transverse processes is enlarged and fused with the sacrum, but there are many variations. Occasionally, the anatomic L5 is completely sacralized, having the appearance of the first portion of the sacrum. Transitional vertebra may become symptomatic, especially after excessive back strain or when there is a *pseudarthrosis* (two bones articulating without a joint between them) as seen in Fig. 6.17. A less common anomaly is an abnormal articulation between the C1 spinous process and the occiput (Fig. 6.17B). A more severe anomaly of the spine is total absence of the posterior vertebral arch as in a meningomyelocele.

An important anomaly is spina bifida (Fig. 6.18), which occurs in approximately 5% of the population. Spina bifida occulta is a midline defect of the vertebral arch (usually posterior), and it is generally asymptomatic. When spina bifida has an associated soft tissue mass associated, it is called a meningocele. Meningoceles contain cerebral spinal fluid, and the sac envelope consists of the meninges. When the sac contains spinal cord and/or nerve roots, it is called a *myelomeningocele* ("myelo-" refers to the cord). A *meningocele* (Fig. 6.19) is a herniation of neural tissue through a bone defect. The size of these herniations is variable, and the herniation direction most commonly is posterior but can be anterior or lateral. The symptoms vary

FIGURE 6.13   A: Thoracic spine posteroanterior (PA) myelogram radiograph. Normal. The spinal cord (*between the straight arrows*) is outlined by the injected subarachnoid contrast media (*curved arrows*). **B:** Lumbar spine oblique and PA myelogram radiographs. Normal. The *straight arrows* indicate the nerve roots surrounded by contrast media exiting the spinal canal. The *curved arrows* indicate nerve roots within the thecal sac. The *double arrows* indicate the L5 lumbar vertebra. **C:** Lumbar spine lateral myelogram radiograph. Normal. The thecal sac contains contrast media (*straight arrow*).

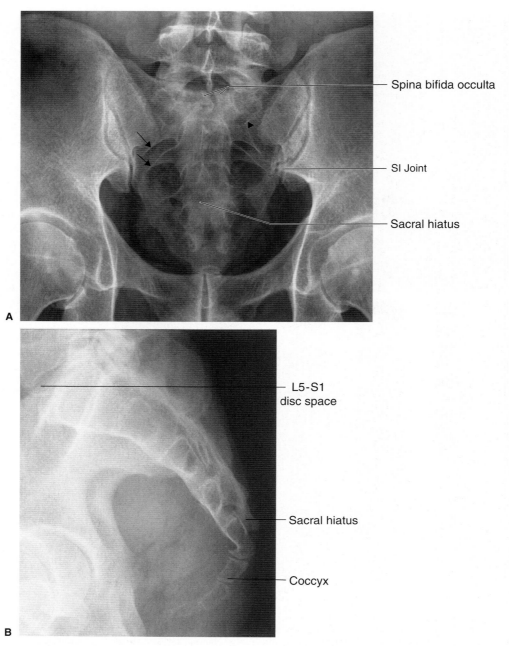

Spina bifida occulta

SI Joint

Sacral hiatus

L5-S1
disc space

Sacral hiatus

Coccyx

FIGURE 6.14 Sacrum AP with cephalad angulation (**A**) and lateral (**B**) radiographs. Normal. The *short arrows* demonstrate the normal arcuate lines of the anterior openings of the sacral neural foramina. The *arrowheads* demarcate the posterior margin of the left S1 foramen. There is a spina bifida occulta. The sacral hiatus represents the termination of the posterior elements at the midline.

FIGURE 6.15   Pelvis AP radiograph. Normal.

- Ilium
- Sacroiliac joints
- Sacrum foramina
- Acetabulum
- Femoral head
- Femur greater trochanter
- Obturator foramen
- Ischium tuberosity
- Superior and inferior pubis rami
- Symphysis pubis

- L2 left transverse process
- L3 superior articular process
- L2 inferior articular process
- L4 right transverse process

A

B

C

FIGURE 6.16 **A:** Cervical spine lateral radiograph. This accessory ossicle is located inferior to the anterior arch of the atlas or C1. This supernumerary bone or os (*straight arrow*) is a normal variant. **B:** Lumbar spine right oblique radiograph. Lumbar spine accessory ossicles (*straight arrows*). This 22-year-old gymnast experienced a sudden onset of back pain. The accessory ossicles are variants of normal and had nothing to do with the patient's back pain. They are usually found around the L2 and L3 levels. **C:** Lower cervical and upper thoracic spine AP radiograph. Bilateral cervical ribs. The small bilateral ribs (*arrows*) arise from the C7 vertebra; hence the name cervical ribs.

Left 12th rib

L4 vertebra

Sacroiliac joint

A   **B**

FIGURE 6.17 **A:** Lumbar spine AP radiograph. Partial sacralization of L5. L5 articulates with the left sacrum in an anomalous fashion (*straight arrows*). There is a pseudarthrosis (*open arrow*). Transitional vertebrae describe a situation in which L5 begins to look like a part of the sacrum or the sacrum begins to look like a part of the lumbar spine. The *curved arrows* indicate calcifications within the cartilaginous portion of the ribs. **B:** Cervical spine lateral radiograph. Partial occipitalization of C1. The spinous process of C1 articulates with the occiput (*arrow*). Normally the spinous process of C1 does not articulate with the occiput.

from nonexistent to extensive and disabling. Visceral innervation of the bladder and/or rectum may be affected as well as sensory and motor nerves. Another unfortunate anomaly in this category is complete absence of the sacrum (sacral agenesis), and it is often associated with a variety of other anomalies. Another severe anomaly is exstrophy of the urinary bladder, which is associated with abnormal widening of the symphysis pubis. This widening of the symphysis pubis, or diastasis, is most often the result of trauma (Fig. 6.20) but can occasionally be as-

sociated with a difficult or large baby birth, some bone dysplasias, epispadias, hypospadias, and the prune belly syndrome (loss or absence of abdominal wall muscles).

One of the most clinically important anomalies of the spine is scoliosis. Some of the many etiologies of scoliosis include idiopathic, disc degeneration and osteoarthritis, neuromuscular diseases, trauma, infections, tumors, radiation therapy, acromegaly, and underlying congenital problems such as hemivertebrae (Fig. 6.21) and pedicle bars. A *hemivertebra* is a

FIGURE 6.18 Pelvis AP radiograph. Spina bifida occulta and developmental dysplasia of the hip. Spina bifida occulta is indicated by the *straight arrow* and represents incomplete fusion of the posterior sacral segments. Right hip developmental dysplasia (*curved arrows*) is characterized by the steep slant of the acetabulum compared to the left. The femoral head remodels as it grows in the shallow socket. Note the presence of a gonadal shield.

FIGURE 6.19   A: Pelvis AP radiograph. Sacral meningocele. This 54-year-old patient consulted a physician because of urinary retention. The lucent areas in the sacrum (*straight arrows*) indicate the bone defect secondary to the meningocele mass. **B:** Pelvis axial CT image. The full extent of the meningocele mass within the sacrum is indicated by the *straight arrows*.

vertebra with formation of only one side secondary to absence of a lateral ossification center. Typically, there is a body, pedicle, lamina, and corresponding rib on only one side (Fig. 6.22). Pedicle bars occur when two or more pedicles on the same side are joined by a bony bridge. While the normal side grows, the absent side of a hemivertebra or side with a pedicle bar cannot grow as much, and a curvature develops. Approximately 10% of scoliosis cases are congenital with associated vertebral and rib abnormalities as shown in Fig. 6.22, but, by far, most cases are idiopathic (Fig. 6.23). Scoliosis may be associated with ab-

normalities of the spinal cord, such as a syrinx. When scoliosis is severe or rapidly progressive, it may be treated by fusion of a long segment of the spine (Fig. 6.24). Degenerative lumbar scoliosis (Fig. 6.25) is an increasing problem in the older population. It is likely multifactorial and may be related to altered load due to compression deformities, degenerative disc changes, leg length discrepancies, and lumbosacral anomalies. This deformity may be slow or rapidly progressive and can lead to back pain, radiculopathy, and spinal stenosis. It is occasionally treated by decompression of the stenosis and fusion.

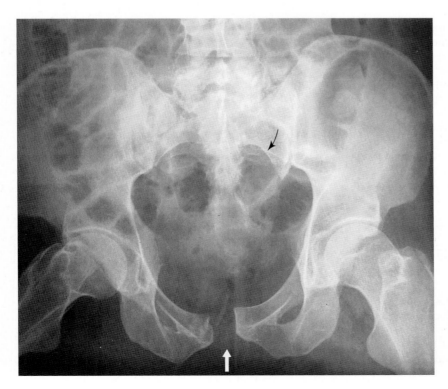

FIGURE 6.20   AP pelvis radiograph. Symphysis pubis diastasis. Widening of the normal close relationship of the left and right pubic bones (*white arrow*) is due to trauma in this patient. Note the irregular margin from fracture of the right side of the symphysis. The disrupted arcuate line of the left sacral foramen (*arrow*) should be searched for since the pelvic "ring" typically breaks in at least two places.

FIGURE 6.21 Lumbar spine lateral radiograph. L1 posterior hemivertebra (*arrow*). This is usually asymptomatic.

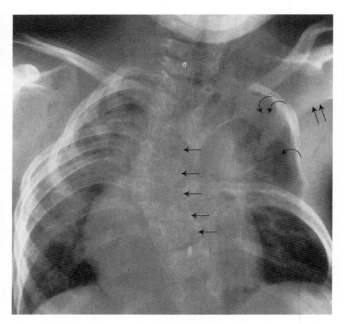

FIGURE 6.22 Thoracic spine AP radiograph. Congenital scoliosis. The thoracic spine is convex to the right, and the thorax is markedly asymmetric. Underlying the scoliosis are multiple hemivertebrae or incompletely formed thoracic vertebrae (*straight arrows*). There are multiple absent left ribs (*curved arrow*), and several left upper ribs are fused (*double curved arrows*). The left scapula is abnormally elevated (*double straight arrows*).

Osteitis condensans ilii (Fig. 6.26) is a well-marginated, triangular-shaped area of increased bone density found predominately in women of childbearing years. It is located in the iliac bone just lateral to the SI joint, but the sacrum and SI joints are not involved. This abnormality may or may not be symptomatic. The differential diagnosis should include osteoblastic metastatic disease, ankylosing spondylitis, and other inflammatory arthritides such as rheumatoid arthritis. It usually can be differentiated from metastatic disease that commonly involves multiple widespread sites. The SI joints are usually narrowed or absent in ankylosing spondylitis and often appear irregular in the other inflammatory arthritides such as rheumatoid arthritis.

A sometimes confusing variant in the pelvis is *os acetabulare*. This is an accessory center of ossification at the superolateral margin of the acetabulum (Fig. 6.27). It is typically triangular in shape. The margins are smooth and corticated, which should allow differentiation from a fracture.

TRAUMA

Fractures

Fractures of the spine and pelvis are common and result from a wide variety of traumas including motor vehicle accidents, sports, falls, and normal activity in those who have osteoporosis or bone loss due to tumor. Fractures of the spine are obviously important as the spinal cord and cauda equina are vulnerable to injury because of their close proximity to the

FIGURE 6.23 Thoracolumbar spine AP radiograph. Idiopathic scoliosis of the thoracic and lumbar spine. The lumbar spine is convex to the left (*curved arrow*), and the lumbar vertebrae are markedly rotated. This rotation component causes the lumbar vertebra to appear oblique on the radiograph. The lower thoracic spine is convex to the right (*straight arrow*), resulting in asymmetry of the ribs and thorax. Interestingly, the foramen magnum and sacrum usually form a vertical line when a line connects the two.

A　　　　　　　　　　　　　　　　　　　　**B**

FIGURE 6.24 AP (**A**) and lateral (**B**) thoracolumbar radiographs. Posterior spinal fusion for idiopathic scoliosis. Fusion rods, screws, and hooks are used to decrease the curvature. Bone graft is usually placed as well to prevent progression of the curves.

FIGURE 6.25 Lumbar spine AP radiograph. Senile scoliosis. The lumbar spine is convex to the left. The discs are asymmetrically narrowed and there is prominent osteoarthritis of facets (*arrows*), which is worse on the concave sides.

FIGURE 6.26 Pelvis AP radiograph. Osteitis condensans ilii. The sharply marginated, bilateral increased densities (sclerosis) involve the iliac sides of the sacroiliac joints and spare the sacrum. This is a benign condition that is usually found in women in their childbearing years and seldom found in older women. This can be an incidental finding on a radiograph, or the patient may present with acute or chronic back pain.

vertebrae. Roughly 40% of cervical spine fractures have neurologic complications, 10% in the thoracic spine and 4% at the thoracolumbar junction.

Cervical Spine Injuries

Most cervical spine fractures occur between C5 and C7, with another peak at C1 and 2. A variety of injuries occur when the cervical spine undergoes acute hyperflexion and hyperextension (Table 6.6). The flexion teardrop fracture (Fig. 6.28) is one type of injury that results from acute cervical spine hyperflexion. The teardrop-shaped fracture fragment is the result of compression at the anterior inferior aspect of the vertebral body. This fracture is usually accompanied by disruption of the interspinal ligaments between the spinous processes, thus making the spine very unstable. Other ligaments that may be involved are the supraspinous ligament and the ligamentum flavum. The involved vertebral body may be displaced posteriorly, and this situation is a good indication for CT imaging to determine the extent of the fracture lines and to determine the precise location of the fracture fragments, especially their relationship to the cervical spinal cord. Particularly with neurologic deficit, MRI may be used to evaluate the spinal cord for injury and the soft tissue structures such as the ligamentum flavum and interspinous ligaments.

FIGURE 6.27   Hip AP radiograph. Os acetabulare. The smoothly marginated, oval density near the superolateral margin of the acetabulum (*arrow*) is a normal variant and should not be confused with a fracture.

Monitoring electrodes

Endotracheal tube

C5 spinous process

C6 spinous process

FIGURE 6.28   A: Lateral cervical spine radiograph. C5 flexion teardrop fracture. This 21-year-old man was involved in a motor vehicle accident. There is mild compression anteriorly of the C5 vertebral body secondary to the comminuted fracture (*straight arrows*), and there is mild separation of the fracture fragments. The major fracture fragment has a teardrop shape (*curved arrow*) due to avulsion at the site of the anterior longitudinal ligament. The hyperflexion injury has resulted in a mild separation or fanning of the space between the C5 and the C6 spinous processes secondary to ligamentous disruption (*double curved arrows*). The disrupted ligaments are the interspinal and supraspinal ligaments and possibly the ligamentum flavum. Also, the hyperflexion injury created minimal widening of the C5-C6 disc space (*double straight arrows*) and mild angulation of the spine at this level with minimal retrolisthesis of C5 on C6. This type of cervical fracture is usually associated with severe cord injury as the vertebral body is often displaced posteriorly into the spinal canal. (*continued*)

A

FIGURE 6.28 (*Continued*) B: Cervical spine axial CT image of the C5 vertebra. The comminuted fracture lines in the vertebral body are separated or distracted (*straight arrows*), and the anterior fracture fragments are displaced anteriorly approximately 3 mm (*curved arrow*). C: Lateral cervical spine radiograph. Posterior wire stabilization of the cervical spine between the spinous processes of C5 and C6 vertebrae (*curved arrow*). The major fracture fragment (*straight arrow*) is in fairly good alignment with mild offset of the fragments (*double straight arrows*), but no attempt is made to reduce this fragment.

Facet locking (Fig. 6.29) is another hyperflexion injury. Locking will occur when the inferior articular process of the upper vertebra moves forward or anteriorly over the superior articular process of the lower vertebra, which results in an anterior dislocation of the upper vertebra. Once again, the spine is unstable as there usually is posterior and sometimes anterior ligamentous disruption, and cervical spinal cord injury is common. The lateral radiograph is usually sufficient to make the diagnosis (see Fig. 6.29A), but occasionally a reconstructed sagittal CT image (Fig. 6.29B, C) is necessary to confirm the diagnosis. Unilateral locked facet (Fig. 6.29C) has a rotational component and does not have the extensive ligamentous disruption as the bilateral form does. Unilateral facet fracture-dislocation may be a difficult diagnosis since there is less displacement as a result of the fracture of the superior articular process. The rotational component may not be manifest until later and should be looked for on subsequent radiographs (Fig. 6.30A–C).

Occasionally, hyperflexion injury results in ligamentous injury without fracture (Fig. 6.31). As with other hyperflexion injuries, this has the potential for spinal instability and cord injury.

Dens or odontoid process fractures are relatively common in the older population, and they may result from hyperflexion or hyperextension injuries. The fractures are often not displaced initially and may be difficult to detect. The best methods for the diagnosis of odontoid process fracture are AP open mouth and lateral cervical radiographs, and, of course, CT imaging. The odontoid fracture in Fig. 6.32 is

TABLE 6.6

CERVICAL SPINE INJURIES

Flexion
Anterior wedge fracture
Facet locking
Ligament disruption
Odontoid process fracture
Teardrop fracture (C5)

Extension
Hangman fracture (C2)
Ligament disruption
Odontoid process fracture
Spinous process fracture
Teardrop fracture (C2)

FIGURE 6.29   A: Cervical spine lateral radiograph. Bilateral facet locking at the C5-6 level. The inferior articular process of C5 (*straight arrow*) is anterior to the superior articular process of C6 (*curved arrow*). The *double straight arrows* indicate the expected normal position for the superior articular process of the C6 vertebra. There is obvious anterior dislocation of the C5 vertebral body referable to the C6 vertebral body. No fractures are apparent. **B:** Cervical spine sagittal reconstructed CT image on a different patient. Bilateral facet lock. The inferior articular process of the upper vertebra (*straight arrow*) is in an abnormal relationship with the superior articular process of the lower vertebra (*curved arrow*). The *double straight arrows* indicate the expected normal location of the displaced superior articular process. A normal apophyseal articulation is visible at the level below (*double curved arrows*). **C:** Reformatted CT image in another patient with unilateral locked facets at C4-5 on the right. Note how the upper cervical spine appears rotated while the lower cervical spine is straight. The left facets are not shown on this three-dimensional reformat but had a normal relationship.

FIGURE 6.30   A: Axial CT image through C6. The left inferior articular process of C5 is broken but not displaced *(arrow)*. **B:** Sagittal reformatted image uses the axial data set from the CT scan to project a sagittal slice through the facet joints. There is a normal relationship between the fractured C5 inferior articular process and the superior articular process of C6 *(arrow)*. **C:** Lateral radiograph of the cervical spine obtained 1 month later demonstrated mild anterolisthesis of C5 on C6 *(arrow)* and rotation of the articular pillar above this level. Note the overlap of bilateral facets below *(curved arrow)* compared to the "bowtie" appearance above with this unilateral interfacet fracture dislocation *(double arrow)*.

probably a hyperextension injury as the odontoid is displaced posteriorly.

Thoracic Spine Fractures

Most fractures of the thoracic (dorsal) spine occur in the lower thoracic region. Fractures of the thoracic spine may result from significant trauma; however, underlying bone diseases can weaken the vertebrae and pathologic fractures may occur with little or no trauma. These fractures are usually wedged-shaped compression fractures, often with no canal compromise and are, by far, the most common thoracic spine fracture. A few of the underlying diseases that may cause pathologic fractures are osteoporosis, primary and secondary bone tumors, Paget's disease, osteopetrosis, and osteomalacia (Fig. 6.33). If there are neurologic symptoms, imaging with MR or CT is usually warranted.

C4 spinous process

C5 spinous process

A

B

C4 spinous process

C5 spinous process

C

FIGURE 6.31 **A:** Cervical spine cross-table lateral radiograph with the patient supine. Posterior ligament disruption at C4-5. There is an increase in the height of the interspinous space between the C4-5 spinous processes (*straight arrow*) secondary to disruption of the C4-5 interspinal ligament, supraspinal ligament, and possibly the ligamentum flavum. Compare the height of the C4-5 interspinous space to those above and below. The mild anterior spondylolisthesis of C4 referable to C5 (*curved arrow*) has resulted in mild kyphotic angulation and reverse of the normal cervical curvature at the C4 level. **B:** Cervical spine extension lateral radiograph in the same patient. When the cervical spine is in full extension, the C4-5 interspinous space (*straight arrow*) is now normal in height and the anterolisthesis of C4 on C5 has been reduced. **C:** Sagittal T2-weighted MRI cervical spine in a different patient. Ligament disruption without fracture. There is widening between the spinous processes at C5-6 and increased signal (white) (*arrowheads*). Disruption of the ligamentum flavum (*arrow*) is also seen. A hematoma (*curved arrow*) can be seen, which would explain persistent widening of spinous processes on radiographs. There is a small amount of high signal within the posterior aspect of the C5-6 disc, which may suggest a disc injury as well.

FIGURE 6.32 Cervical spine lateral radiograph. Displaced fracture through the caudad or inferior aspect of the dens or odontoid process of C2. The actual fracture edges are indicated by the *dotted lines,* and the dens (*arrow*) is displaced posteriorly approximately 8 mm. The *curved arrows* indicate the amount of displacement of the dens.

More than 700,000 osteoporotic compression fractures occur in the United States each year. The peak location for osteoporotic compression fractures is the midthoracic spine and at the thoraco-lumbar junction. They are quite rare in the cervical spine. It may be difficult to distinguish an acute compression fracture from an osteoporotic compression deformity that has developed over time. Back pain is found with an acute compression, but many elderly patients also have arthritis and nerve root irritation, which may become more pronounced. Axial CT images, when viewed without the benefit of sagittal reformatted images, may miss these remote compression deformities altogether. Compression deformity may increase the likelihood of subsequent vertebral body fractures because of the altered weight and force on the spine. Multiple wedge-shaped deformities lead to the development of kyphosis, or an angular deformity of the spine, also called a "Dowager's hump." This can result in chronic pain, decreased lung capacity, and a moderate increased mortality.

Lumbar Spine Fractures

Fractures commonly occur in the lumbar spine and are usually diagnosed by radiography (Fig. 6.34A, B). MRI may be helpful

FIGURE 6.33 Thoracic spine AP (**A**) and lateral (**B**) radiographs. Osteopenia due to senile osteoporosis with secondary pathologic compression fractures of the T7 and T8 vertebral bodies. The compression fractures (*straight arrows*) are manifest by a decrease in the vertical height of the T7 and T8 vertebral bodies when compared to the other dorsal vertebral bodies. Notice the overall decreased density (osteopenia) of all the osseous structures due to osteoporosis.

Intervertebral disc

L3 vertebral body

L4 vertebral body

L5 vertebral body

FIGURE 6.34 Lumbar spine AP (**A**) and lateral (**B**) radiographs. Seat belt fracture of the L3 vertebrae. This 30-year-old patient was wearing a lap seat belt when involved in a motor vehicle accident, and this is a flexion injury caused by the mobile upper body flexing on the lower body that is fixed by the lap seat belt. There is a transverse fracture through the L3 vertebra involving the vertebral body and the transverse processes (*straight arrows in A and B*). A large fracture fragment arising posteriorly from the vertebral body is displaced into the neural canal (*curved arrow in B*). The L3 vertebral body height is less than normal secondary to compression or collapse caused by the fracture. There is mild dorsal angulation of the spine at the level of the L3 fracture. These fractures may be either stable or unstable. The remainder of the lumbar spine is normal. Note the clothing snaps. **C:** Lumbar spine sagittal proton-density MR image. A lap seat belt L3 displaced fracture in another 30-year-old patient. The L3 vertebral body is mildly compressed secondary to a fracture (*straight arrows*), and a posterior fracture fragment resides in the neural canal compressing the neural canal (*curved arrow*). **D:** Lumbar spine axial CT image. L4 vertebra displaced burst-type fracture in a 28-year-old patient involved in a motor vehicle accident. The mechanism of injury is axial compression with or without flexion and/or rotation. There is severe compromise of the neural canal (*asterisk*) with resultant neurologic injury. The *straight arrow* demonstrates a fracture of the right lamina in this unstable fracture. (*continued*)

FIGURE 6.34 (*Continued*) **E:** Sagittal reformatted CT image on the same patient shows the severity of the canal compromise compared to the other levels.

in assessing the effect of the fracture fragments on the thecal sac (Fig. 6.34C). As in other areas of the spine, CT imaging is helpful in evaluating the extent of the fractures and precisely locating the fracture fragments within the neural canal and their relationship relative to the thecal sac (Fig. 6.34D, E).

Spondylolysis and Spondylolisthesis

Spondylolysis and spondylolisthesis are difficult and confusing terms for the beginner. To add to the confusion, many will use the term "spondylosis" to describe degenerative changes in the spine. However, an understanding of these conditions and their clinical significance is necessary as they will commonly be encountered in clinical practice.

Spondylolysis refers to a defect in the pars interarticularis that lies between the superior and inferior articular processes of a vertebra. In other words, the neck of the Scotty dog is missing or some say that a collar has been placed (Fig. 6.10A). The defect occurs in about 5% of the population and, in most cases, is thought to be a stress fracture. It is seen on lateral radiographs but seen particularly well on oblique views (Fig. 6.35). It is seen more often in athletes whose activities require prolonged or forced extension of the lower back.

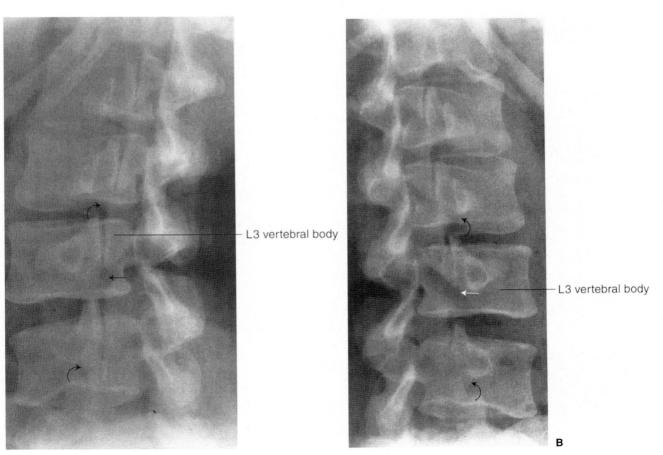

— L3 vertebral body

— L3 vertebral body

FIGURE 6.35 Lumbar spine right (**A**) and left oblique (**B**) radiographs. Bilateral spondylolysis of L3 (*straight arrows*). The pars interarticularis or the Scotty-dog neck is absent bilaterally in the L3 vertebra. Normal Scotty-dog necks or pars interarticulares are present in the L2 and L4 vertebrae bilaterally (*curved arrows*). (*continued*)

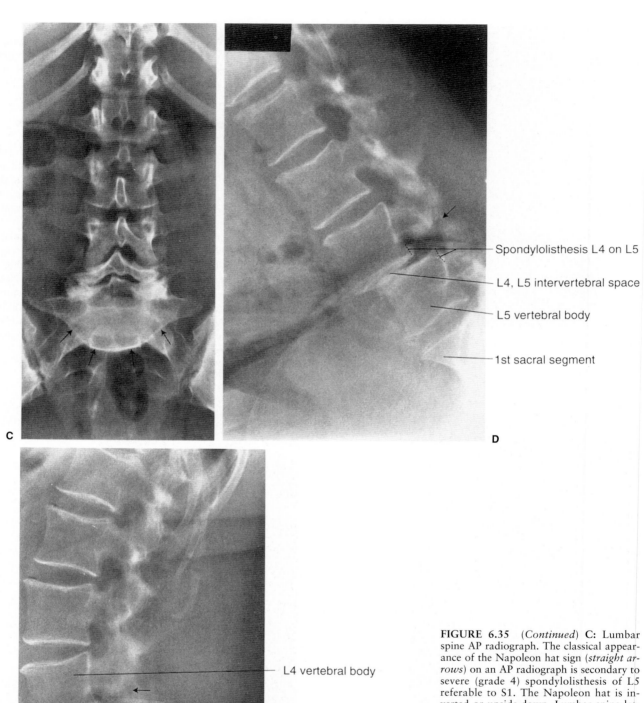

C

Spondylolisthesis L4 on L5

L4, L5 intervertebral space

L5 vertebral body

1st sacral segment

D

L4 vertebral body

L4, L5 intervertebral space

L5 vertebral body

Artery calcification

1st sacral segment

E

FIGURE 6.35 (*Continued*) **C:** Lumbar spine AP radiograph. The classical appearance of the Napoleon hat sign (*straight arrows*) on an AP radiograph is secondary to severe (grade 4) spondylolisthesis of L5 referable to S1. The Napoleon hat is inverted or upside-down. Lumbar spine lateral flexion (**D**) and extension (**E**) radiographs. This is a different patient with L4 spondylolysis and grade 2 anterior spondylolisthesis of the L4 vertebral body referable to the L5 vertebral body. The spondylolysis defect in the pars interarticularis (*straight arrows*) can be visualized on both views, but the flexion radiograph opens the defect for easier visibility. The degree of spondylolisthesis is slightly less on the lateral extension radiograph as extension would counteract the forward slip. Notice the marked narrowing of the L4-5 intervertebral disc space.

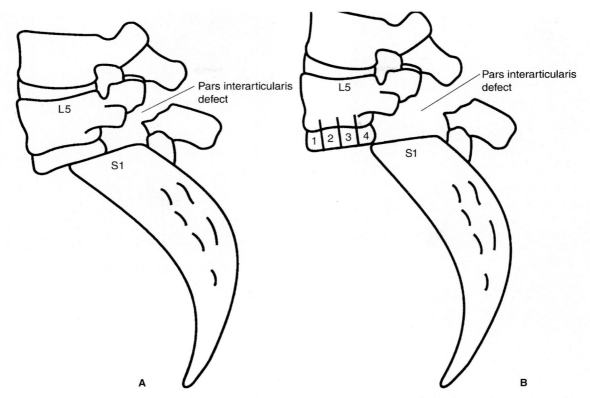

FIGURE 6.36 A: Illustration of spondylolysis and spondylolisthesis on a lateral radiograph. The L5 vertebral body, pedicles, and superior articular processes have moved forward or ventral relative to the sacrum. However, the L5 inferior articular processes, laminae, and the spinous process remain in their normal position. **B:** Illustration of spondylolisthesis classification or grading system. The sacrum is divided into fourths and the forward movement of L5 is simply given a grade of 1–4.

Spondylolisthesis is the forward movement of a vertebra relative to the more stable vertebra below. The forward movement may be made possible by a bilateral spondylolysis defect in the vertebra (Figs. 6.35 and 6.36). Actually, with a pars defect, it is the vertebral body, pedicles, and superior articular processes that move forward or ventrally, whereas the laminae, inferior articular processes, and the spinous process remain in their normal positions (Fig. 6.36). This actually increases the size of the canal at this level. The majority of the spondylolysis with spondylolisthesis cases occur in the lumbar spine, especially at L5-S1 levels, and it is uncommon in the thoracic and cervical spine. Spondylolisthesis may be asymptomatic, and the most frequent symptom is low back pain probably due to muscle spasm and instability. Symptoms, when they occur, are not necessarily related to the severity of the disease.

Spondylolisthesis secondary to spondylolysis must be differentiated from the spondylolisthesis secondary to disc and facet degeneration without spondylolysis. Degenerative spondylolisthesis is best imaged on a lateral radiograph of the lumbar spine (Fig. 6.37), and it most commonly occurs at the L4-5 level. There are degenerative changes in the disc space and the apophyseal (facet) joints *without a defect in the pars interarticularis*. Because there is no defect in the region of the pars interarticularis, however, there is more likely to be en- croachment of bony structures into the neural foramina, which may lead to nerve compression.

Pelvic, Acetabular, and Sacral Fractures

Fractures of the pelvis are common and result from a variety of injuries (Fig. 6.38). Stable pelvic fractures break the "ring" of the pelvis in only one place. These include fractures of unilateral pubic rami, acetabulum, or sacrum. Typically, both superior and inferior pubic rami are broken on one side since the rami form a ring. However, it is virtually impossible to break a ring in only one place and most pelvic fractures are unstable, disrupting the pelvic bones, symphysis, and/or SI joints. This is a common fracture in the older patient with osteoporosis, and a careful look at the pubic rami is important during evaluation for a hip fracture. These fractures may be better evaluated by CT, which when performed with intravenous contrast also allows evaluation of many of the soft tissue structures such as the bladder, urethra, and other pelvis soft tissues that may be damaged by fracture fragments. CT reformatted images are often useful for better evaluating the pelvic fractures.

Acetabular fractures result most commonly from motor vehicle accidents as the femoral head is driven into the

FIGURE 6.37   Lumbar spine lateral radiograph. Degenerative grade 1 spondylolisthesis of L4 on L5 (*straight arrows*). This is a common complication of degenerative spine changes. The pars interarticularis is intact (*curved arrow*). The spondylolisthesis is secondary to the degenerative changes in the intervertebral space and the apophyseal joints that allow L4 to move forward relative to L5.

FIGURE 6.38   Pelvis AP radiograph. Fractures of the left superior and inferior pubis rami (*straight arrows*). Sacral fractures are present but are partly obscured by the overlying intestinal gas. Note how the sacral arcuate lines are poorly seen on the left compared with those on the right.

acetabulum. Depending on the direction of force, the femoral head may dislocate, typically posteriorly, with or without an acetabular fracture. Avascular necrosis is a complication of hip dislocation as the vascular supply to the femoral head is stretched or disrupted during the dislocation. Pelvic oblique, or Judet, views and CT are useful in the evaluation of acetabular fractures (Fig. 6.39).

Sacral fractures may occur with major pelvic trauma but may be an isolated insufficiency-type fracture in the elderly, osteoporotic population. When the fracture enters the sacral foramina, the arcuate lines are disrupted (Fig. 6.20). Sacral insufficiency fractures, which occur in weakened (usually osteoporotic) bone, may occur with little or no trauma. An older patient may present with lower back, buttock, or hip pain. Radiographs frequently will not demonstrate the fracture. Bone scan or MRI may be the next study to evaluate for an occult or developing hip fracture and the sacral fracture discovered (Fig. 6.40). Occasionally, these studies have an atypical appearance, but CT will demonstrate the healing fracture.

Apophyseal avulsion fractures in the adolescent are due to muscle traction in athletes. Several sports are more closely re-lated to these injuries, found in sprinters, long jumpers, cheerleaders, hurdlers, and gymnasts. These are the typical locations and the involved muscles: anterior superior iliac spine (sartorius attachment), anteroinferior iliac spine (rectus femoris attachment), ischial tuberosity (hamstring attachment) (see Fig. 5.77A), and iliac crest (abdominal muscle attachment) (Fig. 6.41). In the more mature athlete, a muscle strain or tear would result from the same type of injury. MRI is useful to evaluate the extent of muscle involvement and degree of muscle retraction, if any.

Herniated Intervertebral Disc Disease

Intervertebral disc herniations may occur at any level in the spine. Although intervertebral discs cannot be visualized on radiographs, disc disease should be suspected whenever there is intervertebral disc space narrowing on radiographs. However, a narrowed disc level identified on radiographs cannot predict whether or not that level is symptomatic. Often the disc spaces are narrowed because of chronic disc degeneration and not an acute herniation. Noninvasive CT and MRI are increasingly being used in conjunction with, or in place of, the myelogram as they are more accurate and have a lower complication rate than myelography.

The normal disc structures are shown in Fig. 6.11. Some confusing terms have developed in the classification of herniated intervertebral discs, but the following is the current most accepted approach to this terminology problem. There is some "normal" drying out of discs with aging, which may lead to decreased disc space height. Disc *degeneration* usually refers to this drying out, narrowing, and/or numerous small tears of the annulus fibrosis in all directions, which allows the nucleus of the disc to spread out. *Annular fissure*

FIGURE 6.39 **A:** Pelvis AP radiograph. Acetabular fracture. There is a left acetabular fracture (*arrows*). The fracture that involves the iliac wing is considered part of the acetabular fracture. **B:** Axial CT at level of the acetabulum. This 23-year-old patient was involved in a motor vehicle accident. The right femoral head is dislocated posteriorly, nicely demonstrating the mechanism for a fracture of the posterior wall of the acetabulum. The *arrow* shows the fracture site from which the posterior wall fragment came. **C:** Posterior view of a three-dimensional CT reformatted image in a different patient with a posterior wall acetabular fracture (*arrow*). These images can sometimes allow better demonstration of the location of fracture fragments.

FIGURE 6.40 **A:** Sacrum AP radiograph. Insufficiency fractures of the sacrum. There is subtle sclerosis in a vertical orientation involving each sacral ala *(arrows)*. Compare this to the normal sacrum in Fig. 6.14A. **B:** Radionuclide bone scan posterior view of the pelvis in this same patient reveals increased activity (black) due to the healing fractures. The vertical orientation of each side with a horizontal connecting fracture line has been termed the "Honda sign." **C:** Coronal T1-weighted MR pelvis in a different patient. The characteristic sacral insufficiency fracture lines are easily seen *(arrows)* but should not be confused with the normal sacroiliac joints *(curved arrows)*.

FIGURE 6.41 Anterior radiograph of the pelvis. Note the increased space between the apophysis and the iliac bone on the right *(arrow)* compared with that of the left *(double arrow)*. There has been an avulsion of the attachment of the abdominal musculature in this young runner following a quick change in direction.

INTERVERTEBRAL DISC HERNIATION NOMENCLATURE

Annular fissure (tear)—focal disruption in the outer fibrous layers of disc

Bulge— ≥50% width of disc displaced beyond vertebral body margin

Herniation

Protrusion—depth of extent of disc < width of base at disc margin

Extrusion—depth of extent of disc > width of base at disc margin

Sequestration—detached disc fragment
  Limbus vertebra
  Schmorl's node
  Scheuermann's disease

(*tear*) usually refers to a focal tear in the annulus allowing nuclear material to extend toward the outer margin of the disc without extending beyond the margin. A *bulging disc* means that 50% or more of the circumference of the disc is mildly displaced outward relative to the margin of the vertebral body. Scoliosis often leads to multiple asymmetric bulging discs due to the change in bony alignment. In this instance, the appearance is not due to structural problems within the discs.

Herniation is a general umbrella term, and it can be divided into three main categories, that is, protruded, extruded, and sequestered discs (Table 6.7). A *protrusion* implies that the depth of disc extension is less than the width of its base at the disc margin. A *broad-based protrusion* involves over 25% of the circumference of the disc, whereas *focal protrusion* involves less than 25% of the disc margin. If the extension of disc material is greater than the width of its base or extends superior or inferior to the endplate, it is termed *extrusion*. If the fragment becomes detached, it is termed a *sequestered fragment*. Herniated lumbar intervertebral disc disease is common, especially at the L4-5 and L5-S1 levels (Fig. 6.42). MRI with the use of intravenous contrast has proved useful in determining whether or not there has been a recurrent disc herniation (Fig. 6.43).

Usually, disc herniations are lateral and/or posterior. However, when the disc herniates anteriorly into the vertebral body, this results in a vertebral defect with a classical appearance called a *limbus vertebra* (Fig. 6.44). When the disc herniates into the vertebral endplate, the resulting defect is called a *Schmorl's node* (Fig. 6.44). There are some people who feel that these are congenital or developmental variants. *Scheuermann's disease* (Fig. 6.44) is osteochondrosis of the epiphyseal plates in teenagers who often complain of back pain. The diagnosis of Scheuermann's disease usually can be made on lateral spine radiographs. The radiographic features include fragmented and sclerotic epiphyseal plates of the vertebrae, wedge-shaped vertebral bodies with increased AP diameter, and narrowed disc spaces. Limbus vertebrae and Schmorl's nodes may be present.

ARTHRITIDES

Because the spine has multiple joints, it is not surprising that most of the arthritides involve the spine in some fashion (Table 6.8).

Osteoarthritis

Osteoarthritis or degenerative arthritis (Fig. 6.45) is the most common arthritis, and the facet joints of the spine are frequently involved. Patients with osteoarthritis will usually complain of pain and/or limited motion in the involved spine. As in the extremities, the typical radiologic features include irregular joint narrowing, sclerosis, and osteophyte formation. The differential diagnosis of degenerative or osteoarthritis must include neuropathic joints and diffuse idiopathic skeletal hyperplasia. Common complications of osteoarthritis are spinal stenosis (Fig. 6.46) and spondylolisthesis.

Spinal stenosis describes a vertebral or neural canal that is too narrow, and the multiple etiologies can be classified as congenital, developmental, and idiopathic. Although myelography dramatically demonstrates this abnormality, CT enjoys excellent patient acceptance and determines the causes and precise location (foraminal, lateral recess, or central) of the stenosis. Often, the stenosis is due to a combination of bulging disc, facet arthritis with osteophytes, and thickened ligamentum flavum (Fig. 6.46B).

ARTHRITIDES

Osteoarthritis
Inflammatory arthritis (rheumatoid arthritis and ankylosing spondylitis, psoriasis, Reiter's disease)
Neuropathic joint (Charcot joint)
Infectious arthritis

FIGURE 6.42   A: Lumbar intervertebral disc illustration. A disc herniation is a tear extending from the nucleus pulposis through all the layers of the annulus fibrosis. There may be compression of the thecal sac and possibly nerve roots. Smaller annular fissures may or may not cause pain. **B:** Lumbar spine lateral radiographs. Herniated L4-5 intervertebral disc. The patient is a 30-year-old woman with bilateral leg weakness greater on the right than on the left. There is significant narrowing of the L4-5 intervertebral disc space (*straight arrows*), suggesting disc disease at this level. Again, the disc is not visible on the radiograph. The disc space narrowing is more apparent when you compare the L4-5 disc space to the other lumbar disc spaces. Normally, the L4-5 disc space height is greater than the other lumbar spine disc spaces. **C:** Lumbar spine axial T1 MR image in the same patient. Large extruded L4-5 intervertebral disc. The disc is extruded posterolaterally to the right (*straight arrows*), and it is creating extrinsic pressure on the neural sac and obliterating the epidural fat on the right side. Normal epidural fat is present on the left (*curved arrow*). **D:** Lumbar spine sagittal T1 MR image in the same patient. Caudally extruded L4-5 intervertebral disc and a protruding L5-S1 intervertebral disc. Notice that the extruded L4-5 disc (*arrows*) has migrated inferiorly to the level of the L5-S1 disc space posteriorly and is severely compressing the neural sac. A bulging disc at L5-S1 does not touch the thecal sac at this level. (*continued*)

FIGURE 6.42 (*Continued*) **E:** Axial T2 MR image at L3-4 in a 43-year-old man. Foraminal disc protrusion. The disc protrusion (*arrow*) narrows the left foramen and displaces the L3 nerve (*curved arrow*). **F:** Sagittal PD (proton density) MR on the same patient. This view shows the disc extension into the neural foramen (*arrow*) and relationship to the nerve (*curved arrow*). There are degenerative disc changes at L2-3 as well with some foraminal narrowing seen at that level. **G:** Lumbar spine axial CT image. Protruded L4-5 intervertebral disc. The *straight arrows* mark the protruded disc with narrowing of the right foramen by the disc and facet arthritis.

FIGURE 6.43 Axial T1-weighted MR images at L5-S1 without (**A**) and with (**B**) intravenous contrast. Scar tissue in a person with recurrent back pain. The *curved arrow* demonstrates an absent portion of lamina from this patient's prior surgery. The *arrow* in **A** shows abnormal signal, which could be a new disc herniation or scar tissue. **B** demonstrates that this area (*arrow*) enhances completely. Disc material does not enhance. The left S1 nerve root (*double arrow*) is displaced and enhances suggesting that it is affected by the scar tissue.

FIGURE 6.44 Lumbar spine lateral radiograph. Scheuermann's disease. The involvement of three or more vertebrae by Schmorl's nodes (*straight arrows*) defines Scheuermann's disease. Anterior wedging and increased AP diameter of the vertebral bodies (*curved arrow*) may result from this process. There is a limbus vertebra (*double straight arrows*). Note the wavy appearance of the endplates.

FIGURE 6.45 Thoracic spine AP (**A**) and lateral (**B**) radiographs. Osteoarthritis or degenerative arthritis. Multiple osteophytes (*curved arrows*) are present and multiple disc spaces are narrowed (*straight arrows*) secondary to degenerative disc disease.

L3 vertebral body

L4 vertebral body

Sacrum

A

B

FIGURE 6.46   A: Lumbar myelogram lateral radiographs. Spinal stenosis. The *straight arrows* indicate multiple levels of neural sac compression secondary to spinal canal narrowing that is in turn secondary to degenerative changes in and around the neural canal. The L3-4 and L4-5 intervertebral disc spaces are also markedly narrowed (*curved arrows*). **B:** Lumbar spine axial CT image with contrast. Spinal stenosis at the L3-4 level secondary to hypertrophic facet changes in this 71-year-old man. The *straight arrows* outline the marked narrowing of the spinal canal, and the *curved arrows* indicate the deformity of the thecal sac secondary to the spinal stenosis.

Ankylosing Spondylitis, Psoriasis, and Reiter's Disease

A group of arthritides that have prominent axial skeleton involvement is collectively known as *spondyloarthropathies*. The three most frequently discussed are ankylosing spondylitis, psoriasis, and Reiter's disease.

Ankylosing spondylitis is a chronic inflammatory arthritis. It is most common in young men and most frequently involves the spine and SI joints (Fig. 6.47). The SI joints become symmetrically narrowed or completely obliterated. Ankylosing spondylitis in the spine often results in squaring of the vertebral bodies and syndesmophytes, ossification between the outer margin of the vertebral bodies and the disc annulus. These changes radiographically simulate a piece of bamboo and have been termed the "bamboo spine" (Fig. 6.47B, C).

Because of the rigidity of the spine and relatively weak fusion across discs, even mild trauma may lead to fractures at the disc levels (Fig. 6.47D). Ankylosing spondylitis may involve other joints, and these joints will have an appearance similar to rheumatoid arthritis.

Psoriasis is probably most known for its characteristic dermatologic manifestations, but its arthritis may coincide or even predate the skin changes. Psoriatic arthritis features both erosions and bony proliferation. When the SI joints are involved, they are asymmetrically involved (Fig. 6.48). Sporadic paravertebral ossification will connect adjacent vertebral bodies.

Reiter's disease consists of a constellation of conjunctivitis, urethritis, and arthritis. The radiographic features are quite similar to psoriasis but more likely to involve the lower extremity rather than upper extremity joints. The spine and SI joint changes are indistinguishable from psoriasis.

FIGURE 6.47   Lateral cervical (**A**), lumbar (**B**), and AP lumbar (**C**) radiographs. Ankylosing spondylitis. *Straight arrows* demonstrate the syndesmophytes that bridge across disc levels forming a solid "bamboo" spine. The *curved arrows* in **B** mark the fused apophyseal joints while the *curved arrow* in **C** is in the expected location of the sacroiliac joint, which has fused. **D:** Lateral radiograph in a man with ankylosis spondylitis following a relatively minor fall. There is anterolisthesis of L1 on L2 and a widened L1-2 disc (*arrow*) due to a fracture through this disc level.

FIGURE 6.48   Pelvis AP radiograph. Psoriasis. There is sclerosis and irregularity of the right sacroiliac (SI) joint (*arrow*) due to sacroiliitis associated with psoriatic arthritis. Compare the appearance to the sharply defined margins of the left (SI) joint (*curved arrows*).

Rheumatoid Arthritis

There are many synovial joints in the spine; thus, rheumatoid arthritis often involves the spine. The severity of rheumatoid arthritis of the spine ranges from mild to severe. There may be only mild narrowing of cervical disc spaces. However, when rheumatoid arthritis involves the odontoid and the atlantoaxial joint, the result can be weakening of the transverse atlantal ligament that holds the odontoid close to the anterior arch of C1. When this ligament becomes involved, subluxation or even dislocation of the atlantoaxial joint may occur (Fig. 6.49). These patients can experience cervical pain either at rest or with head movement. On a lateral radiograph, the normal distance between the anterior border of the odontoid and posterior aspect of the C1 anterior arch is usually less than 2.5 mm in adults. When there is subluxation or dislocation of this joint, the distance becomes greater than 2.5 mm, especially when the cervical spine is flexed.

Flexion and extension lateral cervical spine radiographs are indicated in patients with rheumatoid arthritis when they experience pain with head movement and before undergoing general anesthesia or any other procedure in which their head might be hyperflexed or hyperextended. These precautions help prevent spinal cord injury. As elsewhere, rheumatoid arthritis is often associated with osteopenia and secondary pathologic fractures. The differential diagnosis for osteopenia and vertebral fracture includes osteoporosis, metastatic disease, multiple myeloma, infection, and trauma.

Neuropathic Joints

Charcot joints or neuropathic or neurotrophic joints can occur in the spine as well as the extremities (Fig. 6.50). The joint changes are secondary to lost pain sensation and/or unstable joints found in a variety of neurologic conditions including diabetes mellitus, syringomyelia, and spina bifida with meningocele. The radiographic findings are disc space narrowing, bone destruction and fragmentation, sclerotic subchondral bone, subluxation and dislocation, and marginal bone mass formation. Many of these findings can be found in osteoarthritis, and the appearance is that of severe osteoarthritis of the spine.

INFECTION

Osteomyelitis or bone infection is common and has been discussed in Chapter 5. Spine infections are caused by a wide range of organisms, but staphylococcal infections are the most common. As with osteomyelitis elsewhere, patients with spinal osteomyelitis usually have fever and localized pain. The radiographic findings are subtle, and often poor definition of a vertebral endplate is the only finding (Fig. 6.51). With progression, frank bony destruction may be found. Osteomyelitis is in the differential diagnosis of lytic bone lesions. Radionuclide bone scans are often helpful for detecting osteomyelitis, especially when the radiographs are negative. MRI is sensitive in detecting osteomyelitis (Fig. 6.52). On T1 MR images, the infections have a decreased signal intensity (they appear dark gray), whereas on T2 images the infections have an increased signal intensity (they appear white). Contrast enhancement is fairly intense. The disc is invariably involved, which often helps differentiate infection from fractures and metastases. CT scans may detect bone and joint destruction that is not visible on radiographs (Fig. 6.52B).

C1 anterior
arch (mass)

C2 vertebral
body

FIGURE 6.49   A: Cervical spine AP open-mouth radiograph. Rheumatoid arthritis. The odontoid process (*straight arrows*) is narrowed, osteopenic, and poorly marginated. Note the increased distances between the odontoid process of C2 and the inferior articular processes of C1 (*curved arrows*) due to partial loss of odontoid bone. **B:** Cervical spine lateral tomograph in the same patient. Rheumatoid arthritis. The odontoid (*straight arrows*) is markedly narrowed. The space between the anterior odontoid and the anterior arch of C1 (*curved arrow*) is greater than the normal 2.5 mm or less. This can also occur in ankylosing spondylitis. **C:** Cervical spine lateral flexion radiograph in a different patient than shown in **B.** Rheumatoid arthritis. When the cervical spine is flexed, the space (*straight arrows*) between the anterior surface of the odontoid and the posterior aspect of the anterior arch of C1 (*dotted lines*) is dramatically widened. This widening represents an unstable dislocation of C1 relative to C2. There is grade 1 anterior spondylolisthesis of C3 relative to C4. Note the narrowing of all the cervical disc spaces and the generalized osteopenia. **D:** Cervical spine axial CT image. Rheumatoid arthritis with spinal stenosis in a 55-year-old man. The C1-2 joint is abnormal with 8 mm distance between the anterior arch of C1 and the odontoid (*between the straight arrows*). There are advanced erosive changes in the odontoid (*curved arrow*). Cervical spine CT sagittal reconstruction (**E**) and sagittal CT three-dimensional reconstruction (**F**) in the same patient as shown in **D.** The odontoid is involved with erosive changes and has a distal penciled appearance (*curved arrows*). There is redemonstration of the abnormal C1-2 joint (*between the straight arrows*). **G:** Cervical spine sagittal T2 MR image in the same patient as shown in **D–F.** The odontoid (*double arrows*) is displaced posterior, resulting in spinal stenosis and cervical cord compression (*curved arrow*). The increased signal in the compressed cord (*arrowhead*) probably represents edema and/or chronic reaction to the compression. The *single straight arrows* indicate multiple levels of mild spinal stenosis. (*continued*)

FIGURE 6.49 (Continued)

L2 vertebral body

L4 vertebral body

FIGURE 6.50 Lumbar spine AP radiograph. Diabetic neuropathic arthropathy. The characteristic changes of neuropathic arthropathy are present including sclerotic and destructive changes (*single straight arrows*), fragmentation and marginal bone mass formation (*double straight arrows*), and osteophyte formation (*curved arrow*).

A

B

FIGURE 6.51 Lower thoracic and upper lumbar spine AP (**A**) and lateral (**B**) radiographs. Osteomyelitis of T11 vertebral body. This 41-year-old patient had back pain and a low-grade fever. There is destruction of the posterior portion of the T11 inferior endplate (*straight arrows*), and the marked narrowing of the T11-12 intervertebral disc space (*curved arrows*) suggests disc and joint destruction.

A

B

C

FIGURE 6.52   A: Sagittal T1 MR with intravenous contrast. Discitis. The L2-3 disc appears enlarged because the adjacent endplates have been destroyed by the infection. There is contrast enhancement (white) surrounding the infected disc and of the involved vertebral bodies. **B:** Axial CT during biopsy in the same patient. The tip of the biopsy needle (*arrow*) is in the infected disc. In only about half of biopsies performed for discitis will an organism be identified. **C:** Thoracic and lumbar spine T2 sagittal MR image. Osteomyelitis of the T11 vertebral body and infectious destruction of the T11-12 intervertebral disc space. The white appearance of the T11 vertebral body confirms the clinical impression of osteomyelitis (*straight arrow*). Compare the abnormal density of T11 vertebral body to the normal density of the uninvolved vertebral bodies above and below the T11 vertebra. Notice that a large portion of the T11-12 intervertebral disc is missing (*curved arrow*), compatible with probable disc destruction. Compare the involved abnormal disc space at T11-12 to the normal-appearing discs above and below.

MISCELLANEOUS DISEASES

Diffuse Idiopathic Skeletal Hyperostosis

Diffuse idiopathic skeletal hyperostosis (DISH) or Forestier's disease is best demonstrated on a lateral spine radiograph (Fig. 6.53) and is characterized by ossification involving the anterior longitudinal ligament. It is characteristically accompanied by exuberant osteophytes. The overall appearance is similar to the bamboo spine of ankylosing spondylitis; however, ankylosing spondylitis is usually accompanied by obliteration of the SI joints. Spinal stenosis is a significant complication of DISH (Fig. 6.54). As in ankylosing spondylitis, fractures may occur from a relatively minor trauma. Elsewhere in the body, DISH is manifested by prominent bony projections at ligament attachment sites.

Paget's Disease

Paget's disease is due to an imbalance of osteoclastic and osteoblastic activity that may be metabolic in origin, and this has been discussed in Chapter 5. It often involves the spine and, more frequently, the pelvis (Fig. 6.55). The classic spine appearance is the picture frame vertebra caused by increased peripheral vertebra density and central lucency.

TABLE 6.9
SOME PRIMARY SPINE BONE TUMORS

Benign
  Hemangioma
  Osteoid osteoma
  Osteoblastoma
  Aneurysmal bone cyst
  Osteochondroma
Malignant
  Multiple myeloma (most common)
  Chondrosarcoma
  Osteosarcoma
  Ewing's sarcoma

Tumors

Benign tumors may involve the spine (Table 6.9). One such tumor is the hemangioma. These are usually asymptomatic and an incidental finding in the spine. Hemangiomas in the spine require no therapy unless they become symptomatic. Symptoms may develop when the tumor causes a pathologic fracture or the lesion extends outside the vertebrae and compresses the spinal cord. Hemangiomas can develop in other

FIGURE 6.53 Lumbar spine lateral radiograph. Diffuse idiopathic skeletal hyperostosis, or DISH. Note the large osteophytes (*straight arrows*) along the anterior vertebral bodies that extend anteriorly across the disc spaces and ossification of the anterior longitudinal ligament. The intervertebral disc spaces are normal in height.

FIGURE 6.54 Lumbar myelogram PA radiograph in a different patient. Spinal stenosis secondary to diffuse idiopathic skeletal hyperostosis (DISH). The *straight arrows* indicate multiple levels of spinal stenosis and neural sac compression due to DISH changes in the spinal canal. The overall appearance of the spine is somewhat similar to the bamboo spine of ankylosing spondylitis.

FIGURE 6.55   A: Lumbar spine lateral radiograph. Paget's disease L2 vertebra (*straight arrow*). The L2 vertebra has the classic picture frame appearance secondary to the increased trabecular density in the periphery of the vertebral body. There is mild loss of the L2 vertebral body height compared to the vertical heights of L1 and L3, and this is compatible with a mild compression fracture. The remainder of the lumbar spine is not involved by the Paget's disease. **B:** Pelvis AP radiograph. Paget's disease. The bone trabeculae are coarse (*straight arrows*), with an overall increased density and widening or expansion of the bones.

bones, but in the spine they have a classic appearance with prominent or thickened vertical trabeculae that simulate jail bars or corduroy fabric (Fig. 6.56). The MRI and CT appearances are also quite characteristic and do not pose a diagnostic dilemma.

As previously discussed in Chapter 5, *metastatic disease is the most common neoplasm in bone and this includes the spine.* As in other bones, metastatic disease involving the spine can be osteolytic (Fig. 6.57) with or without destruction and/or osteoblastic activity (Fig. 6.58). The primary neoplasms causing osteolytic and osteoblastic bone lesions are listed in Table 6.10.

The importance of visualizing the vertebral pedicles is emphasized in Fig. 6.59. When one or both pedicles are missing in patients with known or suspected cancer, the first diagnosis that must come to mind is metastatic disease. MRI is very useful for confirming the presence of metastatic disease in a vertebra with a missing pedicle (see Fig. 6.57B) and for assessing the extent and location of the metastases (Fig. 6.60).

Primary tumors of the thecal sac and the spinal cord can mimic bone tumors of the spine. Thus, tumors arising from these structures should be considered in the differential diagnosis when dealing with back pain and abnormal radiographs and myelograms.

Others

Osteoporosis and osteomalacia have been discussed in the metabolic disease section of Chapter 5. The typical patient with osteoporosis (Fig. 6.61) is elderly and complains of back pain, especially if secondary compression fractures are present. Vertebral fractures not only cause back pain but also often result in loss of height and kyphosis. The typical radiographic appearance of osteoporosis in the spine is decreased overall density of the vertebral bodies, and as a result the vertebral endplates appear prominent. As the vertebrae become softer than the discs, the endplates can sag, resulting in fishmouth deformities of the vertebrae.

Sickle cell anemia is a Mendelian-dominant hereditary trait. The disease is variable in severity and characterized by crises that include anemia, fever, severe abdominal and bone

TABLE 6.10

CHARACTERISTICS OF METASTASES

Osteoblastic
  Prostate
  Breast
  Lymphoma
  Carcinoid
  Neuroblastoma (occasional)

Osteolytic
  Breast
  Lung
  Almost all other metastatic tumors

FIGURE 6.56   A: Thoracolumbar spine AP radiograph. T12 vertebral body hemangioma. The prominent vertical trabecular pattern is characteristic of bone hemangioma (*straight arrow*). Compare the appearance of the T12 vertebral body to those above and below that level. **B:** Sagittal T1 MR of the lumbar spine. The round focal area of higher signal (*arrow*) is quite characteristic of hemangioma in the spine since it contains a moderate amount of fat. **C:** Axial CT of a thoracic vertebral body demonstrates the punctate appearance of the cross section of coarse trabeculae (*arrows*), similar to that seen in **A.** Note the very low density of the fat within the hemangioma (black).

A

B

FIGURE 6.57 **A:** Cervical spine lateral radiograph. Osteolytic metastatic disease of multiple cervical vertebrae. The C2, C3, and C4 vertebral bodies are involved by destructive (lytic) metastatic disease from the lung (*straight arrows*). **B:** Pelvis AP radiograph. Osteolytic metastatic carcinoma of the cervix involving the left ilium and ischium (*straight arrows*). The extensive involvement of the left ischium has resulted in left acetabular protrusio. There is a large soft tissue metastatic mass in the left pelvis (*curved arrows*).

pain, and bone infarction. Radiographs may show osteoporosis, bone infarcts, aseptic necrosis, and fish-mouth vertebrae (Fig. 6.62).

Dwarfism and several congenital anomalies have classic or typical appearances of the spine and pelvis, but a discussion is beyond the scope of this introductory text.

APPROACH TO CLINICAL PROBLEMS

Initial evaluation of a patient with back pain requires a thorough history and physical examination. If the patient experienced

pain two or three days after playing in the father–son football game, he is more likely to have a muscle strain or delayed-onset muscle soreness. Acute pain after lifting a heavy object is more likely a herniated nucleus pulposis. Insidious onset of pain may be related to arthritis, developing osteoporotic compressions, or metastatic disease. The level of clinical suspicion will determine what steps to take next. Most patients will undergo a trial of conservative treatment of rest, physical therapy, and pain medications. If there is no improvement, imaging studies may then be considered. However, if the patient has a known primary neoplasm, MRI or radionuclide bone scan may be the initial study because of a higher clinical suspicion of metastases and the importance of the diagnosis.

FIGURE 6.58 Abdomen AP radiograph. Osteoblastic metastatic carcinoma of the prostate. The multiple areas of increased density (*straight arrows*) represent the metastases that involve the pelvis, lumbar spine, dorsal spine, and ribs.

FIGURE 6.59 **A:** Thoracic spine AP radiograph. Osteolytic metastatic lesion of the left T9 vertebral pedicle. The missing left T9 pedicle (*straight arrow*) was destroyed by metastatic disease while the uninvolved normal right T9 pedicle (*curved arrow*) remains clearly visible. This finding prompted further investigation by MRI that proved the missing pedicle was destroyed by a metastatic lesion. **B:** Thoracic spine sagittal T1 MR image in the same patient. Metastatic disease of the T9 vertebra. The metastatic disease involving the T9 vertebral body (*straight arrow*) has replaced almost all of the bone marrow fat, resulting in a low-intensity signal. This abnormality of T9 is quite obvious when compared to the high-intensity signals from the normal bone marrow of the uninvolved vertebral bodies above and below T9.

FIGURE 6.60 Lumbosacral spine sagittal T1 MR image. Metastatic carcinoma of the breast. The patient complained of severe back pain, but the radiographs were negative. The *straight arrows* indicate some of the many metastatic lesions present in the lumbar and sacral spine. The metastatic lesions appear black on the T1 MR image but white or gray on T2 images.

— T11 vertebral body

— T11 ribs

— L1 vertebral body

FIGURE 6.61 Lumbar spine lateral radiograph. Senile osteoporosis. Note the overall decreased density or osteopenia of the spine. There are multiple compression pathologic fractures secondary to osteoporosis (*straight arrows*). The fractures of T12, L2, -3, and -4 are manifest by a loss of the vertical heights of the involved vertebral bodies. Compare the fractured vertebrae to the normal vertical heights of the T11 and L1 vertebral bodies. Note the multiple fish-mouth deformities (*curved arrows*).

FIGURE 6.62 Thoracic spine (**A**) and lumbar (**B**) spine lateral radiographs. Sickle cell anemia. There is overall osteopenia, and the fish-mouth deformities of the vertebral bodies (*straight arrows*) are similar to those in senile osteoporosis (Fig. 6.61). Note the ribs in **A** (*arrowheads*).

KEY POINTS

- Basic observations on spine radiographs should include spinal alignment, the heights of the vertebral bodies and the intervertebral disc spaces, osseous density, presence of the pars interarticularis in the lumbar spine, and presence of the pedicles of each vertebra.

- An absent pedicle is abnormal and should make you suspicious of a destructive process such as primary and secondary bone neoplasms.

- Spine CT is good for bone detail, localization of fracture fragments and their relationship to the spinal canal and cord, and diagnosis of herniated intervertebral disc disease.

- Spine MRI is good for imaging disease processes that involve the bone marrow fat such as tumor and infection. MRI is also valuable for diagnosis and staging of herniated intervertebral disc disease and evaluating the spinal cord.

- Most congenital anomalies of the spine are asymptomatic.

- Hyperflexion injuries include teardrop fractures, posterior ligament injury, and facet locking. Locked facets commonly have associated spinal cord injury.

- Odontoid process fractures are frequent in the elderly and result from both hyperflexion and hyperextension injuries.

- Open-mouth AP radiographs and CT are useful tools for diagnosing odontoid fractures.

- A ring is rarely broken in only one location. At least two fractures are usually present in the pelvis.

- Acetabular fractures are evaluated by AP and oblique (Judet) views of the pelvis.

- Following an acetabular fracture, subsequent studies should closely evaluate for the presence of avascular necrosis in the femoral head.

Further Readings

El-Khoury GY. *Essentials of musculoskeletal imaging.* New York: Churchill Livingstone, 2003.
Renfrew DL. *Atlas of spine imaging.* Philadelphia: WB Saunders, 2003.
Rogers LF. *Radiology of skeletal trauma,* 3rd ed. New York: Churchill Livingstone, 2002.

CHAPTER 7 ■ BRAIN

WILBUR L. SMITH

BRAIN IMAGING

Neuroradiology was a relatively unsophisticated branch of imaging prior to 1970. Plain radiographs of the skull were insensitive for predicting neurologic disorders, and obtaining more useful diagnostic imaging information about the brain and spinal cord was cumbersome, painful, and yielded images that were difficult to interpret without advanced knowledge of neuroanatomy. The early brain imaging techniques were at best minimally invasive and many involved such gruesome activities as injecting air into the spinal canal (pneumoencephalography) and rolling the patient about in a specially devised torture chair. Few patients willingly returned for another one of those examinations! The highest level of comfort that the poor patient who needed brain imaging could anticipate was a direct puncture carotid arteriogram or a spinal tap.

The invention and widespread use of the technique of computerized axial tomography (CAT), or computed tomography (CT), allowed relatively painless access to the processes inside the skull and allowed the field of neuroradiology to become a premier subspecialty within radiology. The early CT scanners were slow, lacking in detail, and hard to manage (Fig. 7.1), but they were such a marvelous advance that they were embraced as a revolution in medical imaging. Indeed, Sir Godfrey Hounsfield, the pioneer of CT imaging, won many international awards and was knighted for his work. While magnetic resonance imaging (MRI) advances have supplanted CT in many applications, CT still is the technique of choice for the majority of the diagnostic studies of the brain and spine and is still the most common neuroimaging study performed in the United States. The CT scanners of today are capable of obtaining simultaneous multiple slices documenting cerebral perfusion and with new image processing techniques can produce reconstructed anatomical images in any plane desired. CT scans are routinely performed either with or without intravenous contrast enhancement, and the enhancement produced coupled with the speed of the new scanners makes real-time vascular mapping of the brain a practical clinical tool (Fig. 7.2). Certain clinical indications are generally predictive of the need for iodinated CT contrast, although there are many variations. Table 7.1 gives the usual indications for contrast use; however, if in doubt, radiologists are always available for consultation on individual cases.

In CT scanning, images of the brain are usually acquired in axial (horizontal) planes and then viewed at different digital levels so that one can see the bones of the face and skull as well as the tissues of the brain itself. Two image acquisitions are not required to get these data, but rather, two different levels of viewing the same digital data. The sections that result from the CT scans depict the anatomy at predetermined intervals depending on the parameters of reconstruction of the slices (thickness) and timing of acquisition of the data. Generally, the thicker the slices the fewer the sections needed to get through the brain, but as the slices are thickened, anatomy is depicted in less detail. In the standard brain CT scan, there are several key landmarks to observe for proper orientation. Figure 7.3 illustrates some of the highlights for which you should look in orienting yourself to the anatomy depicted by the slices.

Let's begin with the caudal sections and work cephalad. The fourth ventricle, a cerebrospinal fluid (CSF) space located dorsal to the brain stem and in the midline of the posterior fossa, is a good marker for identifying the level of the pons, cerebellar vermis, and the base of the anterior cranial fossa (Fig. 7.3A). On the same section lying ventral to the brain stem are the suprasellar cistern and the dorsum sellae. Note that the figures depict the anatomy of the posterior fossa less sharply than some of the more cephalad sections of brain. CT scans in the posterior fossa are often degraded owing to the absorption of x-rays by the large amount of dense surrounding bone; therefore, detail of the cerebellar hemispheres may be obscured. This technique limitation is mitigated to some degree by faster and better scanners, but bone artifact is a limitation of CT scanning.

Proceeding to sections cephalad from the fourth ventricle, one encounters the ambient cistern and cephalad portion of the suprasellar cistern (Fig. 7.3B). The former is an important landmark for the point where the cerebral peduncles (an extension of the brain stem) pass through the tentorium cerebri. Ventral to this landmark and slightly cephalad are located the third ventricle and the anterior horns of the lateral ventricles. At the lateral margins of the anterior horns of the ventricles are the basal ganglia, identifiable as masses of gray matter bordering the lateral and third ventricles (Fig. 7.3C). The caudate nuclei protrude into the anterior horns of the lateral ventricles.

Further cephalad the scans depict the brain cortex and the orderly interfaces between the gray and white matter

Lateral ventricle

FIGURE 7.1 A scan of the brain performed in 1976 on an EMI device. This single section took about 1 minute to acquire. The coarse pixels make anything but the larger brain structures such as the ventricles difficult to appreciate. This was, however, a huge improvement over the pneumoencephalogram.

(Fig. 7.3D). Note that each section of gray matter has an accompanying area of white matter arranged in a predictable pattern. Symmetry is everything in looking at CT scans of the brain. Provided that the patient is properly positioned, structures should match up from side to side.

Despite its immense success, CT has limitations that inhibit its value. For example, CT is inherently limited in its ability to display high degrees of tissue contrast. If two tissues absorb roughly the same number of photons, even though the tissues may be chemically very different, CT cannot discriminate be-

FIGURE 7.2 CT arteriogram of the brain obtained after intravenous contrast shows detail of the intracerebral vessels of the circle of Willis.

TABLE 7.1	

SOME COMMON INDICATIONS FOR CAT SCANNING AND USE OF INTRAVENOUS CONTRAST ENHANCEMENT

Indications for CAT scan	Intravenous contrast
Trauma	No
Infection	Yes
Congenital anomalies	No
Tumor	Yes
Metabolic disorder	No
Multiple sclerosis	Yes
Hydrocephalus	No

tween them. Bone or other high-density items such as aneurysm clips degrade the CT image. Although the time needed to obtain a section by CT has declined substantially in recent years, there are still physical limitations to CT scanning, and motion artifacts abound in uncooperative or combative patients.

The newer major technique in the imaging of the brain and spinal cord is MRI. This technique also had humble beginnings; the first scanners were used to quantify fat in livestock coming to market. MR images are wonderfully detailed and yield unique anatomical and functional data. Generally, the MRI studies require more time and are more expensive to carry out than CT scans. MRI has much better tissue contrast than CT, although special resolution is less. The new imaging sequences and enhanced capabilities of MRI to show metabolic, vascular, and functional changes in tissues suggest that it will ultimately be the imaging modality of choice for many conditions.

MRI imaging depends on alterations in the physical behavior of protons (hydrogen is the most abundant natural proton in our water-filled tissues) when first magnetized, then exposed to a pulse of radio frequency energy. The major variables are, therefore, the strength of the magnetic field, the ability to apply energy to disrupt magnetic equilibrium (gradient coils) the way the radio frequency waves are applied (pulse sequences). Table 7.2 is a very simplified overview of the current major pulse sequences and the color of lesions and the CSF on the currently used 1.5-tesla MRI scans. There are many exceptions to the data in Table 7.2, and new sequences are rapidly being developed; therefore, this table should be used only as a rough (90% accurate) guideline to get you in the ballpark when looking at MRI images. Despite the great potential of MRI and its progression from a research device in the early 1980s to a staple of most imaging departments in the United States, at present CT scans still provide the bulk of diagnostic brain images. Table 7.3 compares the strengths and limitations of CT and MRI. A series of images showing both sequences and typical anatomic structures are demonstrated. (Fig. 7.4A–C)

TRAUMA

Perhaps the most common indication for brain imaging is trauma. Human heads are extremely vulnerable to injury; consequently, the trauma CT scanner rarely lacks sufficient

FIGURE 7.3 A: CT scan of a normal adult at the level of the fourth ventricle. The brain stem structure ventral to the fourth ventricle is the pons. Further anterior lies the five-pointed star representing the suprasellar cistern. Lying within the suprasellar cistern are the vessels of the circle of Willis and the dorsum sellae or back of the sella turcica. **B:** A cut cephalad to **A** demonstrates the ambient cisterns as curved black cerebrospinal fluid densities just posterior to the cerebral peduncles. If you use your imagination, the cistern is the mouth, the anterior horns of the lateral ventricles the eyes, and the third ventricle the nose of a smiling man! This is an important landmark as it is the point where the cerebral peduncles pass through the tentorium. **C:** Proceeding cephalad we leave the posterior fossa and image the lateral ventricles, third ventricles, aqueduct of Sylvius, and the cerebral hemispheres. (*continued*)

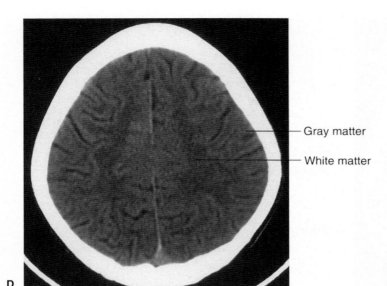

— Gray matter

— White matter

D

FIGURE 7.3 (*Continued*) **D:** A scan near the vertex of the head depicts the white matter (black on CT) and its relationship to the gray matter. Note that each area of gray matter has an associated column of white matter.

business. In assessing a CT performed for trauma, one has a finite number of search parameters for major findings that represent conditions likely to demand immediate intervention. MRI is excellent for subacute trauma detection, but the speed and availability of CT makes it the usual primary imaging device for trauma patients.

The presence of blood in the head but outside the vascular system is often a key to the correct diagnosis. Fortunately, when blood is loose in the head, it usually appears as a conspicuous white blob on the CT scan. Therefore, the first rule of looking at trauma CT scans is to look for the white collections inside the skull (Fig. 7.5). Your diagnosis often can be even more specific because the white (or blood) had characteristic absorption (Hounsfield number) and tends to align in certain predictable ways according to its anatomic location. As an overview, the locations of intracranial bleeding whether by CT or MRI are first separated into intra-axial, meaning within the brain tissues themselves, or extra-axial. The extra-axial hemorrhages occur in spaces with characteristic shapes that can assist in localizing the hemorrhage. Fluid in the epidural space, between skull and dura, usually presents as a crescentic mass, convex to the brain (Fig. 7.6). The subdural space between dura and arachnoid membranes, however, is usually concave to the brain surface, paralleling the surface of the skull; therefore, subdural hematomas are differentiated

from epidural bleeding by their shape (Fig. 7.7). Subarachnoid blood diffuses over the surface of the gyri and fills the CSF cisterns around the brain (Fig. 7.8). Intra-axial bleeding is often confined to the area of the ruptured vessel and is entirely enclosed within the substance of the brain. Intraventricular hemorrhage lies within the ventricles, often pooling in the dependent portion of the ventricle to form a blood–CSF level. By first finding the "white" blood, then looking at its shape and anatomic location, one can be pretty precise about the diagnosis and the location of the blood. As the hematoma ages, the blood assumes different image characteristics. Table 7.4 provides a description of the differing appearances of blood in the head with age of the bleed.

After looking for bleeding in trauma patients, the next step is to look for mass effect, a clue that there is pressure impinging on an area of the brain. For most injuries, the best way to find significant mass effects is to look for asymmetry with displacement of the midline structures, the most prominent of which are the falx cerebri, lateral ventricles, and interhemispheric fissure (Figs. 7.6 and 7.9). A midline shift away from a lesion, for example, an epidural blood collection, is usually an emergent situation, particularly in the context of trauma. However, a word of caution is advisable: Midline shift does not always signal a need to take out your pocketknife to perform emergent, kitchen table–type neurosurgery. Diffuse

TABLE 7.2

MRI PULSE SEQUENCES

Sequence	Cerebrospinal fluid color	Lesion color
T1-weighted	Black	Variable
T2-weighted	White	White
Inversion recovery	Black	White
Diffusion	Black	White
Gradient (susceptibility)	Black	Black

TABLE 7.3

A COMPARISON OF INDICATIONS AND FACTORS AFFECTING THE CHOICE OF CT OR MRI

Factor	CT	MRI
Cost	++	+++
Availability	+++	++
Tissue differentiation	+	+++
Multiplanar sequences	+++	+++
Speed of examination	+++	++
Bone reconstruction	+++	+

7-A

7-B

FIGURE 7.4 A: Axial T1-weighted (left) and T2-weighted MRI images at the level of the foramen of Monro. On T1-weighted images, the cerebrospinal fluid in the ventricles is black and on T2-weighted images it is white. Notice the superb anatomical detail, much better than CT. **B:** Coronal T2-weighted image at the level of the foramen of Monro in the same patients. The anatomical definition rivals that of a brain section in the neuroanatomy laboratory. **C:** Sagittal midline T1-weighted image of the same patient. The midline structures, face and foramen magnum, are seen in fine detail. Note how well you see the cerebellum and brain stem without the beam hardening artifacts of CT.

edema of one hemisphere of the brain (Fig. 7.9) or even atrophy of the contralateral hemisphere can cause apparent (or real) shift. The important concept is midline shift. When the brain structures are shifted away from the side of the evident abnormality, such as a hematoma, increase your level of suspicion and urgency in evaluating your patient.

After searching for blood and mass effects on the brain CT scan or MRI, the next important step is to assess the densities of the brain tissues themselves. Earlier we described how the gray and white matter components of the brain should be visible on the CT scan (Fig. 7.3D). The lateral ventricles and CSF spaces are black and should be easily distinguished as separate from the tissues of the brain. Variations on this theme are generally bad news. The most prominent and dangerous sign is the obliteration of the distinction between the gray and white matter, which indicates profound edema in the area (get focal edema on MRI). If this is a universal pattern, there is a special name for the profound edema that occurs, obliterating all brain landmarks—the "bad black brain" (Fig. 7.10). This

finding usually portends a poor outcome, representing diffuse breakdown of tissue integrity with ensuing cerebral edema. The cause of this catastrophic chain of events is almost always a limitation of the oxygen supply to the brain tissues, owing to either a compromise of the blood supply or a loss of oxygen to the brain cells. In the latter instance, as the brain swells, cerebral blood supply is compromised by loss of the arterial perfusion gradient, and ultimately there is no circulation to the brain. Owing to different tissue densities and less vulnerable perfusion, the basal ganglia and brain stem are often particularly conspicuous against the uniform density of the bad black brain, and their conspicuity results in the so-called reversal sign (Fig. 7.11).

Please note the intentional lack of a detailed discussion of skull fractures in this section on trauma. That is because, in general, skull fractures aren't very important in the immediate outcome of a patient. It is the effect of the trauma on the brain that does your patient harm, not the crack in the bone (Fig. 7.12). A significant important exception is the depressed skull

FIGURE 7.5   A child injured in a severe auto accident shows multiple white areas in the brain as well as disruption of the skull. The white areas are intraparenchymal hemorrhage. Also note the disruption of the normal brain architecture (compare to Fig. 7.3D, which shows a section at roughly the same level), reflecting the severe cerebral edema.

FIGURE 7.6   A large mass of white (blood) density convex toward the brain is characteristic of an epidural hemorrhage. Most of these occur because of traumatic tear of an artery and are surgical emergencies. The brain is shifted by the hematoma as evidenced by the shift of midline.

fracture, a situation in which the bone is driven directly back into the meningeal coverings and the brain itself. CT imaging and bone windows are of great importance in documenting the depth and extent of this type of injury as well as documenting any intracranial air leaks owing to tears of the dura or meninges (Fig. 7.13). In this type of trauma, surgery is usu-

ally needed and the identification of the fracture, depth of the fragment(s), surface brain injury, and pneumocephalus (air inside the skull) are the key observations.

MRI is not to be omitted in any discussion of trauma, but its role, although dramatically increasing, is usually secondary. Because of the limitations of patient access (ventilator limitations,

FIGURE 7.7   MRI of the brain, shown to illustrate that MRI is also effective in showing trauma. This is an abused child who has a subdural space hematoma (*arrows*). Note that the surface is concave, reflecting the contour of the cerebral cortex, but not extending among the gyri. This configuration is typical for a subdural hematoma. Also note that the signal densities are different on MRI. Imaging of bleeding is more complex on MRI than by CAT.

FIGURE 7.8 A CT scan at the level of the ambient cistern showing the cistern as white (blood) instead of black (cerebrospinal fluid; compare to Fig. 7.3B). Note that the white density also surrounds the brain stem. When blood mimics cerebrospinal fluid distribution, it is usually extra-axial and in the subarachnoid space flowing around and over the brain tissues.

FIGURE 7.9 Intra-axial or intraparenchymal hemorrhage of the brain in a trauma patient. The white densities (blood) do not conform to any definable space and are actually within and between the tissues of the brain. A subdural hematoma (*arrows*) is also present in this patient. Note that the lateral ventricle and its temporal horn (*arrowheads*) are displaced by the mass effect.

difficulty in patient observation, etc.) and the longer examination times, MRI is rarely the first imaging modality used for acute trauma. After the acute, life-threatening emergencies have been handled, MRI is extremely sensitive for assessing the extent of parenchymal injury to the brain and for defining more precisely the compartment of localized extra-axial fluid. In each of these instances, the prognosis and etiology of the injury is better defined after MRI. MRI spectroscopy, a study of brain metabolism, holds great promise for predicting the outcome of some injuries. The utility of MRI for finding subarachnoid blood is debatable, but MRI is unparalleled in defining precisely which gyrus was smashed in a previous auto accident (Fig. 7.14). The instances in which MRI is critical in deciding the urgent management of a trauma patient are few, but it is an invaluable secondary tool in selected patients.

TABLE 7.4

CHARACTERISTICS OF INTRACRANIAL BLOOD BY IMAGING

		MRI	
Time of bleed	CT	T1-weighted	T2-weighted
Immediate	White	Black	Black
Acute	White	White	Black
Subacute	Gray–White	White	White

FIGURE 7.10 This severely brain-injured child has neither recognizable ventricles nor gray/white matter differentiation (compare with Fig. 7.3D). In fact, the whole neocortex, except for the areas of hemorrhage, is a uniform shade of black. This severe brain edema portends a poor prognosis.

FIGURE 7.11   A child with diffuse hypoxic injury of the brain demonstrates the reversal sign. Note that the basal ganglia are gray and the neocortex black, particularly in the frontal and parietal regions.

In summary, a CT scan of an acute trauma patient should be evaluated for the following findings: (a) white densities defining bleeding, including the shape and distribution of the blood collection(s); (b) mass effect, particularly with shift of the midline structures; and (c) loss of normal contrast characteristics (or asymmetry) of the normal tissue and CSF interfaces. These rules won't get you every answer on every trauma patient, but they will help you in almost 95% of the cases you see. For the other 5%, you may have to do a radiology or neurosurgery residency!

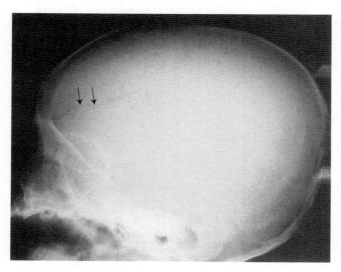

FIGURE 7.12   This child with a linear skull fracture (*arrows*) was completely asymptomatic (except for a palpable bump on his skull) because the brain underlying the skull was not affected. The presence of the skull fracture documents trauma but is of little importance in patient management.

FIGURE 7.13   Bone windows of a CT scan demonstrate the depth of injury in a depressed skull fracture (*arrow*) after this teenager was struck with a hammer.

VASCULAR DISEASE

Just after trauma as an indication for brain imaging is vascular disease, and the most prevalent form is stroke. Stroke results from occlusion of the vascular supply (usually arterial but occasionally venous as well) to a focal area of the brain causing tissue ischemia. Many "strokes" are small and not

FIGURE 7.14   MRI shows a diffusely increased signal (*white indicated by arrow*) in the posterior parietal lobes of a blunt head trauma victim. This is owing to a cortical contusion that was subtle on the CT scan. Although the finding explained the patient's symptoms and documented the severity of injury, the lesion did not require urgent intervention.

FIGURE 7.15 Widely scattered unidentified bright objects (UBOs) on MRI in the basal ganglia of this octogenarian are not of significance. These UBOs are common near the basal ganglia but can be seen anywhere and are assumed to represent small artery disease with lacunar infarctions.

FIGURE 7.16 The low-density lesion in the right cerebellar hemisphere represents an acute stroke owing to arterial occlusion. Note that there is swelling of tissues involved in the stroke as evidenced by effacement of the ambient cistern on the right (*arrowheads*). The lesion does not contain blood because there is no white signal on CT.

even detected clinically. Most people in their fifth or sixth decade have small areas of abnormal signal called unidentified bright objects (UBOs) on MRI of the brain (Fig. 7.15), and there are some who ascribe the origin of UBOs to silent strokes. We have a lot of brain tissue that we don't fully use and so loss of these small areas isn't necessarily perceived as a clinical problem.

Only when either a large or a particularly critical area of brain becomes ischemic do emergent symptoms appear and neuroimaging comes into play. CT scans are often the first examination; however, their use is problematic as there is a significant incidence of false-negative CT scans in the first 24 to 48 hours after a stroke. The size, severity, and presence of hemorrhage clearly affect the CT picture of stroke and so some strokes appear almost immediately; however, the sensitivity of CT scan for the diagnosis is considerably higher after the first 24 to 48 hours, unfortunately outside the window for "clot buster" treatments (Fig. 7.16).

The most reliable finding in stroke on CT scan is the loss of the normal architecture of brain substance. The area of the stroke is depicted as a dark (edematous) blotch obliterating the normal tissue density. Occasional strokes will have associated bleeding, particularly in patients with hypertension, and the blood will show up on CT as a white density within the darker area of infarct (Fig. 7.17). A stroke may also change in nature as the tissue is destroyed and revascularization takes place. Bleeding may ensue such that initially nonhemorrhagic strokes can develop high signal characteristic of internal bleeding. This change often portends a poor prognosis. Newer CT perfusion techniques enabled by faster scanners and better computers may well supersede the current CT for stroke protocols.

FIGURE 7.17 This huge hematoma in the left side of the brain has an irregular margin and edema surrounding the white area of fresh hemorrhage. This is a 53-year-old hypertensive executive who suffered a fatal acute hemorrhagic stroke.

FIGURE 7.18   A: An acute stroke in the anterior portion of the right thalamus in this 50-year-old hypertensive executive was detected promptly by diffusion-weighted MRI. The acute diffusion coefficient image shows a low-density (black) lesion in the thalamus on the T2 sequence. **B:** The same lesion is white on the conventional inversion recovery sequence.

There is a developing body of knowledge suggesting that early treatment of stroke may restore circulation and limit brain tissue damage. This has led to a change in imaging to emphasize early diagnosis. MRI, particularly with diffusion imaging sequences, is more sensitive to the early changes and has assumed a larger role in the imaging of acute stroke. Diffusion imaging is a series of specific inversion recovery sequences that show Brownian motion of the water molecules released from the damaged brain tissue, which roughly correlates with areas of cell death. This finding is very sensitive and appears within minutes of tissue injury in experimental studies, making it the most useful tool for diagnosing acute stroke (Fig. 7.18). Advances in MRI sequencing are rapid, so it is likely that these sequences will be further refined possibly even to anticipate cell death, but for now diffusion is the most accurate and early sequence for stroke. Eight hours or more after a stroke, the MRI of the damaged tissues shows white (on T2 and FLAIR) owing to the large amount of free water

leaked by the ischemic cells (Fig. 7.19). Unfortunately, by this time it is too late to use many of the thrombolytic techniques to limit stroke; therefore, diffusion is critical early in stroke. The use of MRI contrast (gadolinium) has improved detection even further, and MRI may soon be the standard for stroke imaging (Fig. 7.20).

So far we've discussed acute strokes. Chronic strokes result in atrophy of the brain tissue (Fig. 7.21) manifested by either focal or diffuse shrinkage of the brain owing to cell death. Of special note is diffuse multi-infarct dementia, a condition that is difficult to differentiate from Alzheimer's disease. Here the strokes are small and confined to the areas near the ventricles and so the ventricles enlarge at the expense of the dead tissue (Fig. 7.22). The patient's CT scan looks like the ventricles are dilated, with the gyri and sulci appearing unusually prominent, a condition sometimes referred to as *hydrocephalus ex vacuo*. These cases are truly a conundrum because Alzheimer's disease, normal pressure hydrocephalus of the elderly, and

FIGURE 7.19 A diffusion-weighted image of a 2-hour-old left parietal stroke (A and B). Note that the acute stroke is black on the diffusion image (17B) and white on the composite ADC "map" (17A). The patient did not have "clot busters" for other clinical reasons, so a conventional T2-weighted image at 12 hours shows the left parietal stroke as a bright signal.

FIGURE 7.20   The white area in the right temporal lobe on this patient is a newly symptomatic stroke as depicted by gadolinium-enhanced MRI.

FIGURE 7.22   T2-weighted scan at the level of the lateral ventricles demonstrates multiple high-signal periventricular infarcts owing to lack of perfusion of the deep layers of the brain. These patients present with dementia and movement disorders that may mimic a number of degenerative neurologic conditions.

diffuse brain atrophy from any cause all look the same. Functional brain imaging with spectroscopy, blood perfusion analysis, and/or metabolic measurement are of future consideration for this diagnosis. There is no easy imaging answer, and at present there is no specific treatment with good efficacy for any of these conditions. However, this is a rapidly developing area of medicine and exciting imaging developments are to be anticipated.

FIGURE 7.21   This elderly man has diffusely dilated ventricles as well as deep sulci over the brain surface because of atrophy presumably associated with multiple prior infarcts.

TUMOR

The third common application of brain imaging is tumor evaluation. In adults, metastases (Fig. 7.23) constitute the most common tumors, with primary benign or malignant tumors being somewhat less common. The converse is true in children owing to the lower frequency of primary malignancies that metastasize to brain. The location of the tumors also differs with age. A greater proportion of adult tumors are in the cerebral cortex, whereas in children the proportion of tumors originating below the tentorium is much greater (Fig. 7.24).

CT scanning for tumor follows the same general principles as for trauma, with the major exception that most tumor scans are performed after the administration of intravenous contrast. The theory, which works most of the time, is that the abnormal tumor circulation allows contrast to penetrate the blood–brain barrier and enhance the tumor. Because contrast enhancement is white on a CT scan, the tumor becomes conspicuous. However, tumors can bleed, and the white of the contrast may obscure the white of the bleeding. Because the appearance of blood is an important issue in tumor patients, we often have to study them both with and without intravenous enhancement. In defining tumor and

FIGURE 7.23 A contrast-enhanced CT scan of a 59-year-old woman with known lung cancer shows multiple high-and mixed-density lesions. These were metastases from the lung tumor.

FIGURE 7.24 T1-weighted MRI documents a huge tumor that arises from the cerebellar vermis and pushes the brain stem forward. This is typical behavior of a medulloblastoma.

normal anatomy, MRI equals or surpasses CT in efficacy and few neurosurgeons would tackle a brain tumor without the aid of a contrast (gadolinium) MRI (Fig. 7.25).

Just as with trauma, it is important to differentiate intra-axial masses (within the brain tissues) from extra-axial masses, as the differential diagnosis and approach are different. Determining tumor origin is one of the most difficult diagnostic tasks. In general, an extra-axial tumor will display its widest base at the brain surface and will smoothly indent the brain from without (Fig. 7.26). Extra-axial tumors tend to be related to the meninges or the bones of the skull. Occasionally, a parenchymal brain tumor originates at the brain surface and differentiation is impossible. Conversely, extra-axial tumors

sometimes grow from slips of tissues insinuated into the brain, giving the appearance of parenchymal masses.

Tumors that are entirely enveloped within the brain tissues are usually of glial cell origin, with astrocytoma being the most common primary tumor (Fig. 7.27) and metastasis being the most common overall. When the distinction of intra-axial from extra-axial is difficult and critical, using another modality with multiplanar imaging capability, such as MRI, is invaluable. MRI also offers different tissue contrast parameters, and contrast-enhanced MRI adds yet another dimension.

Once the tumor is diagnosed and localized to the proper anatomic location, the next job is to look at the mass effect caused by the tumor and to assess the likelihood of damage to

FIGURE 7.25 **A:** A T2-weighted image of a brain tumor, a glioma in the right occipital lobe. The central tumor (white) is surrounded by a rim of edema infiltrating the white matter. **B:** After intravenous contrast (gadolinium) a collar of enhancement better defines the boundaries of the tumor for the surgeon.

brain tissue? If so, you have to move quickly. Once again, shift away from the tumor and alteration of the normal differentiation of the brain tissues are key to the proper determination.

CONGENITAL ANOMALIES

Although CT is often used for the diagnosis of congenital anomalies of the brain, MRI, with its superior tissue contrast, is invaluable in this area. Congenital anomalies usually present in childhood, either with abnormal physical findings or with seizures. Physical abnormalities most often associated with congenital brain abnormalities include macrocephaly (big head), abnormal appearance of the face (particularly with midline abnormalities such as cleft palate), and meningocele. Each of these findings should tip you off to pursue a specific type of abnormality.

In the case of macrocranium (a big head), the likely diagnosis is hydrocephalus or dilatation of the ventricles because of abnormal CSF circulation. The lateral ventricles stand out so well owing to their CSF content that CT is well adapted to the initial diagnosis and monitoring of treatment for hydrocephalus (Fig. 7.28). The most critical factor is determining the cause of the hydrocephalus so that you can predict whether or not surgical shunting will be of value for the patient. In most instances the method is straightforward: One looks for the most caudal dilated ventricle and assumes that the obstruction is between that site and the most cephalad normal ventricle. For example, if the lateral and third ventricles are dilated but the fourth ventricle is normal, the obstruction

FIGURE 7.26 This large tumor (*arrow*) has a broad base along the roof of the orbit and displaces the frontal lobe of the brain superiorly. This growth is typical of an extra-axial tumor, in this case a meningioma.

critical centers of the brain requiring emergent action. Here, the principles applied in trauma are useful. Does the tumor cause displacement of the normal structures, such that they are sufficiently compressed to cause compromise of the blood supply or direct pressure damage to the cells of the normal

FIGURE 7.27 On gadolinium-enhanced MRI, this cerebellar tumor contains a very bright nidus of tissue within a cystic mass. This is characteristic of a pilocytic astrocytoma.

FIGURE 7.28 This child presented with a large head. Family history documented macrocranium in several other family members including the father. The head CT scan shows the ventricles to be slightly enlarged and the subarachnoid spaces to be prominent. This constellation of findings is diagnostic for benign familial macrocranium.

FIGURE 7.29   Sagittal (**A**) and coronal (**B**) MRIs of an infant with a huge head at birth. The child has severe hydrocephalus involving the lateral and third ventricles but a normal fourth ventricle. This is suggestive of an aqueductal obstruction.

is likely at the outflow area of the third ventricle or the aqueduct of Sylvius (Fig. 7.29).

Often obstructive hydrocephalus can become static owing to equilibration of the CSF dynamics of production and absorption. In this case, it may not be necessary to place a shunt to drain the CSF. Once the dilated ventricles are detected, the need to shunt can be determined by following the ventricular size over time. This should, of course, be coupled with close observation of the patient's clinical status. Don't ever let the imaging hold you back if your patient is deteriorating. CT scans provide sufficient detail for monitoring progression of hydrocephalus. MRI is often of value in the initial evaluation of hydrocephalus, but follow-up monitoring is the domain of CT. Hydrocephalus can occur on other than a congenital basis, but the rules outlined here for evaluation hold for most instances.

MRI is the best method for initial evaluation of most babies with complex defects of the face and brain because of its multidimensional imaging capability. Holoprosencephaly, or failure of division of the embryonic forebrain, is always associated with facial anomalies and is a good prototype for illustrating the value of MRI. This complex series of anomalies ranges all the way from a totally malformed brain, a condition not compatible with life, to agenesis of the septum pellucidum and optic abnormalities (septooptical dysplasia), conditions compatible with long life (Fig. 7.30). Whereas CT scans are sufficient for the gross defects of holoprosencephaly, MRI can show sufficient detail to define the absence of the septum pellucidum as well as showing the midline defects of the optic tracts. If you have one test to do in these children, MRI is the best.

Meningocele is a common condition caused by failure of closure of the embryonic neural tube. This condition is almost invariably associated with a complex series of abnormalities called the Arnold-Chiari II malformation. The reason all of these brain anomalies are associated with what commonly is a spinal abnormality is complex, but the findings are reproducible and best demonstrated by MRI (Fig. 7.31). The tethering of the spinal cord that occurs with meningocele is associated with pro-

FIGURE 7.30   MRI of an infant with septooptical dysplasia documents the minimal abnormality of incomplete septation of the lateral ventricles by showing a deficiency of the septum pellucidum.

—Foramen magnum

—Cerebellar tonsils

—Spinal cord

FIGURE 7.31 MRI from a baby with lumbar myelomeningocele. The posterior fossa is small and the cerebellar tonsil protrudes far below the foramen magnum. This is a constant component of the Arnold-Chiari malformation.

trusion of the cerebellar tonsils below the foramen magnum. As with our other examples, the complex anatomy in developmental brain anomalies is best shown by MRI.

The finding of seizures in a child suggests a congenital defect, either structural or owing to a metabolic problem. In either case, MRI is more likely to yield the correct answers. Structural abnormalities include errors of neuronal migration in which the brain tissues are arrested in their normal growth, leaving focal islands of tissue in abnormal locations throughout the brain (Fig. 7.32). Other structural abnormalities result from abnormal arrests of tissues proliferating and disrupting

the normal brain tissue. A good prototype condition here is tuberous sclerosis (Fig. 7.33), although any other phakomatosis can give similar problems. Metabolic abnormalities causing seizures usually cause demyelination, thereby affecting the white matter either diffusely or as focal lesions (Fig. 7.34). MRI is clearly superior to CT here, although the findings are not specific for one disease process; focal infection or demyelinating disorders such as multiple sclerosis can look the same as metabolic defects.

There are many other potential uses for imaging in neurologic disease. However, if you retain the general principles

Schizencephalic cleft

FIGURE 7.32 A child with seizures. MRI shows a cleft from the posterior portion of the left lateral ventricle all the way to the brain surface. This condition, caused by a failure of proper migration of neurons as the brain is formed, is called *schizencephaly*.

FIGURE 7.33 CT scan of the brain demonstrates calcification in the roof of each lateral ventricle. These calcifications are within the hamartomas or tubers. MRI would also demonstrate the hamartomas as well as showing the lesions that are not calcified.

FIGURE 7.34 Multiple high-density white matter lesions are consistent with a myelodegenerative phenomenon, in this case multiple sclerosis. These findings are not specific and must be combined with the clinical and laboratory results to be diagnostic.

elucidated here, you can make most of the diagnoses needed for patient care, whether or not you completely master all of the nuances of the differential diagnosis.

KEY POINTS

- Computerized axial tomography (CAT), or computed tomography (CT), is the most commonly performed neuroimaging study in the United States. CT scans can depict the brain in horizontal planes that can be viewed at different levels.

- When assessing a CT scan for potential trauma, begin by looking for blood in the head outside the vascular system. Blood appears on CT initially as a white blob.

- Mass effect is a clue that pressure is impinging on an area of the brain. The best way to find significant mass effect is to look for asymmetry with displacement of the midline structures.

- Obliteration of the distinction between gray and white matter in the brain represents profound edema. If the edema is universal, you are witnessing a "bad black brain," which portends a poor outcome and is almost always caused by a limitation of oxygen in the brain.

- On CT, acute strokes often initially appear as a dark edematous blotch obliterating the normal tissue density. On many MRI sequences with inversion recovery or T2 weighting, the damaged tissues are white because of water leaked by the ischemic cells. Diffusion MRI is the most sensitive imaging test for acute stroke.

- Tumors that are entirely enveloped in the brain tissues are usually of glial cell origin, with astrocytoma being the most common primary tumor.

- Complex anatomy in developmental brain anomalies is best shown with MRI.

- Physical abnormalities most often associated with congenital brain abnormalities include macrocephaly (big head), abnormal appearance of the face (particularly with midline abnormalities such as cleft palate), and meningocele.

Suggested Reading

Osborn A. *Diagnostic neuroradiology.* St. Louis, MO: Mosby, 1994.

CHAPTER 8 ■ HEAD AND NECK

YUTAKA SATO

In this chapter, a short overview of head and neck imaging is presented. With the recent advancement and widening availability of sectional imagings, such as computed tomography (CT) and magnetic resonance imaging (MRI), the part played by the plain radiographs has decreased significantly.

As an initial screening of sinusitis or facial trauma, radiographs may be used when more sophisticated sectional imagings are not readily available. For facial bone and paranasal sinus evaluation, routine radiographic views include Waters (Fig. 8.1), Caldwell (Fig. 8.2) and lateral (Fig. 8.3) views. Lack of aeration in the sinus antra is suggestive of sinusitis, and a definitive diagnosis can be made when an air–fluid level is present. CT is the primary modality for the evaluation of sinus infection and facial trauma (Figs. 8.4 to 8.6), because bone detail is best evaluated by CT. Because of multiple horizontally placed buttresses of the facial skeleton, multiplaner reconstructed images in coronal and sagittal planes generated from axial data are essential for the detailed evaluation of facial fractures (Figs. 8.7 to 8.9).

MRI is the modality of choice for the evaluation of neoplastic lesions of the head and neck because of its superior soft-tissue characterization and multiplaner capability. MRI is essential to evaluate skull base involvement by head and neck tumors.

SINUSITIS

Clinical presentation of pain, swelling over the paranasal sinuses, and leukocytosis are sufficient for the diagnosis of sinusitis; and, in the majority of cases, imaging is not necessary. When intraorbital or intracranial extension of the inflammatory process is suspected and surgical intervention is contemplated, imaging becomes necessary. CT is the modality of choice. Acute fluid collection in the sinus cavity is diagnostic, and associated findings include mucosal thickening (Fig. 8.10) and erosive or destructive changes of the sinus wall. Extension of the inflammatory process into the orbits (Fig. 8.11) or cranial cavity may be seen and help determine the therapeutic approach.

For examination of children, the developmental sequence of the paranasal sinus should be taken into consideration. Generally, the ethmoid and maxillary sinuses are present at birth but may not be aerated. The sphenoid and frontal sinuses start to be seen at about 3 and 6 years of age, respectively.

TRAUMA

For the evaluation for facial fractures, CT is also the modality of choice. Nasal fractures are the most common, followed by zygomatic fractures. Zygomatic fractures commonly involve (a) the lateral orbital wall at the frontozygomatic suture, (b) the maxillozygomatic suture, and (c) the zygomatic arch, and is named a "trimalar" or "tripod" fracture (Fig. 8.12). If the facial fracture extends posteriorly and violates the pterygoid plate, the fractured facial bones are detached from the cranium. Depending upon the level of the fracture line traversing the central midface, these fractures are classified as Le Fort I, II, or III fractures (Figs. 8.13 and 8.14).

CT is essential to evaluate the entrapped soft tissue and nerves by the fracture fragments, which may require urgent decompression.

Orbital blowout fracture occurs when an object larger than the orbit, such as a fist or a baseball, hits the eye. The impact is transmitted to the orbital contents and raises the intraorbital pressure enough to shatter the weakest wall of the orbit, either the inferior wall into the maxillary sinus (Fig. 8.15) or the medial wall (lamina papyracea) into the ethmoid sinus, without fracturing the orbital rim. The inferior rectus muscle may be trapped and cause paralysis of the inferior gaze of the affected eye.

CONGENITAL ANOMALIES

Premature fusion of a cranial suture (craniosynostoses) prevents growth of cranium in direction perpendicular to the involved suture. Sagittal synostosis results in a narrow, long head (dolichocephaly, scaphocephaly). Bilateral coronal or lambdoid synostosis results in a broad short head (brachycephaly). Unilateral coronal or lambdoid synostosis results in an asymmetric head (plagiocephaly). CT with three-dimensional reconstruction is useful for evaluation of coexisting intracranial abnormalities and surgical planning (Fig. 8.16).

Thyroglossal cysts occur along the course of embryologic descent of the primordial thyroid from the foramen cecum of the tongue base to the normal cervical paratracheal location and are most commonly seen as an anterior paramedian cystic mass closely related to the strap muscle (Fig. 8.17).

Branchial cleft cysts are prototypical congenital lateral neck masses seen at the bifurcation of the carotid artery anterior to the sternocleid muscle (Fig. 8.18).

— Frontal zygomatic process

— Nasal cavity

— Nasal turbinate

— Maxillary sinus

— Zygomatic arch

— Mandible

FIGURE 8.1 Normal Waters view of the face, showing the good delineation of the maxilla. The maxillary sinuses are optimally displayed, and the anterior portions of the orbit and the nasal cavity are clearly outlined.

Orbit —

— Frontal sinus

— Ethmoid sinuses

— Nasal turbinates

— Ramus of mandible

FIGURE 8.2 A Caldwell, or posteroanterior, view of the face. Note how well the orbits and frontal bone are seen. The maxilla is superimposed on the skull base to some degree. The structures of the internal auditory canals are visible through the orbits.

Frontal sinus

Sphenoid sinus

Anterior wall maxillary sinus

Hard palate

Nasopharynx

FIGURE 8.3 Lateral view of the skull shows the posteriorly located sphenoid sinus and the nasopharyngeal airway. This view complements the others, adding the third dimension to the structures of the head and the neck.

Maxillary sinus

Zygomatic arch

Pterygoid plate

Pterygopalatine fossa

Mandibular chondyle

FIGURE 8.4   Normal axial CT image (inferior plane).

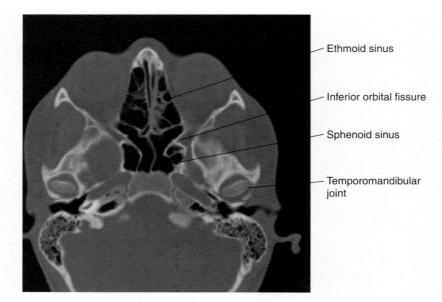

Ethmoid sinus

Inferior orbital fissure

Sphenoid sinus

Temporomandibular joint

FIGURE 8.5   Normal axial CT image (middle plane).

Frontal sinus

Orbit

Optic foramen

Anterior clinoid process

Dorsum sella

FIGURE 8.6   Normal axial CT image (superior plane).

Orbit

Ethmoid sinus

Maxillary sinus

FIGURE 8.7   Reconstructed coronal CT image (anterior plane).

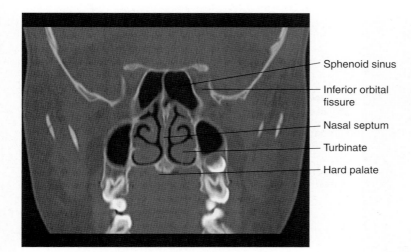

- Sphenoid sinus
- Inferior orbital fissure
- Nasal septum
- Turbinate
- Hard palate

FIGURE 8.8 Reconstructed coronal CT image (middle plane).

- Dorsum sella
- Sphenoid sinus
- Foramen ovale

FIGURE 8.9 Reconstructed coronal CT image (posterior plane).

FIGURE 8.10 Chronic maxillary sinusitis. The right maxillary sinus is opacified by thickened mucosa, and mucosal thickening extends into the right nasal cavity. Also, notice sclerotic thickening of the sinus wall, suggestive of the chronic nature of the sinusitis.

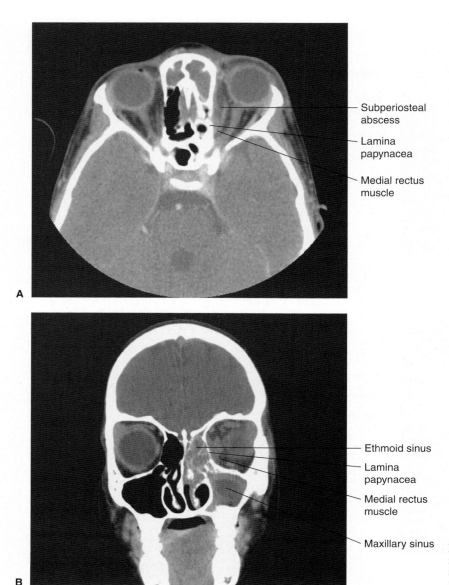

A

B

— Subperiosteal
abscess

— Lamina
papynacea

— Medial rectus
muscle

— Ethmoid sinus

— Lamina
papynacea

— Medial rectus
muscle

— Maxillary sinus

FIGURE 8.11 Orbital cellulitis, **(A,B)** axial/coronal CT. Inflammation of the ethmoid sinus extends into the orbit through the thin wall, lamina papyracea, forming a subperiosteal abscess.

FIGURE 8.12 Tripod fracture. Three-dimensional reformatted CT. Note the fractures involved: (a) the lateral orbital wall, (b) the maxillozygomatic suture, and (c) the zygomatic arch.

FIGURE 8.13 **A:** Le Fort I fracture. **B:** Le Fort II fracture. **C:** Le Fort III fracture. (From Langland OE, Langlais RP, McDavid WD, DelBalso AM, eds. *Panoramic radiology,* 2nd ed. Philadelphia: Lea & Febiger, 1989, with permission.)

FIGURE 8.14 CT scan of an auto accident victim who struck the windshield. There are multiple fractures including disruption of the deeper structures of the face (pterygoid plates illustrated). This is a complex fracture pattern of the Le Forte type and can be defined well only with CT.

Blowout fracture

Entrapped muscle

FIGURE 8.15 A blowout fracture of the orbit caused by a fist to the eye. Note the soft tissue mass protruding into the maxillary sinus. This woman had no gaze abnormality on presentation for care but developed one shortly thereafter. The fracture required surgical reconstruction, but the patient now has a normally functioning eye.

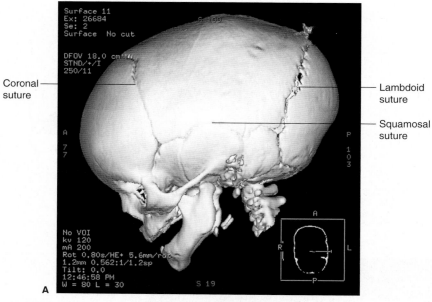

Coronal suture

Lambdoid suture

Squamosal suture

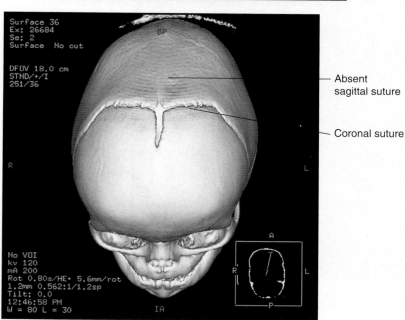

Absent sagittal suture

Coronal suture

FIGURE 8.16 Sagittal synostosis, (A,B) lateral/ anterior view of the three-dimensional reconstructed CT images. The sagittal suture is fused and the head is dolichocephalic.

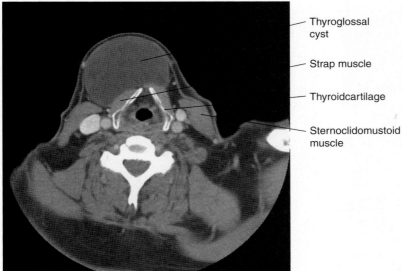

— Thyroglossal cyst

— Strap muscle

— Thyroidcartilage

— Sternoclidomustoid muscle

FIGURE 8.17   Thyroglossal cyst. CT of the infrahyoid neck shows a paramedian cystic mass anterior to the strap muscle.

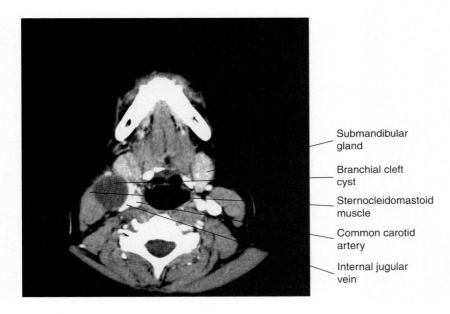

— Submandibular gland

— Branchial cleft cyst

— Sternocleidomastoid muscle

— Common carotid artery

— Internal jugular vein

FIGURE 8.18   Branchial cleft cyst. CT at the hyoid level shows a lateral neck cystic mass anteromedial to the sternocleidomastoid muscle, lateral to the carotid artery and internal jugular vein.

Lymphangioma

A

Sternocleidomastoid muscle

B

FIGURE 8.19 Lymphangioma. MRIs (**A,B,** coronal-/axial-T2-weighted images) show multicystic mass lesion in the base of the neck posteromedial to the sternocleidomastoid muscle extending into the axilla. Also note multiple fluid–fluid levels (*arrow*) caused by intracystic hemorrhage.

Lymphangiomas (aka cystic hygroma) are developmental vascular malformations most commonly seen as a multilocular cystic mass often associated with hemorrhagic fluid–fluid levels in the posterolateral neck centered around the posterior triangle (Fig. 8.19).

TUMORS

MRI is the modality of choice to evaluate the neoplastic lesions of the head and neck. The histologic diagnosis of head and neck neoplasms is usually made by fine-needle biopsy and imagings are primarily used to evaluate the extent of the disease, to delineate the relationship of the tumor to the adjacent anatomic structures, and to evaluate metastasis to the regional lymph nodes. All of this information is essential to determine the optimal mode of therapy. MRI is essential, particularly for the evaluation of skull base involvement by head and neck tumors (Fig. 8.20).

In adults, squamous cell carcinoma is the most common malignant head and neck mass. Among the pediatric age group, benign masses are more common than malignant ones. Benign masses include congenital cystic lesions, such as thyroglossal cysts and branchial cleft cysts. Benign neoplasms seen

Orbital extension

Tumor

Intracranial extension

Tumor

FIGURE 8.20 Rhabdomyosarcoma originating from the nasal cavity. Axial (**A**) and coronal (**B**) contrast-enhanced T1-weighted MRIs show an avidly enhancing tumor extending into the right orbit and into the cranium through the central skull base.

in this age group include teratoma and juvenile angiofibroma. Rhabdomyosarcoma is the most common pediatric head and neck malignancy.

KEY POINTS

- CT is the imaging modality of choice in the evaluation of sinusitis and facial bone fractures.

- Imaging features of sinusitis include (a) acute fluid collection of the sinus cavity, (b) mucosal thickening, and (c) erosion of the bony wall of the sinus.

- "Tripod" fractures involve the (a) lateral orbital wall, (b) maxillozygomatic suture, and (c) zygomatic arch.

- In Le Fort fractures, the facial bones are detached from the cranium by the fracture of the pterygoid plates.

- In orbital blowout fractures, the inferior rectus muscle may be trapped by the fracture fragments of the orbital floor, requiring surgical release.

- Magnetic resonance is the imaging modality of choice in evaluating head and neck tumors. A skull base extension of the tumor requires MRI.

- In adults, malignant mass lesions are common. In children, benign masses are more common.

Suggested Readings

Harnsberger HR, Wiggins RH III, Hudgins PA, et al. *Diagnostic imaging: head and neck*. Salt Lake City, UT: Amirsys, 2004.
Som PM, Curtain HD, eds. *Head and neck imaging*, 4th ed. St. Louis, MO: Mosby, 2003.

CHAPTER 9 ■ NUCLEAR IMAGING

DAVID L. BUSHNELL, JR.

Nuclear medicine is an important medical specialty that uses measurements of radioactive tracer behavior in the body to detect and assess various types of diseases. The physiologic images generated by nuclear imaging procedures reveal less anatomic detail than radiologic studies. It is, therefore, often necessary to correlate the nuclear images with the corresponding radiologic images. Although there are also several therapeutic applications for radioactive agents, the primary emphasis of this chapter will be on diagnostic nuclear imaging.

TECHNICAL ASPECTS OF NUCLEAR IMAGING

When molecules with radionuclide components are prepared for administration to human beings, they are called *radiopharmaceuticals*. The radionuclide portion of the radiopharmaceutical typically emits radiation in the form of gamma rays and/or x-rays that can be detected and used to create the scintigraphic images (often loosely referred to as scans). Radiopharmaceuticals participate in, but do not alter, various physiologic processes. Specific radiopharmaceuticals with particular physiochemical properties are used to study an organ or organ system. Although radiopharmaceuticals can be introduced into the body in several different ways, the most common mode of administration is intravenously through a peripheral vein.

Side effects from the administration of radiopharmaceuticals for diagnostic imaging are extremely rare. The probability of an adverse reaction from the radiation exposure received by a patient or technologist during a diagnostic nuclear medicine procedure is so small that it has not been measurable to date.

Gamma ray imaging systems are used to detect the radiation emitted from the patient and to create images that depict the regional distribution of the radiopharmaceutical within the body. The most common of these imaging systems is the gamma camera. Gamma cameras use a sodium iodide crystal to detect the gamma rays and x-rays. Photons striking the crystal produce light scintillations that are converted to a digital signal. This digital information is stored in a computer

and can be transferred to film or interpreted directly from the computer screen (Fig. 9.1). The resultant picture is often referred to as a scan or more appropriately a scintigraphic image. The image is essentially a physiologic map of the radiopharmaceutical distribution within the body. Table 9.1 presents the radiopharmaceuticals and the corresponding imaging procedures that are discussed in this chapter.

VENTILATION AND PERFUSION LUNG IMAGING FOR DIAGNOSIS OF PULMONARY EMBOLISM

Pulmonary thromboembolism (PTE) is a common disorder associated with significant mortality, which can be reduced with the appropriate detection and treatment. Establishing the diagnosis of PTE is often very difficult. Although dyspnea, tachypnea, and sinus tachycardia are present in the large majority of individuals with acute PTE, these symptoms and signs may result from any number of cardiopulmonary disorders. *The diagnosis of pulmonary embolism cannot be made with a high degree of reliability based on clinical findings alone.*

A chest radiograph should be obtained in all patients suspected of having pulmonary embolism. The chest x-ray is needed to rule out other causes of the patient's symptoms such as pneumonia, pneumothorax, heart failure, and so on. However, the radiograph may appear entirely normal even when PTE is present. Even if the chest radiograph is abnormal and consistent with PTE, the results are never adequately predictive to form the basis of a therapeutic decision. Consequently, more specific diagnostic procedures are necessary for the workup of individuals who fall into this category.

Perfusion lung imaging is an important tool in the workup of PTE in which it has a very high sensitivity for detecting this condition. Images of regional pulmonary perfusion are obtained by intravenously injecting several hundred thousand tiny particles of macroaggregated human albumin that are radiolabeled with technetium-99m (Tc-99m). These particles have diameters of 10 to 40 μm. Because the diameter of pulmonary capillaries and precapillary arterioles is less than 10 μm, the radioactive particles lodge in these vessels throughout the

FIGURE 9.1 The basic gamma camera imaging system. The gamma rays that exit the patient perpendicular to the surface of the camera are not absorbed by the collimator and reach the scintillation crystal where they are detected. The pattern of the gamma ray photons striking the crystal is used to create a digital image on the computer. NaI, sodium iodide.

lung fields in concentrations that are directly proportional to the regional pulmonary blood flow (Fig. 9.2). Because less than 0.1% of the total cross section of the pulmonary vasculature is occluded by the injected radiolabeled particles, complications are extremely rare.

Figure 9.3 shows an example of the normal pulmonary blood flow pattern. Patients with PTE often display diminished or absent blood flow to one or more lung segments (Fig. 9.4A). The emboli are often large enough to occlude the segmental pulmonary arteries, and hence the flow defects on the images will often appear segmental in configuration. However, thromboembolic occlusion of smaller arteries may occur, and the perfusion pattern may, therefore, reveal defects that are somewhat smaller.

Lung pathology other than thromboemboli may cause alterations in the regional pulmonary blood flow pattern as well. Disorders of the lung parenchyma such as pneumonia, chronic obstructive lung disease, and regional atelectasis may lead to abnormalities of lung perfusion due to reflex vasoconstriction in the region of the pathology. As a result, the presence of one or more focal blood flow abnormalities is not necessarily specific for a diagnosis of pulmonary thromboemboli. It is for this reason that scintigraphic ventilation imaging of the lungs is typically combined with the perfusion study in the evaluation of PTE. Determination of the ventilation status of a lung region that shows abnormal perfusion improves the specificity of the test for the diagnosis of PTE. Diseases of the lungs that lead to abnormal regional perfusion and

TABLE 9.1

RADIOPHARMACEUTICALS DISCUSSED IN THIS CHAPTER

Radiopharmaceutical	Imaging procedure
Tc-99m macroaggregated albumin	Lung perfusion
Xenon-133, Tc-99m diethylenetriamine pentaacetic acid (DTPA) aerosol	Lung ventilation
Rubidium-82 (Rb-82)	Myocardial perfusion
Tc-99m iminodiacetic acid	Hepatobiliary dynamics
Tc-99m diphosphonate	Skeletal
Tc-99m DTPA	Renal glomerular filtration rate
Thallium-201, Tc-99m sestamibi, Tc-99m tetrofosmin	Myocardial perfusion
F-18 fluorodeoxyglucose (FDG)	PET tumor imaging

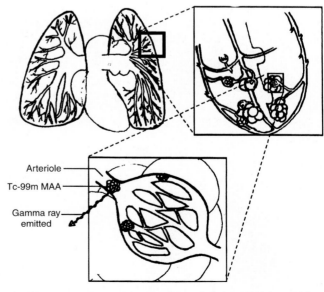

FIGURE 9.2 A Tc-99m macroaggregated albumin (MAA) particle as it becomes trapped in the pulmonary capillaries and emits gamma rays.

FIGURE 9.3 Normal perfusion lung images in six projections. Ant, anterior; Post, posterior; LPO, left posterior oblique; RPO, right posterior oblique; LL, left lateral; RL, right lateral. "H" designates area of absent activity due to the heart.

corresponding abnormal regional ventilation are summarized in Table 9.2.

Images of regional pulmonary ventilation are obtained by having the patient breath either radioactive xenon gas or an aerosolized form of Tc-99m diethylenetriamine pentaacetic

TABLE 9.2

PULMONARY DISEASES THAT CAUSE DECREASED REGIONAL LUNG PERFUSION WITH CORRESPONDING ABNORMAL VENTILATION

Pneumonia
Chronic obstructive lung disease
Atelectasis
Asthma

acid. A normal ventilation pattern with xenon is shown in Fig. 9.5.

Areas of the lung with diminished perfusion secondary to nonembolic lung pathology are associated with matching ventilation defects (Fig. 9.6). In contrast, ventilation usually appears normal in regions of the lung that show perfusion defects caused by thromboemboli (Figs. 9.4 and 9.7).

Typically, results from the ventilation/perfusion (V/P) study are used to estimate the probability that acute PTE has occurred. An entirely normal perfusion pattern indicates virtually no chance that the patient has emboli, and the clinician should then focus on a search for other causes of the patient's symptoms. Multiple vascular appearing perfusion defects with correspondingly normal ventilation indicate a very high probability that the patient has PTE.

A

B

FIGURE 9.4 **A:** Six-view perfusion scan showing numerous bilateral segmental flow defects. **B:** Single-breath ventilation images showing normal ventilation. This pattern is essentially diagnostic for PTE.

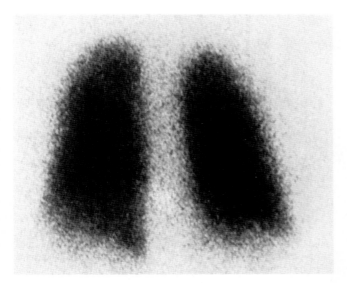

FIGURE 9.5 Normal xenon ventilation study. Posterior view of the initial breath hold image.

A computed tomography (CT) chest scan with contrast angiography is now considered the examination of choice (Fig. 2.49) to establish the diagnosis of pulmonary embolism. CT angiography has a sensitivity of 95% for the diagnosis of pulmonary embolism. It is considered by most as the gold standard although perfusion/ventilation scans continue to be performed under special circumstances such as when patients are allergic to intravenous contrast.

HEPATOBILIARY IMAGING

Patients with acute cholecystitis classically present with right upper quadrant pain/tenderness, fever, and leukocytosis. However, the signs and symptoms of acute cholecystitis often vary, and there are a number of pathologic conditions that occasionally present in a similar fashion. Consequently, the provisional diagnosis of acute cholecystitis typically requires confirmatory testing with ultrasound and/or hepatobiliary scintigraphy.

Hepatobiliary scintigraphic imaging is performed using a Tc-99m-labeled iminodiacetic acid derivative that is an analog of bilirubin. This radiopharmaceutical is actively transported into hepatocytes by the same system that transports bilirubin and is excreted unchanged into the biliary tract.

FIGURE 9.6 Patient with chronic obstructive pulmonary disease showing matching ventilation and perfusion defects in upper lobes (*arrows*). **A:** Posterior perfusion image. **B:** Posterior initial breath hold ventilation image. **C:** Later equilibrium ventilation image showing eventual filling in of defects seen on the initial ventilation image.

FIGURE 9.7 Top two images are posterior ventilation images with xenon-133 showing uniform ventilation to both lungs. Bottom four images are from the perfusion study showing multiple segmental defects. *Arrow* points to region of absent perfusion in what is probably all three segments of the right upper lobe. Note that the lung regions with flow defects have normal ventilation. This pattern indicates a very high probability for PTE.

In normal individuals, the hepatobiliary radiotracer will flow into the gallbladder within the first hour after intravenous administration (Fig. 9.8). However, in acute cholecystitis the gallbladder fails to fill with the radiotracer because of cystic duct obstruction by a stone. This test is extremely sensitive, and a normal result (i.e., visualization of the gallbladder) virtually excludes the possibility of acute cholecystitis. It is important to note that there are certain conditions that predispose to false-positive results. The most common false-positive result occurs in prolonged fasting of more than 2 or 3 days. Under this condition, the gallbladder rarely contracts and its contents begin to partially solidify into a gelatinous material that can impede or block the entry of the radioactive bile into the gallbladder. The gallbladder also fails to visualize in many patients who have ingested food within 2 hours of the hepatobiliary study as a result of the high level of circulating cholecystokinin causing gallbladder contraction, which limits entry of the radioactive bile. For this reason, scintigraphic hepatobiliary imaging should not be performed within 2 hours of a meal. Conditions that lead to false-positive (gallbladder nonvisualization) results are summarized in Table 9.3.

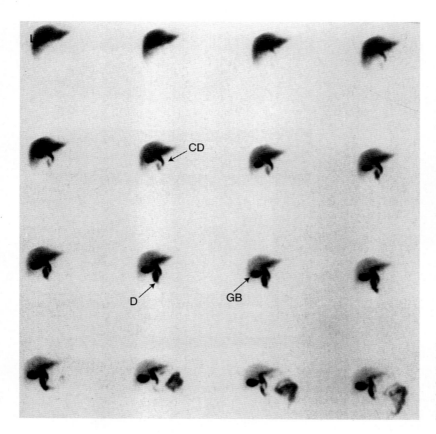

FIGURE 9.8 Normal hepatobiliary study. Images obtained in the anterior view every 2 minutes (moving from left to right and top to bottom) following injection of the hepatobiliary radiotracer show good extraction of the agent by the liver (L). The common bile duct (*arrow* CD) is seen along with the duodenum (*arrow* D) and gallbladder (*arrow GB*).

The use of morphine with hepatobiliary imaging has been found to be helpful in reducing the number of false-positive results, thereby improving the specificity of the test. Morphine causes constriction of the sphincter of Odi and leads to a rise in biliary system pressure. This augments bile movement through the cystic duct, improving gallbladder visualization. For this reason, the use of morphine has become standard practice with this procedure. Figure 9.9 shows a case in which a normal gallbladder became visible only after administration of morphine. Figure 9.10 shows a patient with acute cholecystitis and gallbladder nonvisualization both before and after administration of morphine.

SKELETAL IMAGING

Skeletal scintigraphic imaging, more commonly referred to as the bone scan, is a valuable tool for investigation of a number

TABLE 9.3

CONDITIONS THAT MAY YIELD FALSE-POSITIVE RESULTS WITH HEPATOBILIARY IMAGING IN THE EVALUATION OF ACUTE CHOLECYSTITIS

Prolonged fasting (3 days)
Ingestion of food within 2 hours of the study
Chronic cholecystitis
Chronic alcohol abuse
Pancreatitis

of disorders of the skeletal system. A Tc-99m-labeled diphosphonate derivative is used to perform skeletal scintigraphy because this radiolabeled agent is adsorbed onto the surface of newly forming hydroxyapatite crystal in the bone. New bone formation occurs in response to the presence of almost all skeletal pathology. Consequently, scintigraphic images will demonstrate increased gamma ray emissions localized to the site of bone abnormality.

It is important for clinicians to know whether skeletal metastases are present in patients with malignant tumors. Examination of patients for possible metastases is carried out predominantly in those individuals who have tumors that tend to metastasize to the bone, such as breast, lung, prostate, and renal carcinomas. Well-differentiated thyroid cancer is also prone to disseminate to sites in bone, but these lesions are probably better detected with iodine-131 imaging.

The normal bone scan appearance is shown in Fig. 9.11. The bone scan in a patient with skeletal metastases typically reveals numerous foci of excessive tracer accumulation, most commonly in the axial skeleton but also to a lesser extent in the appendicular skeleton (Fig. 9.12). Skeletal metastases usually arise as a result of hematogenous seeding of tumor cells in the bone marrow. Because most of the adult marrow resides in the axial skeleton, it makes sense that *the large majority of metastatic lesions are detected in the axial skeleton.*

The bone scan is very sensitive for detecting metastatic lesions and in general will identify a metastasis before a conventional radiograph or even CT can detect it. However, it is often not possible to ascertain whether lesions seen on a bone scan are malignant or benign, and this is particularly true for a single lesion, which often is caused by a benign

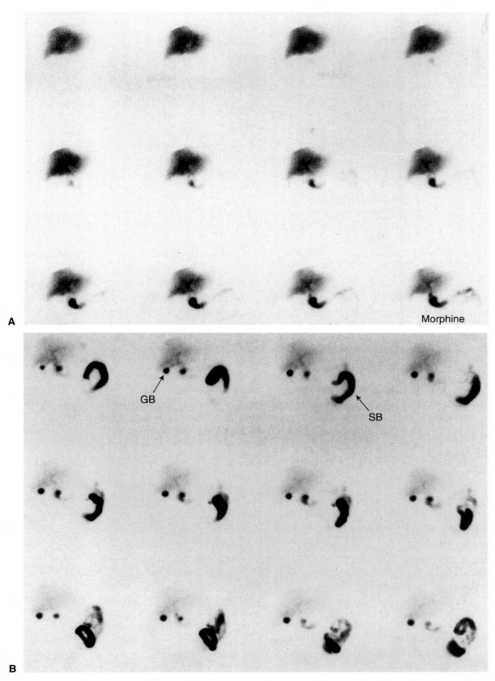

FIGURE 9.9 Hepatobiliary examination in a patient with right upper quadrant pain. **A:** Initial set of images show normal uptake and excretion by the liver, but over time the gallbladder is not visualized and consequently morphine is given at approximately 40 minutes into the study. **B:** Images obtained immediately following administration of morphine show the gallbladder visualization (*arrow* GB), which effectively rules out acute cholecystitis. Note activity in the small bowel (*arrow* SB).

process. *Numerous focal lesions are much more often due to metastatic disease.*

Other skeletal abnormalities are also readily detected with a bone scan. Like metastases, osteomyelitis can be detected earlier with a bone scan than with a radiograph (Fig. 9.13). The bone scan is particularly useful in childhood osteomyelitis in which early treatment is very important. The bone scan

may also be useful to detect a nondisplaced fracture or traumatic lesion of a type not easily seen on radiographs. For example, lesions that originate from intense physical activity, such as stress fractures (Fig. 9.14) and shin splints (Fig. 9.15), are readily detected on a bone scan and may not be seen on a radiograph. In most cases, fractures through the full thickness of the bone cortex are readily detected by a plain radiograph.

FIGURE 9.10   Hepatobiliary study in a patient with fever and right upper quadrant pain. **A:** Initial set of images show normal uptake and excretion by the liver, but the gallbladder is not visualized and consequently morphine is given at approximately the time of the image at bottom right. **B:** Images obtained immediately following injection of morphine continue to show absence of gallbladder activity, indicating cystic duct obstruction and very probably acute cholecystitis. Note the reflux of radioactive bile into the stomach (*arrow S*). The patient was taken to surgery and found to have acute cholecystitis.

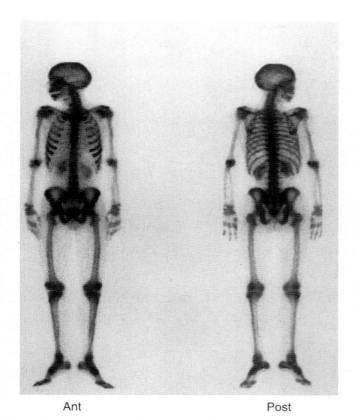

Ant   Post

FIGURE 9.11   Anterior and posterior whole-body images of a normal bone scan.

Ant   Post

FIGURE 9.12   Whole-body bone scan in anterior and posterior projections of a 65-year-old man with diffuse skeletal metastases from prostate carcinoma. Images reveal numerous metastatic lesions (black foci), primarily in the axial skeleton on both anterior and posterior views. However, lesions are also seen in the proximal femurs and humeri (*arrows*).

Some full-thickness fractures, such as those in the sacrum, scapula, femoral neck, and small bones of the wrist and ankle, are occasionally difficult to visualize on a radiograph but are detectable by a bone scan.

ANGIOTENSIN-CONVERTING ENZYME INHIBITOR RENAL SCINTIGRAPHIC IMAGING

Scintigraphic imaging procedures can be used to evaluate renal perfusion and various aspects of renal function. Technetium-99m-labeled molecules that are filtered by the renal glomerulus can be used to assess glomerular filtration rate (GFR). Scintigraphic imaging of GFR combined with administration of an angiotensin-converting enzyme (ACE) inhibitor, such as captopril, is used to identify patients with hypertension caused by renal artery stenosis.

In patients with renal vascular hypertension, renin secretion is enhanced secondary to the hemodynamic effects of a functionally significant stenosis in the renal artery (Fig. 9.16). Decreased perfusion pressure as a result of the stenosis causes the juxtaglomerular cells to increase secretion of renin. Renin acts on angiotensinogen to form angiotensin I. Angiotensin I is converted to angiotensin II by ACE. Angiotensin II stimulates release of aldosterone and also acts as a potent vasoconstrictor of the peripheral vasculature, including vasoconstriction of the efferent renal arterioles distal to the glomerulus in the under-

perfused kidney with the stenosis. The efferent vasoconstriction acts to preserve the transglomerular pressure gradient and, therefore, helps preserve the GFR in the affected kidney. If an ACE inhibitor such as captopril is administered in this setting, angiotensin II levels will drop and the efferent arterioles will dilate, leading to a fall in GFR in the stenotic kidney.

In patients with renal vascular hypertension, scintigraphic images of the kidneys obtained during ACE inhibition demonstrate this deterioration in GFR in the stenotic kidney (Fig. 9.17). In contrast, patients with essential hypertension will have no effect from captopril on the renal scintigraphic images.

Patients with a strongly positive scintigraphic ACE inhibitor study are very likely to experience improvement or cure in their hypertension if the stenosis is repaired. Conversely, patients with a completely normal result are very unlikely to respond to repair of the renal artery stenosis.

MYOCARDIAL PERFUSION IMAGING

Perfusion imaging of the myocardium can be performed using intravenous injected thallium-201 chloride or Tc-99m-labeled agents known as sestamibi or tetrofosmin. These substances

FIGURE 9.13 Skeletal scintigraphic images (whole body, **A**; regional view, **B**) from an 18-year-old girl with diabetes who presented with 3 to 4 weeks of low back pain. Radiographs of the vertebra were unremarkable. The images show abnormally increased technetium-99m methylenediphosphanate (MDP) activity in the L3 vertebral body (*arrow*). Biopsy of the site confirmed osteomyelitis. Notice the normal intense uptake of Tc-99m MDP at the growth plates in the lower extremities (*arrowhead*) on the whole-body images.

accumulate in the myocardium in direct proportion to the regional myocardial blood flow and the number of viable myocytes. Single photon emission computed tomography (SPECT) imaging is used to obtain perfusion images of the heart in three dimensions using one of these agents (Fig. 9.18). SPECT is a technique that yields a three-dimensional pattern of radiopharmaceutical distribution in the body with images displayed in cross section much like CT or MRI. A normal cardiac SPECT thallium-201 study shows uniform perfusion throughout the myocardium (Fig. 9.19).

Myocardial perfusion stress imaging can be performed with either exercise or a pharmacologic agent such as adenosine or dipyridamole. Use of cardiac stress improves the sensitivity of myocardial perfusion imaging for detecting coronary artery disease (CAD). Arterioles distal to a normal coronary artery will dilate substantially in response to either exercise or pharmacologic stimulation. As a result, perfusion (and, therefore, radiotracer concentration) will increase considerably in the myocardium distal to a normal vessel, whereas myocardial perfusion will change little if at all distal to a significant stenosis (Fig. 9.20). Therefore, significant CAD will result in a perfusion defect on the cardiac images immediately following the stress (Fig. 9.21).

Perfusion defects seen on the stress images that become less severe or normalize on delayed images are referred to as reversible and almost always contain viable myocardium

(Fig. 9.21). Defects that do not change from stress to the delayed images (termed "fixed") usually contain scar tissue. However, in some instances fixed defects might still contain viable tissue. This information is very important for making decisions about possible coronary bypass surgery. Figure 9.22 shows an example of a fixed thallium defect representing scar tissue from previous infarction.

Myocardial stress imaging can be used to select appropriate candidates with suspected CAD for coronary arteriography or coronary CT angiography. In addition, this technique can provide information on the hemodynamic severity of coronary lesions already seen on the CT or standard angiogram and thus assist in selecting patients for coronary revascularization procedures.

AS discussed below under positron emission tomography (PET), myocardial stress perfusion imaging is now being conducted routinely with PET and rubidium-82 (Rb-82).

POSITRON EMISSION TOMOGRAPHY AND PET/CT

PET differs somewhat from the more conventional nuclear medicine procedures because the radioisotopes that are used emit positrons and the PET imaging machine is consequently

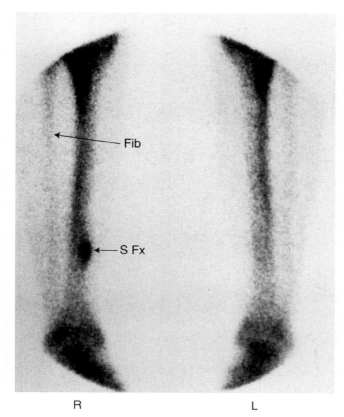

FIGURE 9.14 A 20-year-old woman with pain in the right distal lower extremity. Patient was an athlete in training with an extensive running regimen. Radiographs shortly after the onset of pain were normal. Scintigraphic images of the distal lower extremities show focal lesion in the posterior medial aspect of the right distal tibia consistent with a stress fracture (*arrow*). Notice that the lesion does not involve the full thickness of the tibia. Fibula indicated by *long arrow*.

FIGURE 9.15 Bone scan in a patient with shin splints showing linear pattern of increased radiopharmaceutical concentration (*arrows*) along the posterior aspect of the tibia.

FIGURE 9.16 **A:** Without ACE inhibitor. Effect of angiotensin-converting enzyme (ACE) inhibitor, such as captopril (**B**), on glomerular filtration rate (GFR) in the setting of renal artery stenosis and renal vascular hypertension.

FIGURE 9.17 **A:** Scintigraphic images of the kidneys in the posterior projection, 1 to 3 minutes and 3 to 5 minutes following intravenous injection of a Tc-99m-labeled agent that is filtered by the glomerulus. **B:** Repeat images following administration of captopril show a significant decrease in the concentration of this agent (and, therefore, decrease in GFR) in the left kidney compared to the precaptopril study. This finding indicates renal artery stenosis causing renal vascular hypertension.

designed differently. After a positron is emitted, it travels a very short distance in body tissue (a few mm), combines with an electron, and the mass of the positron and electron are converted into energy in the form of two gamma rays that travel in opposite directions along a line. These gamma rays are detected by the PET machine, which then creates a three-dimensional image set of the distribution of the radioisotope in the body.

Positron-emitting radioisotopes include C-11, N-13, O-15, and F-18. These radioisotopes can in theory be labeled to virtually any organic molecule. Currently, the primary PET radiopharmaceutical used in clinical practice is F-18-labeled fluorodeoxyglucose (FDG). PET imaging with FDG depicts the distribution of glucose metabolism in the body.

The large majority of malignant tumors demonstrate enhanced metabolism of glucose relative to normal organs, and consequently PET imaging with FDG can be used to detect sites of malignancy throughout the body. A PET image of a patient with primary non–small cell lung cancer (NSCLC) is shown in Fig. 9.23, and images of a patient with lymphoma are presented in Fig. 9.24. In both examples, the malignancies demonstrate intense image signal as a result of high FDG tumor concentration.

Although the absolute level of tumor glucose metabolism can be quantified on PET, in practice this is time consuming and requires arterial blood sampling of FDG levels. Consequently, an alternative, semi-quantitative measurement, is used and referred to as the standardized uptake value, which

FIGURE 9.18 Single photon emission computed tomography (SPECT) short-axis cross section from the left ventricle. The short-axis cross-sectional view is obtained by slicing the three-dimensional image of the heart muscle in planes perpendicular to the long dimension of the heart.

FIGURE 9.20 Diagram showing the effects on the caliber of coronary arterioles from a pressure gradient. Blood flow through the stenosed artery, F1, is essentially the same as flow through the normal artery, F2, at rest due to arteriolar vasodilatation. However, in the presence of a stress (exercise or pharmacologic), F2 increases to a greater extent than does F1, creating a discrepancy in regional myocardial perfusion.

FIGURE 9.19 Stress (dipyridamole) and delayed SPECT thallium images showing normal distribution of thallium-201 in the left ventricular myocardium. A: All short-axis images from the apex of the heart to the base of the heart. B: Selected short-axis images from the midregion of the heart.

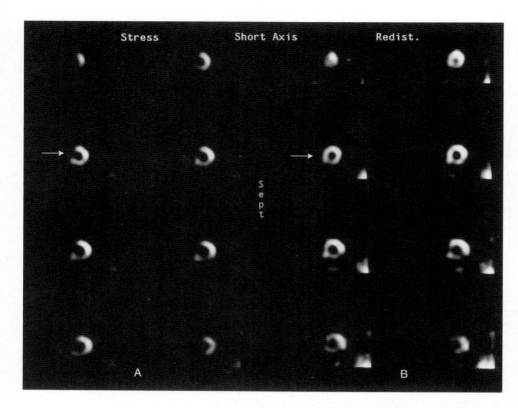

FIGURE 9.21 Thallium SPECT images from a patient with tight stenosis of the left anterior descending coronary artery; short-axis stress images (**A**) showing a severe perfusion defect in the septum, which is reversible on rest/redistribution images (**B**).

is directly related to glucose metabolism and much simpler to determine from PET images. In general, lesions associated with standardized uptake value levels above 2.5 are likely to be malignant, whereas uptake levels below 2.5 are more likely to be physiologic in origin or caused by benign lesions.

To improve the ability to localize lesions detected on PET images, current state-of-the-art machines combine both PET and CT into one unit. *Fused images from both the CT and the PET data sets improve both the sensitivity and the specificity for malignant tumor detection.* Figure 9.25 A and B shows an example of a patient with NSCLC being staged for possible surgery where it is easy to appreciate the value of the fused

PET/CT images for localizing a subtle focal abnormality of FDG uptake to an adrenal gland. The presence of the adrenal metastasis indicates stage 4 disease.

There are many clinical applications now for FDG-PET/CT imaging in oncology including initial staging, detection of recurrent tumor, and evaluation of response to chemotherapy. *Tumor types commonly referred for PET/CT evaluation in clinical practice include NSCLC, head and neck cancers, lymphomas, colon cancer, breast cancer, and melanoma.* Figure 9.26 shows an example of a patient who presented with a neck mass that was biopsied and found to be a squamous cell cancer that had metastasized to a neck

FIGURE 9.22 Thallium SPECT images from a patient with past infarction of the anterior wall of the heart. Short-axis images show severe defects in the anterior wall (*arrows*) and lateral wall, both of which are fixed (unchanged from stress to rest/redistribution images). These findings are consistent with scarring in the anterior and lateral walls.

FIGURE 9.23   Tomographic coronal plane FDG-PET images of a patient with primary lung cancer. The tumor has metastasized to numerous locations (white/bright foci). The primary lung tumor is noted by the *black arrow* in the right lung. Metastatic lesions are located in the proximal left humerus, posterior right third rib, left adrenal, mediastinum, and left lung base. Note the intense FDG metabolism in the brain (marked with a "B").

lymph node. PET/CT was used in this case to identify the primary head/neck tumor site.

As the number of PET/CT machines in medical facilities has increased, myocardial perfusion PET imaging is being used more and more for the examination of patients with known or suspected CAD in place of SPECT. The radioisotope Rb-82 acts physiologically just like thallium in the heart yet unlike thallium or technetium it emits a positron. Image resolution is enhanced with Rb-82 PET compared to SPECT. Figure 9. 27A and B depicts a patient with CAD imaged with Rb-82 PET/CT.

RADIONUCLIDE THERAPY

Although a detailed discussion of the therapeutic applications of internally administered radionuclides is beyond the scope of this chapter, it is important to recognize this aspect of nuclear medicine. Generally, the radioactive isotopes being used now

for therapy emit beta particles, and in the future alpha particle emitters may also be used. Currently, the most common radioisotope used in therapy is I-131. In its elemental form this agent is used to treat thyroid disorders such as Graves disease and thyroid cancer. Because the iodine is trapped by the abnormal thyroid cells, the radiation effect is concentrated at the desired site. A relatively new way of delivering a radioisotope to a selected target in the body is through the use of radiolabeled monoclonal antibodies (MoAb). The MoAb carrying the radioisotope will bind to a particular tumor cell surface antigen and thus deliver the radioactive beta emissions directly to the tumor site. Two radiolabeled MoAbs are now available for clinical use in treating patients with non-Hodgkin's lymphoma. One is labeled with I-131 and the other is labeled with Y-90. Treatment with these agents, after standard chemotherapy has failed, leads to disease remission in 60% to 70% of patients with follicular or diffuse large cell non-Hodgkin's lymphoma. Table 9.4 lists some of the therapeutic uses of internally administered radioisotopes.

FIGURE 9.24 Tomographic coronal FDG-PET images of a patient with non-Hodgkin's lymphoma prior to therapy. Widespread disease is seen in the chest and abdomen and other lymph node sites. *Horizontal arrow* indicates very large mass of tumor in retroperitoneal lymph nodes. Note the high FDG metabolism in the heart (marked with an "H"). Liver (L) and left kidney (K) are also marked.

FIGURE 9.25 **A, B:** FDG-PET/CT images of a patient with non–small cell lung cancer (NSCLC) referred for staging. **A:** A subtle focus of increased FDG uptake on the axial PET image (top left) and coronal PET image (bottom right) localized by the image cross-hairs to a slightly enlarged right adrenal gland seen on axial CT (top right) and fused axial PET/CT image (bottom left). The axial fused PET/CT image in this figure depicts the CT in black and white overlying the FDG signal from PET typically shown in an orange/yellow color scale but seen here as white. **B:** Further image evaluation of this patient reveals intense FDG signal in lumbar vertebra (LM), seen on the coronal whole-body image (bottom right), indicating widespread skeletal metastases. Closer inspection of the axial PET images (top left) reveals an intense abnormal focal uptake of FDG in the left lobe of the prostate gland (black focus identified by grey arrow) indicating a previously unknown prostate cancer, which in this case was responsible for the skeletal metastases. The fused axial PET plus CT image (bottom left) depicts the FDG signal of the tumor in white localized to the left lobe of the prostate gland as seen on the overlay black/white CT image. Also notice the multiple small FDG positive foci in the chest on the coronal PET images (bottom right) in both A and B indicating mediastinal and right hilar lymph node metastases from the patient's lung cancer. The primary prostate tumor is depicted by the red arrow on the whole-body coronal PET image. The primary lung tumor is not seen on these images (Br, brain; B, bladder; L, liver on coronal PET image).

FIGURE 9.26 FDG-PET/CT images in a patient who presented with a left neck mass which was biopsied and found to be metastatic squamous cell carcinoma to a neck lymph node ("N" on coronal CT, coronal PET, and coronal fused PET plus CT, all in the first column). Coronal, sagittal, and axial images are in the first, second, and third columns, respectively, as labeled. The first row is the CT from the PET/CT examination. The second row is PET only, and the third row represents fused images of PET plus CT with the PET signal depicted typically in color (but in white on these images). The primary tumor (light grey arrows in the second row PET images) was detected by PET and localized to the left lingular tonsil based on the findings from the fused axial PET plus CT image in which the primary tumor is seen as the white FDG focus (PT) overlying the left tonsil on the fused PET/CT image (bottom right image).

TABLE 9.4

SOME RADIOISOTOPES USED IN THERAPEUTIC APPLICATIONS

Radioisotope	Disease
Iodine-131, yttrium-90-labeled monoclonal antibodies	Lymphoma
Samarium-153, strontium-89	Skeletal metastases
Phosphorus-32	Polycythemia vera
Iodine-131	Thyroid cancer, Graves disease

FIGURE 9.27 A, B: Rb-82 cardiac PET images from a patient with suspected CAD ultimately found to have a high-grade stenosis of the circumflex artery which supplies the lateral wall of the left ventricle. The short axis (**A**) tomographic stress images reveal decreased perfusion (white arrows on one of the slices) to the lateral wall of the left ventricle (LV) in the top row, which then appears "reversible" (the signal improves) on rest images in the bottom row (light grey arrows). The horizontal long-axis images (**B**) from same patient demonstrate the same defect in perfusion by revealing much diminished rubidium signal coming from the lateral wall (white arrows on one of the images) in the stress images which again shows significant improvement on the rest images (reversibility) as depicted by light grey arrows. S, septum; StrAC, stress attenuation corrected; RstAC, rest attenuation corrected.

KEY POINTS

- Nuclear imaging is performed using radiolabeled molecules injected into the body to create images of organ physiology.
- CT is considered the gold standard for detecting pulmonary embolism.
- Ventilation–perfusion lung imaging may play a role in the workup of special patients with suspected PTE.
- Visualization of the gallbladder with hepatobiliary scintigraphy almost always rules out the diagnosis of acute cholecystis.
- Bone pathology (e.g., metastases) causes increased bone hydroxyapatite formation, leading to increased uptake of the bone scan radiopharmaceutical.
- Bone scintigraphy is a sensitive test for detecting skeletal metastases, osteomyelitis, and fractures.
- Captopril renal imaging accurately detects hemodynamically significant renal artery stenosis in patients with renovascular hypertension.
- Myocardial stress perfusion imaging is an accurate technique for detecting CAD and can be performed with either SPECT or PET.

- PET imaging with FDG can detect many types of malignant tumors.
- PET/CT fused imaging improves the accuracy for detecting malignancy with FDG.

Acknowledgments

The author thanks Brian Clarke, CNMT, for his original drawings of Figs. 9.1, 9.2, 9.18, 9.21, and 9.23; Dr. Parvez Shirazi for supplying the images for Fig. 9.17; and Ms. Maryann O'Brien, MA, CNMT, for her assistance in preparing this manuscript.

Suggested Readings

Henkin RE, Boles MA, Dillehay GL, Halama JR, Karesh SM, Wagner RH, Zimmer AM, eds. *Nuclear medicine*. St. Louis, MO: Mosby, 1996.

Wagner HN, Szabo Z, Buchanan JW, eds. *Principles of nuclear medicine*. Philadelphia: WB Saunders, 1995.

CHAPTER 10 ■ BREAST IMAGING

JEONG MI PARK, WILLIAM E. ERKONEN, AND LAURIE L. FAJARDO

This chapter is short, but its importance is unrelated to its length. There are a number of good textbooks on this subject that are more encyclopedic, and you can and should refer to these (1–3). The purpose of this chapter is to stress the importance of mammography, ultrasound (US), and magnetic resonance imaging (MRI) in the management of breast disease and the screening for early cancer detection.

Approximately one in eight females in the United States will develop cancer of the breast during her lifetime, and this incidence appears to be increasing. Breast cancer currently involves over 180,000 women per year in the United States, and it causes approximately 40,000 deaths per year. An effective strategy to decrease the mortality associated with this disease is to find the lesions at an early and curable stage. Mammography can detect early invasive lesions or carcinomas *in situ* that measure only a few millimeters before they become symptomatic and/or palpable. It is generally believed that the earlier breast cancer is diagnosed, the smaller the chance of metastases. Consequently, mammography is widely used as a routine screening tool to detect occult breast cancer in the general asymptomatic female population. *However, screening mammography must always be used in conjunction with monthly breast self-examination and an annual breast examination performed by a physician.* A National Cancer Institute review showed that this approach significantly reduces breast cancer deaths for women of all ages.

Mammography is also a key tool in the evaluation of known or suspected breast disease in both males and females. A variety of special diagnostic mammographic studies such as spot compression or magnification mammography are used to supplement a routine screening examination when symptomatic patients are examined.

There is little doubt that mammograms must be interpreted by qualified radiologists, and the radiologist's role in breast disease continues to increase. Radiologists are more frequently being called on to perform breast procedures such as percutaneous breast biopsies. Given the prevalence of breast problems, all physicians should be aware of the basics of breast imaging, including the limitations of mammography.

GUIDELINES FOR MAMMOGRAPHY

Diagnostic mammography should be performed whenever the patient has any symptom, the physician finds a problem, or a radiologist finds some abnormality on a screening mammogram. Screening mammography can be performed for normal, nonsymptomatic patients under recommended guidelines. Some generally accepted guidelines for screening mammography are listed in Table 10.1. These guidelines provide you with something on which you can hang your hat, but there isn't unanimous agreement about them. As indicated in the guidelines in Table 10.1, risk factors are important and influence the timing for mammography. Some of the common risk factors are listed in Table 10.2. Depending on the risk factors, the time tables may be advanced to younger ages.

MAMMOGRAPHY TECHNIQUE

The importance of a well-performed mammogram cannot be overemphasized. A standard screening mammogram consists of a *mediolateral oblique* (MLO) view with the central x-ray beam traversing the breast obliquely in a medial to lateral direction (Fig. 10.1A) and a *craniocaudal* (CC) view (Fig. 10.1B) with the central x-ray beam traversing the breast in a head-to-foot direction. It is necessary to compress the breast during the examination to optimally image all the breast tissue, and this may cause mild to moderate discomfort.

A diagnostic mammogram uses many different views according to the patient's specific problem. The most frequently used diagnostic views are magnification compression views for microcalcifications and spot compression views for mass or focal asymmetry. The technical aspects of mammography are very complicated, and it is extremely important that the mammographer be properly trained and qualified. Mammography quality controls are mandatory and regulated by the federal government under the Mammography Quality Standards Act of 1993.

Normal MLO and CC views of the breast are shown in Fig. 10.2. Notice that breast images are a combination of fat

TABLE 10.1

GENERAL SCREENING MAMMOGRAPHY GUIDELINES[a]

1. Yearly mammograms are recommended starting at age 40; baseline before age 35 if mother or sister had premenopausal breast cancer. The age at which screening should be stopped should be individualized by considering the potential risks and benefits of screening in the context of overall health status and longevity.
2. Clinical breast examination should be part of a periodic health examination about every 3 years for women in their 20s and 30s and every year for women 40 and older.
3. Women should know how their breasts normally feel and report any breast change promptly to their health care providers. Breast self-examination is an option for women starting in their 20s.

[a]Screening MRI is recommended for women with breast cancer (BRCA) gene mutation, women with an approximately 20%–25% or greater lifetime risk of breast cancer.

TABLE 10.2

RISK FACTORS THAT CAN INFLUENCE THE TIMING FOR SCREENING MAMMOGRAPHY

1. Prior personal history of breast cancer
2. Family history of premenopausal breast cancer in mother, sister, or daughter
3. Presence of mutated BRCA-1 and/or BRCA-2 genes
4. Biopsy-confirmed atypical hyperplasia
5. Age (incidence increases with age)
6. Years of menstruation: early age menarche (<12 y), late age menopause (>55 y)
7. Nulliparous, late age first birth (>30 y)
8. Never breast-fed a child
9. Postmenopausal obesity
10. High-dose radiation to chest
11. Long-term use of hormone replacement therapy
12. Others

(black) and soft tissues (gray to white). This background of black and gray, especially the black, enhances visualization of the white calcifications and masses. Breast tissue is composed predominately of fibroglandular tissue in young women and gradually replaced with adipose tissue in older women.

WHAT WE SHOULD SEE ON A MAMMOGRAM

Normal mammograms show a mixture of fat and fibroglandular tissue. Other normal structures such as blood vessels and lactiferous ducts are also seen. Lymph nodes are mainly seen in the axillary areas; however, they can also be seen within the breast parenchyma (intramammary lymph nodes).

The two main mammographic findings suggesting abnormalities are masses and microcalcifications. Other abnormalities include focal asymmetry, architectural distortion, and skin or nipple deformity. Any structural changes over time require attention and further workup, unless otherwise explained such as surgical scar.

The Breast Imaging Reporting and Data System (BIRADS) is a guideline developed by the American College of Radiology for radiologists to describe the mammographic findings, provide conclusions, and make appropriate recommendations for further workup in a well-structured manner. Initially, BIRADS was developed for mammography only; however, it now includes US and MRI according to a recently published version (4). The BIRADS guidelines are continuously revised and updated on the basis of experts' opinions and evidence-based findings.

FIGURE 10.1   A: Illustration of how the patient is positioned for a mediolateral oblique (MLO) mammogram. The x-ray beam passes obliquely through the breast in a medial to lateral direction. The breast is routinely compressed between the compression device (*straight arrows*) and the radiographic cassette (*curved arrow*). The cassette contains a radiographic film on which the image will be recorded. Compression improves the diagnostic quality of the images by thinning the breast to a more homogeneous thickness. **B:** Illustration of how the patient is positioned for a craniocaudal (CC) mammogram. The x-ray beam passes through the breast in a head-to-foot or cephalad to caudad direction. The compression device (*straight arrow*) is more easily visualized in this illustration. Again, the image will be recorded on the film in the radiographic cassette (*curved arrow*).

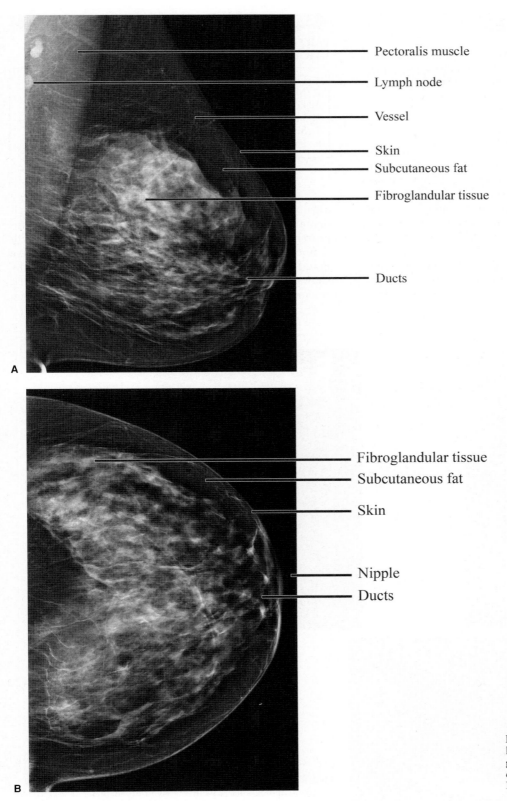

Pectoralis muscle

Lymph node

Vessel

Skin

Subcutaneous fat

Fibroglandular tissue

Ducts

Fibroglandular tissue

Subcutaneous fat

Skin

Nipple

Ducts

FIGURE 10.2 A: Left breast mediolateral oblique (MLO) digital mammogram. Normal. **B:** Left breast craniocaudal (CC) digital mammogram. Normal.

MASSES

Using BIRADS terminology, a mass seen on a mammogram is described in terms of its shape, border (margin), density, location, size, and associated findings. Associated findings may include microcalcifications and architectural distortion.

Benign

Benign disease (Table 10.3) may or may not be symptomatic or have associated masses. A fibroadenoma (Fig. 10.3) is a benign lesion that must be differentiated from a malignant mass. It generally occurs in young women and may be multiple or single. On physical examination, fibroadenomas are often movable. The mammographic appearance is an oval circumscribed mass sometimes associated with coarse "popcorn" calcifications. On sonography, these fibroadenomas will usually appear isoechoic.

Another common clinical problem is benign cystic disease. This problem occurs at all ages. Cysts may present as

TABLE 10.3

PARTIAL LIST OF BENIGN BREAST DISEASE ETIOLOGIES

1. Cystic disease
2. Mastitis, abscess
3. Fibroadenoma, benign phyllodes tumor
4. Lipoma, hamartoma
5. Sclerosing adenosis, fibrocystic changes
6. Fat necrosis

a palpable mass that may or may not be tender or an incidental mammographic finding. The mammographic appearance of a cyst is usually a mass of isodensity with well-defined sharp borders (Fig. 10.4A). Rarely, cysts have mural calcifications. Ultrasonography (Fig. 10.4B) usually shows a well-defined anechoic mass with posterior acoustic enhancement. Cysts may require aspiration depending on

FIGURE 10.3 Right breast mediolateral oblique (**A**) and craniocaudal (**B**) mammograms. Calcified benign fibroadenoma. The fibroadenoma mass is only faintly visible (*single straight arrows*). The benign calcifications within the fibroadenoma are typically globular, coarse, and variable in size (*curved arrows*). Note the single benign globular calcification incidentally found without a mass associated (*double straight arrows*). **C:** Another patient's fibroadenoma. Ultrasound image. A 30-year-old woman. Ultrasound of the right breast shows a well-circumscribed homogeneous isoechoic solid mass which is corresponding to a palpable mass (*arrows*).

FIGURE 10.4   A: Right breast mediolateral oblique digital mammogram. A simple cyst. The isodense cyst (*arrows*) has sharp borders and no calcifications. Note the difference between the smooth sharp borders of this benign cyst compared to the irregular and poorly defined borders of the carcinoma in Fig. 10.7. **B:** Right breast ultrasound of the lesion in **A.** This is the classic appearance of a benign simple cyst. The cyst is a round well-circumscribed anechoic mass with very thin cyst-parenchymal transition. Posterior acoustic enhancement (*arrows*) is commonly found immediately posterior to a cyst.

the clinical situation, and aspiration under US guidance is quite effective.

Although a cyst is usually rounder and much better circumscribed than a solid mass on a mammogram, mammography is frequently not diagnostic enough to differentiate a solid mass from a cystic mass. However, mammography can show diagnostic findings in some lesions such as hamartoma (Fig. 10.5).

Breast augmentation implants (Fig. 10.6) are relatively common; over 2 million women now have them (1). The augmentations may be for cosmetic reasons or for postsurgical reconstruction. Special views, called implant displaced views, are required to visualize the breast tissue surrounding the implant. Breast implants vary in appearance from less dense saline to dense silicone.

Malignant

Common mammographic/ultrasonographic findings of malignancy are listed in Table 10.4. Malignant masses are usually irregularly shaped and of high density and have ill-defined or spiculated borders (Fig. 10.7A–C). Microcalcifications are frequently associated within and/or outside of the mass. When these suspicious findings are present, it is important to evaluate the extent of the disease such as multifocality/multicen-

tricity on the imaging studies. Multifocality means that there are other disease foci in the same breast quadrant. Multicentricity means that there are other disease foci in a different breast quadrant.

Asymmetric densities and architectural distortions are also suspicious for malignancy, especially if they have appeared recently.

TABLE 10.4

MAMMOGRAPHIC/ULTRASONOGRAPHIC FINDINGS SUSPECT FOR MALIGNANCY

1. Developing mass on a mammogram with:
   a. Ill-defined or spiculated borders
   b. Associated malignant calcifications
   c. High density relative to the volume
   d. Skin retraction or thickening
2. Microcalcifications with or without a mass
   a. Pleomorphic
   b. Linear or branching
   c. Clusters
3. Architectural distortion or focal asymmetry
4. Irregular hypoechoic solid mass on ultrasound with ill-defined/spiculated border, thick boundary echogenicity, and/or surrounding architectural distortion

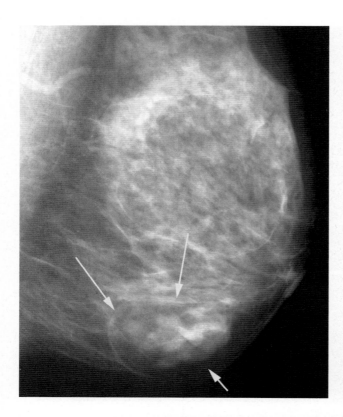

FIGURE 10.5 Benign hamartoma. The MLO view of the left breast shows a well-defined mass with heterogeneous internal density which is not different from the surrounding normal breast tissue except it is confined within a thin wall in the lower left breast (*arrows*). Patients usually don't feel this mass due to its soft nature. The other name of hamartoma is fibroadeno-lipoma. This mammographic appearance is diagnostic.

FIGURE 10.6 Left breast mediolateral oblique (**A**) and craniocaudal (**B**) digital mammograms. Bilateral breast augmentations. The bright white areas represent the surgically implanted silicone augmentation implants (*straight arrows*). (*continued*)

C   D

FIGURE 10.6 (*Continued*) Implant displaced MLO (**C**) and CC (**D**) views show breast parenchyma better than routine views.

MICROCALCIFICATIONS

Calcifications are important as they may represent the first sign of malignancy, especially if they are new, pleomorphic, or branching (Fig. 10.7D). It should be emphasized that most calcifications are benign. Therefore, it is essential that the radiologist distinguish between benign and malignant calcifications. Some calcifications are so small that a magnifying glass is needed when viewing mammograms. After being detected on a screening mammogram, calcifications are frequently evaluated in more detail, using special magnification mammography images. Once suspicious calcifications have been biopsied, the biopsy specimen can be radiographed to make sure that the calcifications have been adequately sampled and/or removed. The description of microcalcifications using BIRADS terminology includes the shape, distribution, location, and associated findings. Associated findings may include mass. Benign microcalcifications are usually homogeneously punctate or round shaped and more diffusely scattered in a wide area. Malignant microcalcifications are more heterogeneous in shape and size (pleomorphic), more clustered in a small area, or linearly/segmentally distributed.

INDICATIONS FOR BREAST ULTRASOUND

Ultrasound has been an important adjunct imaging modality for breast diseases. The main advantage of US initially was differentiation between cystic and solid masses; however, current advanced technology introduced more complicated techniques such as harmonic imaging, compound imaging, elastography, three-dimensional image acquisition and reconstruction, and automatic scanning. Ultrasound is also widely used for image-guided intervention such as percutaneous core biopsy and cyst/abscess drainage. Real-time monitoring of the process during the entire examination is a main advantage of US.

The ultrasonographic description of mass using BIRADS terminology includes its shape, orientation, margin, boundary

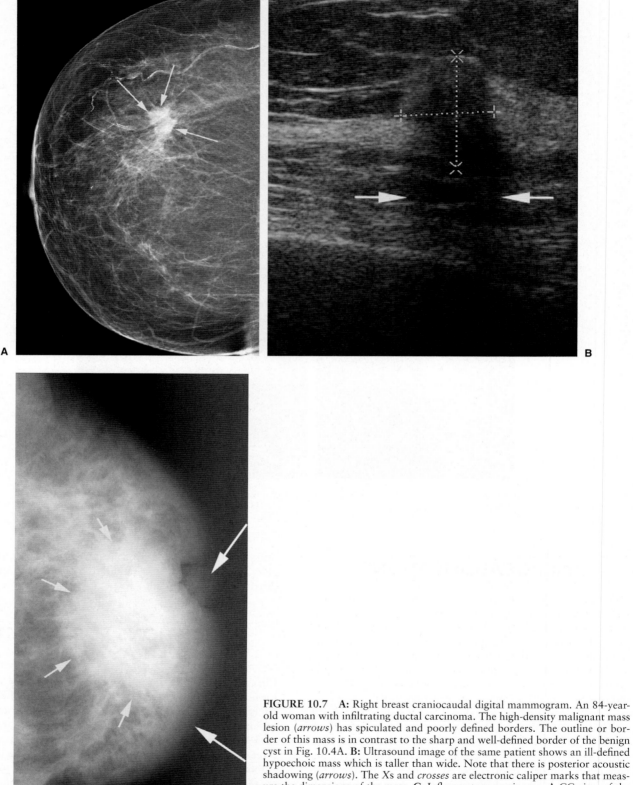

FIGURE 10.7   A: Right breast craniocaudal digital mammogram. An 84-year-old woman with infiltrating ductal carcinoma. The high-density malignant mass lesion (*arrows*) has spiculated and poorly defined borders. The outline or border of this mass is in contrast to the sharp and well-defined border of the benign cyst in Fig. 10.4A. **B:** Ultrasound image of the same patient shows an ill-defined hypoechoic mass which is taller than wide. Note that there is posterior acoustic shadowing (*arrows*). The Xs and *crosses* are electronic caliper marks that measure the dimensions of the mass. **C:** Inflammatory carcinoma. A CC view of the left breast shows a large ill-defined high-density mass (*short arrows*) with surrounding thickened trabeculation. Note the markedly thickened skin and retracted nipple (*long arrows*). (*continued*)

D

FIGURE 10.7 (*Continued*) **D:** A 38-year-old woman with infiltrating ductal carcinoma. Left breast digital MLO magnification compression view demonstrates the classical appearance of malignant calcifications (*short arrows*) in the mass (*long arrows*). Note the difference between the coarse benign calcifications in Fig. 10.3 and these pleomorphic malignant calcifications. Also, the high density and poorly defined borders of the associated mass are more obvious in this magnification compression view. A marker (white dot) indicates that this mass is palpable.

of the mass, internal echo pattern, and posterior acoustic features. Characteristics suggesting benignity include circumscribed round/oval shape, being wider than tall, thin capsule, and gentle lobulation. Characteristics suggesting malignancy include irregular shape, spiculated/angular/microlobulated border, being taller than wide, and surrounding architectural distortion (Fig. 10.7B).

MALE BREAST

All of the diseases that occur in the female breast can potentially occur in the male breast. The incidence of male breast carcinoma was approximately 2,000 cases in the year of 2007 in the United States or approximately 1% of all breast cancers. This, of course, is dramatically lower than that in the female population. Thus, mammography has no medical use as a screening examination in males. The indications for male diagnostic mammography and the image obtained are similar to those for females. Men tend to be diagnosed in advanced disease status and thus have poorer survival. The reasons for these late-stage diagnoses are they may not be aware of changes in their breasts, slow response to discovered changes, and they are not screened for breast cancer (5).

One benign male breast clinical situation that can be confused with breast cancer is gynecomastia (Fig. 10.8). The etiologies for male gynecomastia are listed in Table 10.5. Usually, adult men present with a tender subareolar breast mass, and it may be unilateral or bilateral. On mammography, there is breast tissue in the subareolar zone that may rarely contain calcifications. The need for biopsy will be determined by a combination of symptoms, physical findings, and mammo-

FIGURE 10.8 Left male breast CC digital mammogram. Benign gynecomastia. The *arrows* indicate the typical increased but normal appearing subareolar fibroglandular tissue without calcification. Normal male patient should not show any fibroglandular tissue in his mammogram.

graphic or ultrasonographic findings. There is probably no correlation between gynecomastia and carcinoma.

Male breast carcinomas are similar in appearance to female breast carcinomas. They most commonly present as irregular or ill-defined solid masses. Pathologically, invasive lobular carcinomas are rarer in men than in women due to less developed lobular structures in men.

SUGGESTED WORKUP OF COMMON CLINICAL PROBLEMS

Suggested algorithms for the workup of two common clinical scenarios are shown in Fig. 10.9.

TABLE 10.5

SOME CAUSES OF MALE GYNECOMASTIA

1. Common in the neonatal male
2. Common in pubertal males
3. Adult men
   a. Any underlying disease causing hormone imbalance (e.g., liver cirrhosis)
   b. Drugs (digitalis, steroids)
   c. Androgen deficiency as in aging

OTHER TECHNOLOGIES

Magnetic resonance (MR) is used to image implants and to evaluate for rupture and the extent of disease in women diagnosed with breast cancer, especially those with dense breast tissue that is not well imaged by mammography. MR is also used for screening purposes in high-risk patients (6). Advantages of MR include better evaluation of the three-dimensional extent of the disease, dynamic kinetic evaluation of the disease using intravenous contrast media and specific software (Fig. 10.10), follow-up evaluation of the cancers following chemotherapy to determine whether the tumor has responded to treatment, diagnosis of otherwise invisible malignancies in the same or opposite breast, differentiation between scar and recurrent cancer, and presurgical planning in a known cancer patient. MR is also used for MR-guided invasive procedures such as MR-guided core biopsy for lesions seen only on MRI.

Small field-of-view digital imaging is used to guide biopsy probe placement for stereotactic core biopsies. Full-field digital mammography is being used in approximately 40% of the United States as of 2008 in filmless radiology departments.

Advantages of digital mammography include the ability to use image-processing techniques to aid in evaluating the images, apply computer-assisted diagnostic techniques (CAD) to aid in detecting abnormalities, transmit images rapidly to another location for a second opinion, and store images electronically so that they cannot be lost or misplaced as may occur with film images. The advantages of digital screening mammography over traditional film-screen analog mammogram were evaluated and published in 2005 from a study of

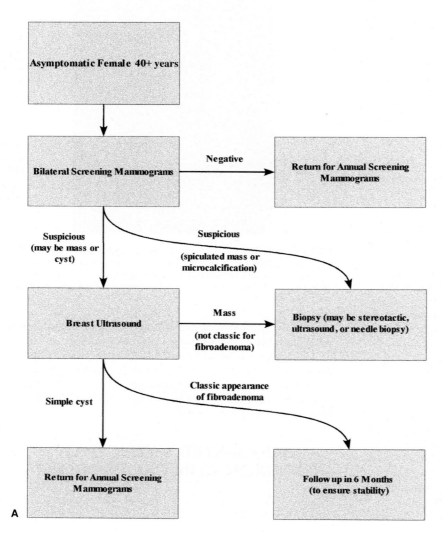

FIGURE 10.9 Examples of possible workup algorithms. **A:** Screening for breast carcinoma. (*continued*)

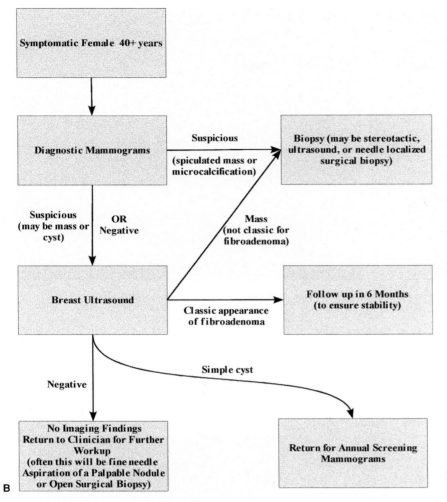

FIGURE 10.9 (*Continued*) **B:** Workup of a palpable breast mass.

FIGURE 10.10 A 39-year-old woman with invasive ductal carcinoma in the right breast. The rounded mass (*arrows*) in the central right breast shows iso-signal intensity on T1-weighted image (**A**) and heterogeneous high-signal intensity on T2-weighted image (**B**). (*continued*)

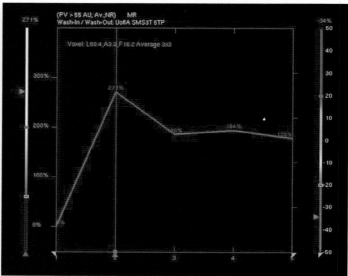

FIGURE 10.10 (*Continued*) The mass shows early rimlike enhancement on postcontrast subtraction image (C) with washout kinetic pattern (D).

42,760 patients (7). The purpose of this study was to verify whether the use of digital mammography would overcome the limitations of film-screen mammography or not. Compared with film-screen mammography, digital mammography was superior in detecting breast cancer in women younger than 50 years, pre- or perimenopausal women, and those with dense breasts.

Tomosynthesis is a modification of two-dimensional digital mammography to three-dimensional digital mammography. This technique provides better visualization/characterization of lesions by removing overlapping structures present in the other planes than the plane the lesion is located. This new technology is still considered experimental and is not yet widely used for imaging the breast.

Positron emission tomography (PET) is a functional or molecular imaging technique that is performed after the intravenous injection of fluorodeoxyglucose. Fluorodeoxyglucose is taken up by cancer cells because of their increased metabolic activity and is detected on the PET scan. In some centers, PET imaging is being evaluated as a technique for staging breast cancer and/or detecting distant metastases. Recently, clinical trials are being conducted to evaluate compact PET imaging devices that mimic standard mammography units and generate mammography-like images (positron emission mammography).

Computed tomography (CT) has not been widely used in the breast imaging because of the low contrast between different tissues in the breast parenchyma and the relatively high radiation doses used in CT imaging. However, investigators have been working on better visualization of the abnormalities of the breast lesions, using novel CT systems and techniques that reduce radiation dose (8).

Galactography is an imaging technique which visualizes the intraductal structures and related abnormalities by injecting radioopaque contrast material into the ducts and then imaging the breast. Active nipple discharge is necessary to perform this examination because the diseased duct must be identified prior to cannulation and contrast injection. An in-traductal abnormality is seen as a "filling defect" in a contrast-filled duct or as abrupt cutoff of the visualized duct (Fig. 10.11). An extraductal abnormality can also be seen indirectly as compression effect from an extraductal mass.

FIGURE 10.11 Galactography. A 48-year-old woman with intraductal papilloma in the left breast. Left CC view shows a small rounded filling defect (*arrows*) in the contrast-filled duct in left subareolar area.

KEY POINTS

- Approximately one in eight females in the United States will develop carcinoma of the breast at some time.

- Mammograms must be interpreted by qualified radiologists. Mammograms of high quality are imperative.

- A routine mammogram consists of mediolateral oblique and craniocaudal views.

- Screening mammography and annual breast examinations by a physician can improve the survival rate of breast cancer.

- Mammographic findings suspect for malignancy include an irregularly shaped mass, pleomorphic microcalcifications, skin retraction or thickening, architectural distortion, or focal asymmetry (asymmetric compared to opposite breast).

- Calcifications that are suspicious for malignancy include new calcifications, pleomorphic calcifications, and small branching calcifications.

- Ultrasonography is often useful in differentiating solid from cystic breast masses.

- MR is useful in evaluating the extent of known diseases, differentiation between scar and recurrent cancer, implant rupture, and screening for high-risk patients.

References

1. Cardenosa G. *Breast imaging companion.* Philadelphia: Lippincott-Raven Publishers, 1997.
2. Berg WA, Birdwell RL, Gombos E, et al. *Diagnostic imaging: breast.* Altona: Amirsys, 2006
3. Conant E, Brennecke C. *Breast imaging: case review series (case review).* Philadelphia: Mosby, 2006.
4. D'Orsi CJ, Bassett LW, Berg WA, et al. Mammography. In: *Breast imaging reporting and data system (BI-RADS),* 4th ed. Reston, VA: American College of Radiology, 2003.
5. Giordano SH, Cohen DS, Buzdar AU, Perkins G, Hortobagyi GN. Breast carcinoma in men: a population-based study. Cancer 2004;101(1):51–57.
6. Saslow D, Boetes C, Burke W, et al. American Cancer Society guidelines for breast screening with MRI as an adjunct to mammography. CA Cancer J Clin 2007;57(2):75–89.
7. Pisano ED, Gatsonis C, Hendrick E, et al. Diagnostic performance of digital versus film mammography for breast-cancer screening. N Engl J Med 2005;353:1773–1783.
8. Keyriläinen J, Fernández M, Karjalainen-Lindsberg ML, et al. Toward high-contrast breast CT at low radiation dose. Radiology 2008;249(1):321–327.

CHAPTER 11 ■ INTERVENTIONAL RADIOLOGY

THOMAS A. FARRELL

OVERVIEW

Interventional radiology (IR) is a diverse practice of patient care using minimally invasive, imaging guided procedures to diagnose and treat disease nonoperatively. Percutaneous diagnostic and therapeutic procedures are performed using fluoroscopy, ultrasound, computed tomography (CT), or magnetic resonance (MR) imaging for guidance. These procedures, which may be categorized as vascular (i.e., arteriography, venography) and nonvascular (e.g., decompression and drainage of obstructed kidneys and bile ducts), are performed in an IR suite and are often done on an outpatient basis. Many procedures that were previously performed surgically are now accomplished by an interventional radiologist with less morbidity and a shorter hospital stay.

Since 1958, when Dr. Seldinger described a method of percutaneous vascular access using a hollow core needle, guidewire, and catheter, IR has continued to evolve, as new techniques and devices are developed to enhance patient care. Technical advances have led to significant improvements in patient safety and procedural diversity. As these rapid changes in endovascular technologies continue to expand, so will the possibilities of image-guided, minimally invasive procedures.

Because IR is procedural, interventional radiologists tend to be more involved in patient care. Referred patients are routinely worked up by the IR service and are subsequently followed up postprocedure. The preprocedure workup consists of patient assessment as well as evaluation of previous imaging studies (Table 11.1). Postprocedure follow-up is essential to determine whether the procedure has been successful and free of complications. This all-inclusive clinical service underlines that there is more to IR than simply doing procedures. Many IR practices offer an active inpatient and outpatient consult service and also employ specially trained nurse practitioners and physician's assistants as physician exten-

ders. Because procedures performed by interventional radiologists are invasive, there are associated risks for developing complications. It is important that the patient be aware of these risks so that an informed decision can be made by weighing the possible risks of a procedure against its benefits. A physician should never place a patient in a position of risk unless the risks, benefits, and alternatives of the planned procedure have been discussed, understood, and consented to before the procedure. It is in the physician's best interest to be honest and forthright when dealing with patients and their expectations about the outcomes of a procedure.

The aim of this chapter is to explain the background, indications, and basic techniques of the procedures commonly performed in IR so that the reader will gain an understanding of how IR contributes to patient care.

INSTRUMENTS AND TOOLS OF THE TRADE

Interventional radiologic procedures are performed in imaging suites with fluoroscopy and digital subtraction angiography. Ultrasound, CT, and MR imaging are also utilized by the interventional radiologist.

Each angiography/interventional suite is staffed by the operating radiologist and at least one assistant. A radiology technologist provides imaging expertise and a nurse provides patient sedation, monitors vital signs, and attends to patient needs during the procedure.

Endoluminal procedures require administration of a contrast agent. Nonionic iodinated contrast is most frequently used to delineate, radiographically, the lumen of an artery, vein, and biliary duct, gastrointestinal (GI) or urinary tract. Carbon dioxide or gadolinium can be used in patients with renal insufficiency or allergy to radiographic contrast agents.

TABLE 11.1

INTERVENTIONAL RADIOLOGY PREPROCEDURE CHECKLIST

Indication for procedure/question(s) to be answered from procedure

Contraindications for procedure

Review prior imaging and noninvasive studies

Check for contrast allergy

Written informed consent

Check coagulation parameters and serum creatinine

Need for prophylactic antibiotics

Patient should be fasting and well hydrated

Discontinue heparin infusion

There is a variety of commercially available catheters, sheaths, guidewires, balloon catheters, vascular stents, and caval filters. Familiarity with these instruments requires significant training and experience. There are numerous preformed shapes and types of angiographic catheters, most of which are made from flexible plastic material such as polyethylene or polyurethane. Wire braiding may be incorporated into the catheter shaft to increase stiffness and improve its torque. Catheter diameters are measured in French (F) size, where 3F = 1.0 mm (outside diameter). Most angiographic catheters are in the 4F to 7F range. Aortic angiography is performed with pigtail catheters that have several side holes proximal to the tip allowing rapid flow of a contrast bolus while the pigtail loop stabilizes the catheter preventing recoil (Fig. 11.1A, B). Selective angiography (renal, celiac, and superior mesenteric arteries) is performed with a curved end-hole catheter such as a Cobra C2 (Fig. 11.1C). A variety of catheters and guidewires may be necessary during a procedure, and placement of a vascular sheath with a hemostatic valve at the site of access reduces vessel trauma and facilitates rapid catheter and guidewire exchange.

Catheters used in the drainage of abscesses, obstructed kidneys (percutaneous nephrostomy), and bile ducts are made of polyurethane and are of greater diameter than angiographic catheters (8F to 12F). These drainage catheters are usually placed using the Seldinger technique after which they are secured in position by deploying a locking pigtail mechanism formed by pulling on a suture that runs in most of the catheter shaft and is attached to its tip. The pigtail loop itself contains large side holes for drainage. The smaller diameter catheters occlude more easily with debris and should be routinely changed over a guidewire every 6 to 8 weeks when continued drainage is required.

Guidewires increase the ease and safety of catheter placement. The outer shell of a guidewire consists of a very tightly wound but flexible metal spring coil. A stiff central core provides rigidity over a variable length of the guidewire. The balance between these two components dictates the handling characteristics of the guidewire. For example, the distal 15 cm of a Bentson guidewire is floppy, allowing easy coiling (Fig. 11.1E). A J-tipped guidewire reduces the risk of damaging the vessel wall because of its blunt tip (Fig. 11.1D). Guidewires usually range in diameter from 18 thousandths of an inch (0.018 in.) to 38 thousandths of an inch (0.038 in.). The standard length for most wires is 145 cm, whereas longer guidewires (260 cm) are available to facilitate catheter exchange.

Needles used in arteriography range in size from a 21-gauge needle through which a 0.018-in. guidewire will pass to an 18-gauge needle that accepts a 0.035-in. guidewire (Fig. 11.1F).

ANGIOGRAPHY

Angiography is a technique of imaging blood vessels, usually by injecting contrast material via an intraluminally placed catheter. Blood vessels may also be visualized noninvasively using computed tomography angiography (CTA) or magnetic resonance angiography (MRA), which takes advantage of the inherent contrast between flowing blood and stationary tissue.

Diagnostic Percutaneous Arteriography

Diagnostic arteriography begins by catheterizing an artery using Seldinger technique (Fig. 11.2). This technique of vascular catheterization was initially described by a radiologist, Sven Seldinger. After placing a hollow core needle into an artery (femoral or brachial), a guidewire is inserted through the needle and into the artery. Sonographic and fluoroscopic guidance is often necessary. The needle is exchanged for a vascular catheter or vascular introducing sheath. Subsequent catheter movement and exchange is performed over a guidewire. Large vessel arteriography is performed using flush catheters (pigtail). Smaller arteries are selectively cannulated using catheters of various shapes and sizes. Microcatheters are used for sub- or superselective arteriography.

After the catheter is safely positioned in the artery of choice, the guidewire is removed and a contrast agent injected through the catheter during image acquisition. Mask images obtained before injection of contrast allow for subtraction of nonvascular structures. Many images are acquired as the contrast agent flows through the lumen of the vessel producing the arteriogram. The catheter can be exchanged or repositioned for additional imaging. After completion of the procedure, the

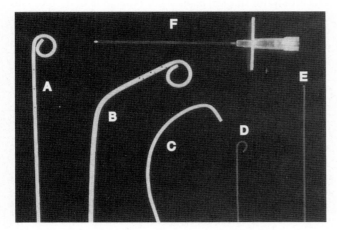

FIGURE 11.1 A–F: Tools of the trade. **A:** Pigtail catheter. **B:** Angled pigtail catheter. **C:** Cobra catheter. **D:** J-tipped guidewire. **E:** Straight (Bentson) guidewire. **F:** An 18-gauge needle for vessel puncture.

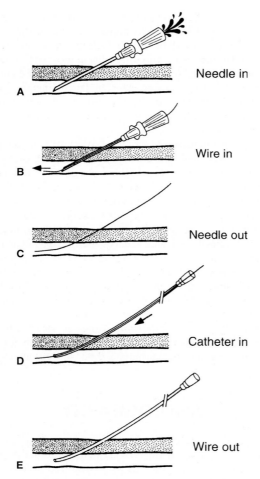

FIGURE 11.2 A–E: Seldinger technique. **A:** The vessel is punctured with the needle. **B:** A guidewire is advanced through the needle into the vessel. **C:** The needle is removed leaving the guidewire in place. **D:** A catheter is advanced over the guidewire into the vessel. **E:** The guidewire is removed and the catheter flushed.

catheter is removed and hemostasis obtained at the arteriotomy site using manual compression or a percutaneous closure device. Recovery time for the patient is 2 to 6 hours.

Noninvasive angiography (MRA/CTA) is replacing most percutaneous diagnostic arteriography, except where intervention is expected or other examinations are indefinite. Pulmonary arteriography performed by venous catheterization and crossing the right side of the heart has largely been replaced by CTA, which has an acceptably high specificity and sensitivity. Both CTA and MRA are widely used in the evaluation of aortic, visceral, renal, and peripheral arterial disease (PAD). However, the administration of gadolinium chelates, commonly used in MR angiography, is associated with a higher incidence of nephrogenic systemic sclerosis in patients with renal impairment.

Peripheral Arterial Disease

Generally, the diagnosis of PAD, or peripheral vascular disease, has already been made by the time an arteriogram is requested. The evaluation includes an assessment of the patient's symptoms, a physical examination, and a review of the non-invasive imaging tests, such as CT, MR, duplex ultrasonography, and segmental limb pressures before proceeding to angiography. Rather than being an end point, the angiogram helps formulate a comprehensive plan in the patient's subsequent treatment as it evaluates the extent and severity of disease and provides a road map for intervention (balloon angioplasty, stenting, surgery, etc.). Patients with diabetes may present with a more advanced stage of ischemia as they are prone to developing peripheral neuropathy that may mask the above symptoms. They also tend to have a greater prevalence of small vessel disease, which is more difficult to treat surgically and contributes to a less favorable long-term prognosis compared to other causes of PAD.

Arteriographic examination of patients with PAD may be divided into three anatomic regions: aortoiliac, infrainguinal, and infrageniculate. Aortic aneurysms occur most commonly below the level of the renal arteries. The number of renal arteries should also be noted, as should the presence of stenoses in these vessels. Bilateral oblique views of the pelvis should be obtained during the arteriogram, as hemodynamically significant stenoses can be missed if only a frontal view is performed.

In general, arterial stenoses are not regarded as significant unless they reduce the lumen diameter by 50% angiographically. Measuring a pressure gradient across it can more accurately assess the significance of a stenosis. The presence of a 10 mm Hg gradient or greater across a stenosis is regarded as significant and worthy of further treatment such as angioplasty or stenting. If the gradient is less than 10 mm Hg, a vasodilator such as nitroglycerin may be given intra-arterially to simulate exercise and possibly unmask a significant stenosis. Most endovascular interventions are performed in the carotid, renal, aortoiliac, and femoropopliteal arteries.

In the absence of satisfactory femoral pulses bilaterally, either the brachial or the axillary arteries can be used for percutaneous access.

Venography

Diagnostic venography is performed in all extremities, as well as centrally, for surgical planning or evaluation of deep venous thrombosis when vascular ultrasound is indeterminate. Most venography is performed in conjunction with interventional procedures (placement of caval filters and central venous catheters, renal vein sampling).

VASCULAR INTERVENTIONS

Thrombolysis

Thrombolysis is the process of dissolving blood clot in order to establish patency of an occluded (thrombosed) vessel, using drugs such as urokinase and tissue plasminogen activator (t-PA). These drugs are infused directly into the thrombosed grafts and vessels to ensure a very high local concentration of the drug. Active internal bleeding, recent intracranial hemorrhage, or surgery is absolute contraindication for thrombolysis (Table 11.2).

Complications of thrombolysis include bleeding and distal embolization of thrombus. The cumulative probability of

TABLE 11.2

CONTRAINDICATIONS FOR ARTERIAL THROMBOLYSIS

Absolute
  Active gastrointestinal (GI) or genitourinary (GU) bleeding
  Recent (<12 months) cerebral hemorrhage/infarct/surgery
  Irreversible limb ischemia
Relative
  History of GI or GU bleeding
  Recent thoracic/abdominal surgery
  Recent trauma
  Severe uncontrolled hypertension

major complications increases with duration of infusion, rising from less than 10% after 16 hours to more than 30% at 40 hours. Once thrombolysis is complete, balloon angioplasty or surgery can be used to treat any underlying vessel stenoses that contributed to the occlusion.

Balloon Angioplasty

Percutaneous transluminal balloon angioplasty (PTA) has become an established technique in the treatment of vascular stenoses due to atherosclerotic plaque and fibromuscular dysplasia. The precise pathophysiologic mechanism of PTA in atherosclerotic plaque is controversial. However, most agree that PTA results in a controlled plaque and intimal fracture with localized dissection into the underlying media thereby increasing the intraluminal diameter. The plaque, intima, and media are subsequently remodeled to give a smoother endoluminal surface. The appropriate angioplasty balloon catheter should be chosen so that its inflated diameter is the same size or slightly larger than the adjacent nondiseased vessel. Initially, the stenosis is crossed with a guidewire that is left across the lesion until the procedure is finished. Heparin and nitro-

glycerin may be given intra-arterially to prevent thrombosis and vessel spasm, respectively. The angioplasty balloon is advanced across the stenosis, inflated, and deflated slowly under fluoroscopic guidance. Repeat angiography and pressure measurements should be obtained to evaluate the results of angioplasty. Suboptimal angioplasty results may require placement of an endovascular stent.

Iliac artery angioplasty improves inflow to the lower limb and requires balloons that are 7 to 10 mm in diameter. Again, a guidewire is left across the stenosis during the procedure, the success of which is judged on angiographic and hemodynamic criteria. Stent placement should be considered if the postangioplasty pressure gradient is greater than 10 mm Hg, there is residual stenosis of greater than 30%, or if a flow-limiting dissection is present (Fig. 11.3). Simultaneous PTA of both common iliac arteries, known as the kissing-balloons technique, is effective in treating bilateral proximal common iliac artery stenoses.

Infrainguinal angioplasty (superficial femoral and popliteal arteries) is gaining clinical acceptance as patency outcomes for PTA and stenting rivals outcomes of surgical bypass procedures (Fig. 11.4A, B).

Infrageniculate angioplasty (anterior/posterior tibial and peroneal arteries) is usually performed for limb salvage or to reduce the extent of an impending below-the-knee or forefoot amputation for ischemia. This technique requires a fine diameter guidewire (0.010″ to 0.018″) and angioplasty balloon (2 to 3 mm in diameter) because of the smaller vessel size.

Renal artery angioplasty is usually performed with a 5- to 7-mm-diameter balloon. Atheromatous disease usually involves the proximal or ostial portion of the vessel in contrast to fibromuscular dysplasia that usually affects the midportion of the vessel. The improvement in renal function and hypertension following renal artery angioplasty is equivalent to that obtained after surgical revascularization (Fig. 11.5). Renal artery stenting is performed if there is a residual stenosis or significant dissection postangioplasty (Fig. 11.6). Ostial renal

A　　　　　　　　　　　　　　　　　　　　　　　　**B**

FIGURE 11.3   A–G: Thrombolysis, balloon angioplasty, and stenting of a common iliac artery occlusion. **A:** Aortogram/pelvic angiogram shows occlusion of the right common iliac artery (*arrow*). **B:** Partial recanalization of the right common iliac artery following thrombolysis performed via an infusion catheter (*arrow*). (*continued*)

FIGURE 11.3 (*Continued*) **C:** Balloon angioplasty was performed showing residual narrowing of the balloon (*arrow*). **D:** The common iliac stenosis persisted postangioplasty (*arrow*). **E, F:** A balloon expandable stent was deployed across the stenosis. The undeployed stent (*arrow*) can be seen on the distal portion of the angioplasty balloon. **G:** Poststenting, no residual stenosis is present.

FIGURE 11.4   **A, B:** Balloon angioplasty. This left knee angiogram shows tandem stenoses (*arrows*) and multiple collateral formation in the popliteal artery. After angioplasty of the stenoses with a 3 mm × 2 cm balloon there is improved flow in the popliteal artery.

FIGURE 11.5   **A, B:** Renal artery angioplasty. **A:** Flush aortogram showing right renal artery stenosis (*curved arrow*). **B:** Residual stenosis persists postballoon angioplasty. Note that the guidewire (*arrow*) is left across the stenosis.

FIGURE 11.6   Renal artery stenting. A Palmaz stent (*arrow*) has been placed across a left renal artery stenosis.

FIGURE 11.7   Palmaz stent mounted on an angioplasty balloon and in its expanded form. (Photograph courtesy of Cordis Corporation.)

artery stenoses are often stented primarily, without balloon predilatation.

Endovascular Stents

Peripheral Endovascular Stents

There are two main indications for endovascular stent placement: (a) a residual pressure gradient of more than 10 mm Hg postangioplasty, which is regarded as an indication for either repeat angioplasty or stent placement; and (b) postangioplasty flow-limiting dissection, in which the goal of stent placement is to appose the dissected flap against the wall and improve flow. The balloon–stent combination is placed across the stenosis and the balloon is inflated, thus opening and deploying the stent. The balloon is then deflated and removed (Fig. 11.7). There are two general types of metallic endovascular stents, balloon-expandable and self-expanding. Deployment of the balloon-expandable stent is described above. Deployment of the self-expanding stent, which does not require delivery on an angioplasty balloon, involves withdrawal of a covering sheath, after which the stent expands. Postdilatation with an angioplasty balloon may be necessary. Self-expanding stents are usually more flexible than balloon-mounted stents, which is an advantage when stenting tortuous vessels (Fig. 11.8). Covered (polytetrafluoroethylene (PTFE), Dacron) stents are available for treatment of vascular injury resulting in pseudoaneurysm, hemorrhage, or arteriovenous fistula. Drug eluting stents are currently being investigated to determine efficacy in treatment of arterial stenosis. These stents are designed to reduce neointimal hyperplasia which develops and covers the inside of the stent.

Aortic Stent Grafts

Stent grafts have revolutionized the treatment of abdominal aortic aneurysms (AAA), reducing the severity and duration of the procedure and postprocedure morbidity and hospital stay. Ninety percent of patients are discharged within 48 hours of the procedure, which is usually done in the operating room or combined operative/fluoroscopy suite, under general or epidural anesthesia. Through bilateral femoral artery surgical cutdowns, the various components of the aortic stent graft are

FIGURE 11.8   The Wallstent is self-expanding and flexible. (Photograph courtesy of Boston Scientific.)

introduced and deployed in the abdominal aorta and iliac arteries, under fluoroscopic guidance. A preprocedure CT scan of the aorta is essential for precise vessel measurement and localization of arterial branches. The device, which is composed of woven polyester on a wire exoskeleton frame, is placed in the infrarenal aorta and extends down to the common or external iliac arteries (Fig. 11.9). Postprocedure follow-up with

FIGURE 11.9   Aortic stent graft device is composed of three components—a main body and two iliac extensions, which can be custom made to suit each patient. The components are placed through femoral artery cutdowns (Courtesy of Cook Medical, Inc.)

FIGURE 11.10   A–D: Aortic Endograft Follow-up. Serial CT studies show an infrarenal abdominal aortic aneurysm (AAA) measuring 4.5 cm in diameter (**A**). Six months post-AAA endograft placement, the excluded aneurysm sac now measures 4.0 cm (**B**) and at 18 months postendograft, it has further reduced to a diameter of 3.2 cm (**C**). CT abdomen in a patient post-AAA endograft shows contrast within the aneurysm sac but outside the endograft (*arrow*) (**D**). This is an endoleak which occurs because of persistent blood flow into the aneurysm which in this patient is due to retrograde flow from a lumbar artery.

CT scans every 6 months is important for the detection of an endoleak, which is a leak into the aneurysm sac. In the absence of such an endoleak, the aneurysm sac should reduce in size (Fig. 11.10A–D).

Complications (Table 11.3)

Complications of diagnostic angiography are infrequent, with access site vascular injury and hematoma comprising the overwhelming majority. Risk factors for this complication include hypertension and obesity. Prevention involves meticulous technique including vessel puncture over the femoral head and constant manual pressure directly over the puncture site after removal of the catheter until hemostasis is achieved. The hematoma may extend into the retroperitoneum when the puncture site is above the inguinal ligament (Fig. 11.11A).

TABLE 11.3

COMPLICATIONS OF ANGIOGRAPHY

Systemic
  Allergic contrast reaction
  Renal failure
Local
  Puncture site
    Hematoma
    Pseudoaneurysm
    Arteriovenous fistula
Intraluminal
  Subintimal dissection
  Thrombosis
  Distal embolization

FIGURE 11.11 **A–D:** Complications of arterial interventions. **A:** This CT scan shows a **hematoma** occupying most of the right hemipelvis. The retroperitoneal hematoma could be traced down to the right external iliac artery where the physician performing an angiogram had made the initial arterial puncture. **B:** The well-defined focal bulge (*arrow*) is a **pseudoaneurysm** which has formed at the site of a previous common femoral arterial puncture. **C:** The vertically oriented well-defined curvilinear filling defect (*arrow*) in the right external iliac is a **dissection** flap. **D:** The well-defined intraluminal filling defect in the distal popliteal artery (*arrow*) is an **embolus** which migrated there after balloon angioplasty of a stenosis containing atherosclerotic plaque upstream in the superficial femoral artery.

Incomplete or intermittent compression over the puncture site may also result in the formation of a pseudoaneurysm (Fig. 11.11B). Dissection of vessel wall may occur if the needle/wire or catheter is introduced subinitmally (Fig. 11.11C), and distal embolization of mural plaque or thrombus is a risk following any endovascular manipulation (Fig. 11.11D). Complications following brachial or axillary arterial puncture are more common than with femoral artery puncture because of the smaller vessel size and the close proximity of the vessels to nerves within a common sheath in the arm. Dissection, thrombosis, or pseudoaneurysm of the access artery may require endovascular intervention or surgical repair.

Contrast-induced nephropathy refers to transient renal insufficiency, and occasionally, acute renal failure, that is a result of iodinated contrast. This complication is usually mild and self-limiting, with serum creatinine levels peaking by 3 to 5 days and returning to normal within 2 weeks. The pathophysiology of this complication is thought to be due to a combination of vasoconstriction and direct toxicity of contrast on the renal tubules. Patients with diabetes and patients with preexisting renal impairment (serum creatinine greater than 2 mg%) are at increased risk for developing contrast-induced renal failure. Clinical judgment, adequate hydration, isoosmolar iodinated contrast, or alternative contrast agents (CO_2, gadolinium) should be used in high-risk patients (elderly, creatinine (Cr) >1.5, DM). Transient renal insufficiency usually returns to baseline in 10 to 14 days. Systemic allergic or idiosyncratic reactions to radiographic contrast media are rare, with severity depending on the type, dose, route, and rate of contrast delivery. Allergic reactions may be categorized as mild, moderate, or severe (Table 11.4). The prevalence of most reactions is greater with the intravenous route. Many studies suggest a lower incidence of severe reactions when

TABLE 11.4

ALLERGIC CONTRAST REACTIONS

Type	Mild	Moderate	Severe
Incidence (%)	5–15	1–2	0.1
Clinical features	Nausea	Bronchospasm	Laryngospasm
	Vomiting	Dyspnea	Facial edema
	Urticaria	Vasovagal reaction	Cardiorespiratory arrest
		Hypertension	Seizures
Treatment	Monitor vital signs	Oxygen	Oxygen/IV fluids
	Observe for clinical deterioration	β^2 agonist	Epinephrine SC or IV
			β^2 agonist
			Diazepam

nonionic iodinated contrast is used. The mortality, which is equivalent for high and lower osmolar contrast agents, is approximately 1 per 45,000 examinations. Moderate contrast reactions characterized by hypertension, hypotension, wheezing, and laryngospasm occur in 1% to 2% of examinations. Allergic reactions are usually mild (nausea, cough, hives, and flushing), are even more common, and can be treated symptomatically. Premedication with steroids for 24 hours prior to angiography has reduced the incidence of contrast reactions.

Therapeutic Embolization

Gastrointestinal Hemorrhage

Selective angiography and therapeutic embolization have become important techniques in the management of patients with GI bleeding. Initially, a nuclear medicine study using radiolabeled red cells is helpful to confirm the presence and anatomic location of the bleeding vessel. Selective angiography of the celiac, superior mesenteric, or inferior mesenteric arteries is then performed. Once a bleeding site has been demonstrated, the catheter can be used to control bleeding by injecting embolic materials such as gelatin sponge pledgets or coils to mechanically occlude flow (Fig. 11.12A–C).

Hemoptysis

Patients with massive hemoptysis may be successfully treated by embolizing the appropriate bronchial arteries, which arise directly from the thoracic aorta or from intercostal branches, with fine particles. Great care should be taken to avoid nontarget embolization of the arterial supply to the spinal cord which may result in paralysis.

Uterine Fibroid Embolization

Fibroids commonly present as pain, menorrhagia, or pressure symptoms related to mass effect. Traditionally, patients were treated with hysterectomy or myomectomy. Uterine fibroid embolization offers an effective and less invasive treatment option. After selective catheterization of the uterine arteries, inert particles up to 900 microns (0.9 mm) in size are injected, infarcting the fibroids, eventually reducing their size and improving symptoms. The fibroid size reduces by 60% at 6 months and up to 90% of patients notice an improvement in their pain, menorrhagia, or pressure symptoms.

FIGURE 11.12   A–C: Embolization of a GI bleed. **A:** This superior mesenteric angiogram (*arrow*) shows extravasation of contrast, which represents hemorrhage into the colon at the hepatic flexure (X). **B:** This extravasation (*white arrow*) is confirmed on selective angiography of the right colic artery performed with a microcatheter (*black arrow*). (*continued*)

FIGURE 11.12 (*Continued*) **C:** Several stainless steel coils 2 to 3 mm in diameter were deployed through the microcatheter occluding the right colic branch at the bleeding site.

Tumor Embolization

Arterial embolization is also utilized for regional cancer therapy. Bland embolization of primary or metastatic tumors is performed to decrease blood flow to a tumor, depriving the tumor of nutrients. Bland embolization is usually performed for vascular tumors, bleeding from tumor or adjacent invaded

organs, and for palliation. In the case of renal cell carcinoma, the kidney or metastatic lesion is often embolized prior to surgery to decrease bleeding during nephrectomy or resection (Fig. 11.13A–C). Chemoembolization is performed in cases of primary or metastatic liver cancer, subselectively embolizing the tumor with chemotherapeutic drugs and inert particles. Chemoembolization has the advantage of prolonging the tumor exposure to a high concentration of drug(s) while also infarcting the tumor (Fig. 11.14A–C).

Trauma

The interventional radiologist has an important role in the management of trauma patients. Most emergent trauma procedures referred to IR involve bleeding or injury to the vascular system. Vessel injury with bleeding, intimal injury, pseudoaneurysm, or fistula can be diagnosed and immediately treated in the angiography suite, often using covered stents or embolization techniques (Fig. 11.15A, B).

Hemorrhage Associated with Pelvic Fracture

Prior to the introduction of external fixation devices, much of the early mortality associated with pelvic fractures was due to

FIGURE 11.13 **A–C:** Preoperative embolization of a renal carcinoma. **A:** The CT scan shows a large hypervascular right renal carcinoma. **B:** Abdominal aortography confirms it hypervascular nature (*arrows*). **C:** Postembolization of the renal artery branches and nonrenal branches (lumbar and inferior phrenic arteries) with stainless steel coils. The prophylactic embolization reduced the operative morbidity and blood loss as the surgeon was operating in a "bloodless" field (Courtesy of Dr. D. Warner.)

FIGURE 11.14   A–D: Chemoembolization of a hepatoma. **A:** CT shows a hypervascular hepatoma (*arrow*). **B, C:** Selective hepatic angiography confirms the tumor's hypervascularity (*arrow*) and more clearly defines its arterial supply. **D:** Angiography postchemoembolization of the hepatoma confirms occlusion (*arrow*) of its main hepatic arterial branch.

FIGURE 11.15   A, B: Embolization of a leaking pseudoaneurysm. This patient presented with a rapidly expanding thigh hematoma shortly after hip replacement surgery. A thigh angiogram shows a pseudoaneurysm (*arrow*) in the distal profunda femoris artery. Several stainless steel coils were deployed through the angiographic catheter occluding the arterial branch proximal to the pseudoaneurysm.

internal hemorrhage. Presently, up to 20% of patients with pelvic fractures require the services of IR for the diagnosis and treatment of hemorrhage. In general, surgery is not a satisfactory treatment option for this problem as exploration will decompress the pelvic hematoma, reduce the tamponade effect, and lead to further blood loss. A diagnostic pelvic angiogram is performed with a pigtail catheter placed above the aortic bifurcation. Active hemorrhage is diagnosed by extravasation of contrast. The bleeding vessel may then be embolized with either a stainless steel Gianturco coil or pledgets of gelatin sponge, both of which can be placed through a selective 5F angiographic catheter. Gelatin sponge results in temporary vascular occlusion that recanalizes within 2 to 3 weeks, whereas a Gianturco coil usually results in a permanent occlusion. Pelvic ischemia following selective arterial embolization is unusual due to the extensive collateral blood supply.

FIGURE 11.16 **A–D:** Traumatic aortic injury. Thoracic aortograms: (A-C) are performed in the left anterior oblique (LAO) view for optimal visualization of the aortic arch. **A:** Normal aortic arch. **B:** Ductus bump, normal variant (*arrow*). **C:** Aortic transection distal to the origin of the left subclavian artery. **D:** This CT scan of the chest shows an intramural hematoma (*arrow*) of the aortic arch consistent with aortic transection.

Traumatic Aortic Injury

Eighty percent of those who sustain a laceration to the thoracic aorta following blunt trauma die at the scene of the accident, en route to the hospital, or shortly after arriving in hospital. The cause of death in most cases is exsanguination from aortic transection. The precise mechanism of aortic transection is uncertain. It may be due to sudden deceleration where the mobile descending aorta shears from the relatively fixed aortic arch, as the most common site for aortic transection is just distal to the origin of the left subclavian artery. As in all trauma patients, rapid clinical evaluation is important, but up to 50% of patients surviving accidents with blunt aortic injuries have no external physical signs of injury. Multidetector CT of the chest has replaced catheter aortography as the gold standard for diagnosing aortic arch injury. One should be aware of a normal anatomic variant in the aortic arch that may be misdiagnosed as traumatic aortic injury—the so-called ductus bump, which lies proximally on the inferior surface of the aortic arch and represents the site of attachment of the ductus arteriosus (Fig. 11.16A–D).

Venous Access

Central Venous Access

Central venous catheters are placed for a variety of indications including administration of antibiotics, chemotherapy, and hemodialysis. There are essentially two types of catheters: tunneled and nontunneled. Tunneling refers to the creation of a subcutaneous tract in which the catheter lies before it enters the vein. The tunnel acts as a physical barrier reducing the in-cidence of catheter-related infection and also enhances catheter security. A Dacron cuff is present on some catheters causing a localized fibrotic reaction, stabilizing it within the subcutaneous tissues. Most long-term catheters are made of polyurethane, a biocompatible material. The optimal position for placement of the catheter tip is at the junction of the superior vena cava and the right atrium. The right internal jugular vein is the preferred site for these catheters. Another type of tunneled venous access is a port device consisting of a subcutaneously implanted reservoir in the chest wall or upper arm to which the catheter is connected. Ports can be accessed percutaneously with a noncoring needle.

For short-term venous access (less than 90 days) a nontunneled catheter, such as a peripherally inserted central catheter is appropriate. A peripherally inserted central catheter is inserted by direct percutaneous puncture of either arm or forearm veins and advanced under fluoroscopic guidance until the tip lies in the superior vena cava (SVC).

Venous Interventions

Vena Cava Filters

The purpose of an inferior vena cava (IVC) filter is to prevent pulmonary embolism by trapping a clot before it gets to the lungs. Filter placement is indicated in patients in whom anticoagulation for deep venous thrombosis/pulmonary embolism (DVT/PE) is contraindicated or ineffective. Currently, there are several types of permanent filters available (Fig. 11.17A, B), all of which are made from either stainless steel or nitinol, an alloy of nickel and titanium and which are introduced

FIGURE 11.17   A, B: Permanent inferior vena cava filters. **A:** Greenfield filter. **B:** Braun Venatech filter. This filter has side struts to prevent tilt.

FIGURE 11.18   **A–C:** IVC filter retrieval. **A:** Under fluoroscopy a retrieval snare has been advanced from the right internal jugular vein to the retrievable IVC filter. **B:** The snare is then used to retrieve the filter by its hook and the filter is collapsed by advancing a sheath (*arrow at tip of sheath*) down over it. **C:** The snared filter and sheath are then removed from the internal jugular vein access site.

percutaneously through the common femoral or internal jugular vein. The filter depends primarily on its legs to trap clot in the infrarenal IVC to reduce risk of renal vein thrombosis. Retrievable IVC filters may be placed in trauma patients or others at short-term risk of PE. These devices may be retrieved within 3 months of initial placement in the IVC. Their design is similar to existing filters apart from a hook at it top to facilitate retrieval with a loop snare (Fig. 11.18A–C). If the indication for filter placement remains at the end of this time then the filter may be left in place as a permanent filter.

Venous Thrombolysis

Deep venous thrombosis can be treated using catheter-directed thrombolysis in a manner similar to arterial thrombolysis. Complete thrombolysis may take several days of continuous thrombolytic infusion. An underlying venous stenosis can be subsequently treated with angioplasty and stent placement.

Foreign Body Retrieval

Occasionally, it may be necessary to retrieve an object—regarded as a foreign body—from within the vascular system. These procedures sometimes necessitate the full use of the interventionalist's armamentarium of skills as well as equipment (Fig. 11.19).

Hemodialysis Access Interventions

Using the percutaneous skills described above, including thrombolysis, angioplasty, and stent placement, hemodialysis access (arteriovenous) fistulae and grafts are declotted and maintained, preserving graft function and longevity. Proper graft or fistula maintenance can add many years to the life of a dialysis-dependent patient. When a dialysis fistula fails to mature, venous collaterals can be embolized to help mature the surgically created dialysis fistula.

NONVASCULAR INTERVENTION

Urological Interventions

Percutaneous nephrostomy is a valuable tool in the treatment of urinary obstruction, which is most commonly caused by calculi, neoplasms, and benign strictures. With the patient in the prone position, the obstructed renal pelvis is accessed using the Seldinger technique during which an 8- or 10F pigtail drainage catheter is passed over a guidewire and the loop formed and secured in the renal pelvis. Further intervention such as ureteral stenting or stone removal (nephrolithotomy) may be performed through this renal access. Mild hematuria

A   B

FIGURE 11.19   A bullet is lodged deep in the subcutaneous tissue below the right clavicle after deflect-
ing off the patient's chin. Attempted removal of the bullet in the emergency department pushed it deeper
into the subcutaneous tissue. A chest radiograph (**A**) showed that the bullet (*arrow*) had migrated to the
right atrium. A 24F (8-mm diameter) vascular sheath (*arrow*) was advanced into the right atrium via the
right internal jugular vein and a loop snare (*curved arrow*) was placed through this to retrieve the slug
(**B**). This case demonstrates the usefulness of interventional radiology in a situation that would otherwise
have required cardiac surgery.

is not uncommon after percutaneous nephrostomy and usually resolves within 72 hours.

Percutaneous Biliary Drainage and Stenting

Obstructive jaundice may be further evaluated by a percutaneous transhepatic cholangiogram whereby a long 22-gauge
needle is advanced through the liver parenchyma from a site in
the eleventh intercostal space in the right midaxillary line or
through the left lobe, using a subxiphoid approach and ultrasound guidance. The needle is then slowly withdrawn while injecting contrast to opacify any bile ducts that may have been
traversed. Successful percutaneous transhepatic cholangiogram
is more likely if the ductal system is dilated. Once a duct is
opacified, a larger (21- or 18-gauge) needle is then used to percutaneously access one of the opacified ducts peripherally. The
tract is dilated over a guidewire and an attempt to traverse the
biliary obstruction is made, followed by placement of an
internal–external biliary drainage catheter (PTBD) to decompress the ductal system. Permanent self-expanding metallic
stents may be placed percutaneously or endoscopically when in-
ternalized biliary drainage is desired, as in the case of a malignant obstruction. Alternatively, temporary short plastic stents
may be placed in the common duct when surgery is planned or
in patients with benign strictures.

Percutaneous Feeding Tubes

Radiologically guided placement of percutaneous gastrostomy
and gastrojejunostomy tubes for enteral nutrition has gained

widespread acceptance in the management of patients who cannot eat or swallow because of stroke, head injury, and head and
neck tumors. The stomach is accessed percutaneously under fluoroscopic guidance using the Seldinger technique and the tract
dilated over a guidewire. A 12- or 14F self-retaining pigtail feeding tube is placed over a guidewire and secured within the stomach. If delivery of liquid feeds directly into the small bowel rather
than the stomach is preferred, then a gastrojejunostomy tube can
be placed in a transgastric fashion as described above and the tip
directed through the pylorus to the distal duodenum (Fig. 11.20).

FIGURE 11.20   Double-lumen gastrojejunostomy tube allows delivery of enteral nutrition through the distal tip of the catheter into small
bowel while the gastric contents are drained through the proximal portion (*arrow*) preventing aspiration of gastric contents into the lungs.

FIGURE 11.21 Radio frequency ablation. CT pelvis shows a RFA needle in a bony metastasis in the right iliac bone, with the patient in the prone position. The heat generated locally will kill the pain fibers improving the patient's symptoms.

Regional Oncology Therapy

Radio Frequency Ablation of Tumors

This minimally invasive technique is often used in the treatment of liver, lung, and bone tumors and results in a reduced hospital stay and complication rate. Under CT or ultrasound guidance, a radio frequency ablation (RFA) needle is percutaneously inserted into the tumor. RFA involves the deposition of energy at 480 KHz causing coagulation necrosis by heating the tissue to 60° C at which temperature cell death occurs (Fig. 11.21).

Vertebroplasty

In the United States, there are more than 1.5 million osteoporosis-related fractures a year of which 700,000 are vertebral compression fractures. Vertebroplasty is the percutaneous injection of bone cement into a vertebral body fracture thereby

FIGURE 11.22 Vertebroplasty. **A:** MR of lumbar spine shows a compression fracture of L1. **B:** Bilateral transpedicular needle placement and injection of bone cement into the vertebral body. **C:** Postvertebroplasty CT shows cement within the vertebral body.

stabilizing it and rendering it less painful. With the patient in the prone position and under fluoroscopic guidance an 11- or 13-gauge needle is advanced percutaneously through each pedicle into the vertebral body, where 3 to 5 cc of liquid bone cement is then injected. The cement hardens and stabilizes the fracture, rendering it less painful (Fig. 11.22A–C).

KEY POINTS

■ Interventional radiology is a specialty of medicine that provides patients diagnostic and therapeutic minimally invasive procedures using imaging guidance.

■ Written informed consent is necessary for most angiographic and interventional procedures. The benefits, risks, and possible complications must be discussed with the patient.

■ The Seldinger technique describes a method for gaining vascular or visceral access using a needle, a guidewire, and a catheter.

■ Most arteriograms are performed via the common femoral artery, which should be punctured over the femoral head.

■ Iodinated contrast is nephrotoxic, particularly in patients with diabetes and patients with preexisting renal impairment.

■ Computed tomography angiography (CTA) has superceded pulmonary angiography and ventilation–perfusion scintigraphy in the diagnosis of pulmonary embolism. CTA is also essential in the diagnostic workup of abdominal aortic aneurysms and their follow-up postendograft placement.

■ Some IVC filters are retrievable within 90 days of placement.

■ A positive nuclear medicine scan is helpful in patients with GI bleeding because it not only confirms the diagnosis but also directs the angiographer to the site of bleeding.

■ Arterial embolization is an important therapy for traumatic vascular injury, GI bleeding, uterine fibroids, and certain tumors.

Suggested Readings

Baum S, Pentecost MHJ, eds., *Abrams Angiography. Interventional Radiology* 2nd ed. Philadelphia: Lippincott, 2005.

Kadir S. Teaching Atlas of Interventional Radiology. *Nonvascular Interventional Procedures.* New York: Thieme, 2006.

Kadir S. Teaching Atlas of Interventional Radiology. *Diagnostic and Therapeutic Angiography.* New York: Thieme, 2005.

Kandarpa K, Aruny JE. *Handbook of interventional radiologic procedures,* 3rd Ed. Philadelphia Lippincott, 2001.

Kaufman J, Lee M. *Vascular and interventional radiology: the requisites,* 1st Ed. Mosby, 2003.

■ INDEX

Page numbers followed by f denote figure; page numbers followed by t denote table.